Normal Child and Adolescent Development

A Psychodynamic Primer

Normal Child and Adolescent Development

A Psychodynamic Primer

by

Karen J. Gilmore, M.D.
Pamela Meersand, Ph.D.

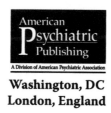

American **P**sychiatric Publishing

A Division of American Psychiatric Association

Washington, DC
London, England

Quantities of 25–99 copies of this or any other American Psychiatric Publishing title may be purchased at a 20% discount; please contact Customer Service at appi@psych.org or 800-368-5777. For 100 or more copies of the same title, e-mail bulksales@psych.org for a price quote.

Copyright © 2014 American Psychiatric Association
ALL RIGHTS RESERVED

Manufactured in the United States of America on acid-free paper
19   5   4   3   2
First Edition

Typeset in Trade Gothic and Warnock Pro.

American Psychiatric Publishing
A Division of American Psychiatric Association
1000 Wilson Boulevard
Arlington, VA 22209-3901
www.appi.org

Library of Congress Cataloging-in-Publication Data
Gilmore, Karen
   Normal child and adolescent development : a psychodynamic primer / by Karen Gilmore, Pamela Meersand. — 1st ed.
       p. ; cm.
   Includes bibliographical references.
   ISBN 978-1-58562-436-2 (pbk. : alk. paper)
   I. Meersand, Pamela. II. American Psychiatric Publishing. III. Title.
   [DNLM: 1. Adolescent Development. 2. Child Development. 3. Adolescent Psychology.
4. Child Psychology. WS 105]
   RJ503
   618.92′8914—dc23
                                                              2013010863

British Library Cataloguing in Publication Data
A CIP record is available from the British Library.

Contents

Video Access: www.appi.org/Gilmore

About the Authors

Karen J. Gilmore, M.D., is Clinical Professor of Psychiatry, Columbia University College of Physicians and Surgeons, and Senior Consultant, Columbia University Center for Psychoanalytic Training and Research. She is in private practice in Manhattan.

Pamela Meersand, Ph.D., is Assistant Professor of Psychology, Department of Psychiatry, Columbia University College of Physicians and Surgeons, and Director, Child Division, Columbia University Center for Psychoanalytic Training and Research. She is in private practice in Manhattan.

Disclosure: The authors affirm that they have no financial interests or affiliations that present or could appear to present a conflict of interest with regard to the content and publication of this book.

Preface

As teachers of human development to psychiatric residents, psychology doctoral students, and psychoanalytic candidates for over a decade, we have been faced with the absence of accessible literature that presents a comprehensive picture of mental development, informed by contemporary research and psychodynamic thinking. Although there are excellent texts from the 1990s about theory (e.g., Tyson and Tyson 1990) and about the broader psychology of development (Gemelli 1996), these perforce do not offer a twenty-first century integration of recent findings in the psychodynamic literature and psychology research that have introduced new ideas, new data, and even a new developmental phase (see Chapter 10). Moreover, there has always been a dearth of readable literature that presents an overview of development as a dynamic interaction of the growing mind (including the unconscious mind), the maturing body, and the evolving demands of environment. Observing our students' struggle to "pull it all together," we felt the need for a straightforward primer that gives the reader a picture of how development unfolds as a complex transactional process progressing through the first three decades of life, retaining both individuality and universality.

As our students labored to envision an organic process of development that was infinitely diverse and yet comprehensible as a coherent set of universal propositions, they educated us as to what was needed to synthesize their thinking while maintaining their receptivity to new ideas. Even as we grapple with current controversies about concepts such as developmental phases and the importance of past experience in present-day functioning, the educational value and usefulness of such a picture for the mental health clinician seem irrefutable to us. For these reasons, we are grateful to the generations of students whose observations, ideas, and challenges helped us realize this project with confidence in its heuristic merit.

Our conviction of the project's value also grows from our belief that understanding development is a building block of clinical thinking. In every encounter with a patient, a clinician with a developmental education can better recognize that the past and present are inextricably woven together; that present consciousness is an amalgam of all experience; and that the relationship that emerges in a therapeutic encounter is a "condensed, co-ordinated, and timeless version of past and present" (Schafer 1982, p. 78) wherein defenses and perceptions from the entirety of the patient's personal history may be invoked (Dowling 2004).

A developmental text such as ours can be likened to an illuminating travel guide to a complex city such as Rome or Berlin, where historical ruins, evidence of traumatic disruption, and modern life create a disorienting jumble. The multiple historical narratives, the impact of environmental catastrophes and when they occurred, the scars they left behind, the new technologies that built on ancient foundations, the changes in function of historical city-planning, the purposes and accommodations that arose to manage all these events and foresee the unknown future—all this is clarified and made more coherent by a multifaceted guidebook to the city of today. This remains true even if we know that historical periods are never neatly delineated, that we can never really "begin at the beginning," and that there are an infinite number of perspectives to consider, each telling a different story. This volume is intended as such a guidebook, one that can be used by the reader, in its entirety or selectively for an epoch of particular interest, to illuminate the remarkable complexity of human mental life in process.

In offering a book organized according to conventional developmental phases, we are not minimizing the contemporary disenchantment with phases that emanates from systems theorists, postmodern analytic schools, and other disciplines interested in new thinking about development. Phases are currently viewed as forming a rigid mold that forces developmental thinking into linear pathways and normative outcomes—concepts that are increasingly in disfavor in psychology (Demos 2007; Hendry and Kloep 2007) and in psychodynamic literature (Chodorow 1996; Galatzer-Levy 2004). Nonetheless, we believe that such time-hallowed categories as infancy and adolescence, while certainly subject to contemporary revision, remain meaningful and useful. However more complex our understanding of individual development becomes; however more recognizable the impact of environment (including the input and expectations of family and culture); and however more intricately parsed our recognition of unevenness and interpenetration of levels, we still all readily identify children as toddlers or latency age or preadolescent. We do this with relative ease not only because we know their chronological ages and because society places them in age-determined settings, but also because we see evidence of emergent capacities and vicissitudes of emotional, relational, intellectual, and self-regulatory processes that make them similar, even while infinitely variable.

For these reasons, our book is sectioned according to the familiar cohorts of childhood: following an introduction to our theoretical orientation in Chapter 1, we cover each developmental epoch in Chapters 2–10. These are infancy (Chapter 2), toddlerhood (Chapter 3), oedipal age (Chapters 4 and 5), latency (Chapter 6), preadolescence (Chapter 7), early and mid-adolescence (Chapter 8), late adolescence (Chapter 9), and finally, emerging adulthood (Chapter 10). We end with a brief reprise of the importance of developmental thinking in clinical practice (Chapter 11).

The fact that we devote two chapters (Chapters 4 and 5) to the oedipal-age child is directly related to our estimation of the importance of this phase, which marks a momentous transition in mental development. An unprecedented number of new capacities emerge in the time frame between ages 3 and 6, including a revolutionary blossoming of symbolization (language and play), a widening range of namable affect, a marked increase in the intensity of passionate feelings, a quantum shift in the complexity of human relationships, and the appearance of a new mental agency, the superego, which consolidates precursors into a functional (albeit immature) whole. Such a comprehensive transformation poses a tremendous challenge to the very young child and his or her environment. Furthermore, the important developmental transformations of this period carry forward into future development in terms of self-regulatory capacities; superego; loving, hateful, and rivalrous feelings and their management; customary defenses; and the nature of personal relationships. This phase represents "the initiation of the child into an adult world, into the moral order, in short, into becoming an individual" (Loewald 1985, p. 439). It is not by any means the end of developmental transformation, but it is a critical juncture in mental life.

Despite our use of these traditional markers, we do not believe that children develop in lockstep in a rigid and universal sequence: they differ markedly both internally, in terms of unevenness of various capacities, and externally, in comparison to their peers. Nonetheless, we continue to find these commonsense traditional divisions useful, something like a guidebook's identification of the Old City, the widening commercial district, and the newly developed hotel strip. Everyone understands that although not arbitrarily defined, these areas have undoubtedly served other functions at other times, are not sharply demarcated, and do not predict or enlighten us as to the organization and function of any single block or building within them. We know an oedipal-age child when we see one, even while fully expecting to encounter a singular, remarkable individual who has integrated inner life, new capabilities, and environmental impingements in an entirely unique way.

We believe that the mental health professional armed with developmental knowledge makes a better clinician, because the here and now is an irreducible amalgam of the individual's whole life up to and including the arrival at the clinician's consulting room. Although childhood events per se may figure only minimally in the clinical encounter, the clinician's awareness of the complex transactions over the life span that have produced this person, in this moment, forms a beacon of orientation that makes meaning out of chaos and coherence out of confusion. Developmental awareness inevitably organizes clinical thinking and enhances our capacity to help our patients by restoring or establishing their ability to reflect on experience in the moment and in the past. We hope our readers will take away an enlightening perspective on clinical material, with a more informed understanding of how the human being before them came to be the person they see there.

REFERENCES

Chodorow N: Reflections of the authority of the past in psychoanalytic theorizing. Psychoanal Q 65:32–51, 1996

Demos V: The dynamics of development, in Self-Organizing Complexity in Psychological Systems. Edited by Piers C, Muller JP, Brent J. New York, Jason Aronson, 2007, pp 135–164

Dowling S: A reconsideration of the concept of regression. Psychoanal Study Child 59:192–210, 2004

Galatzer-Levy RM: Chaotic possibilities: toward a new model of development. Int J Psychoanal 85:419–441, 2004

Gemelli R: Normal Child and Adolescent Development. Washington, DC, American Psychiatric Publishing, 1996

Hendry LB, Kloep M: Conceptualizing emerging adulthood: inspecting the emperor's new clothes? Child Dev Perspect 1:74–79, 2007

Loewald H: Oedipus complex and development of self. Psychoanal Q 54:435–443, 1985

Schafer R: The relevance of "here and now" transference interpretation to the reconstruction of early development. Int J Psychoanal 63:77–82, 1982

Tyson P, Tyson R: Psychoanalytic Theories of Development: An Integration. New Haven, CT, Yale University Press, 1990

Acknowledgments

This book is the fruit of many years of collaboration and of our joint teaching of the lively, intelligent, and challenging candidates in the Columbia University Center for Psychoanalytic Training and Research. We are very grateful to them for their stimulating questions and useful feedback; they have made us better teachers and thinkers.

We are also grateful to the wonderful children and parents, teens, and emerging adults who participated in our video project. Their generous gifts of time and personal reflection are beautifully recorded therein. We hope they will enjoy revisiting their images and thoughts as they move on to their next developmental adventure.

We thank our editors for their attentiveness, support, encouragement, and enthusiasm. We are also grateful to our mentors, too many to name, who have been inspirations for thinking in depth about the wonderful process that is human development.

Finally, we are indebted to our families for their patience and sustenance throughout the process of writing this book.

Video Guide

THE VIDEO LEARNING EXPERIENCE

The companion videos can be viewed online at
www.appi.org/Gilmore

A series of brief videos of parents, children, adolescents, and young adults portrays distinct modes of playing, thinking, and relating that characterize different periods of development. When viewed in tandem with reading the book, these short clips provide a tangible learning experience, further clarifying the complex, often abstract developmental and psychodynamic concepts presented in the text.

In our classroom teaching, we have found that video illustrations make the child of a particular phase "come alive" in a way that reading, discussion, and even case vignettes cannot fully achieve; for example, nothing quite conveys the immediacy and absorption of a preschool child's immersion in imaginary play like watching the youngster's facial expressions and spontaneous actions.

Similarly, the visual dimension of learning helps to concretize major developmental transitions: the mother-infant dyad's shift from bodily intimacy to more distal forms of affective sharing, the latency child's gradual passage from concrete to more reflective thinking about social dilemmas, and the adolescent's dawning sense of self-reliance and personal responsibility are conveyed vividly by the individuals on these clips through their age-typical actions and conversation. Moreover, the viewer can compare children of different ages, achieving a sense of the palpable contrasts between developmental periods, such as the oedipal child's affinity for fantasy versus the latency youngster's embrace of rule-bound play. Multimodal learning is particularly helpful to readers who have limited familiarity with specific age groups and who lack an available set of personal examples and experiences to link with the text.

Although the book provides a sampling of clinical vignettes designed to help the reader contrast typical with more problematic functioning, the chief goal of the videos is to illustrate normal development. With that in mind, we selected individuals who reflect a range of age-expected cognitive, social, and emotional capacities, and we relied on their spontaneous, unscripted comments and behaviors. We interviewed older children, teens, and adults by using open-ended questions; younger children were engaged in play with their parents or with one of us. The children who appear in the videos were recruited from among a group of generous friends and colleagues; for all under the age of 18, parental permissions were obtained.

Using the Book and the Videos Together

We recommend that readers use the • **boldface video prompts** embedded in the text as signals for viewing the associated clips in the online viewer at **www.appi.org/Gilmore.** *(The videos are optimized for most current operating systems, including mobile operating systems iOS 5.1 and Android 4.1 and higher.)* There are no videos for Chapters 1, 5, 7, and 11. Readers who are unfamiliar with a particular developmental period may wish to read a chapter in its entirety first and then return to the prompts, reviewing those particular sections of the text before watching the related videos. Each video begins with a brief oral narration that identifies the age and phase of the individual, previews the content of the tape, and highlights the major concepts to be illustrated. The specific purpose of each video clip is further elaborated below.

Descriptions of the Videos

These 14 clips were designed to exemplify age-salient issues—such as attachment and exploration for the older infant, learning for the latency child, social connection for the young teen, autonomy and self-reliance for the emerging adult—while highlighting the social, emotional, and cognitive capacities that characterize distinct developmental phases. In order to capture the rapid motoric and cognitive growth of such periods as infancy, the more subtle shifts in phases of lengthy duration (e.g., latency), and the range of diverse yet normally functioning boys and girls, we have provided multiple video vignettes for several of the phases.

Chapter 2: Infancy

- **Pregnant Woman (4:27)**
- **3-Month-Old Infant and Mother (1:49)**
- **10-Month-Old Infant and Mother (2:27)**

The first three videos should be viewed in tandem with reading Chapter 2 ("Infancy: Parenthood, the Mother-Infant Relationship, and the Mind of the Infant"). **"Pregnant Woman"** features a working mother in her 30s as she reflects on the bodily and psychological transformations of her second pregnancy. She describes the inwardly focused experience of the final trimester, reflects on a deepened connection to her own mother, and envisions the impact of the newborn on her intimate relationship with her toddler. Her expectations and fantasies about the new baby illustrate the powerful and potentially shaping influence of maternal history and mental state on the infant.

The next two videos, **"3-Month-Old Infant and Mother"** and **"10-Month-Old Infant and Mother,"** demonstrate the mother's empathic identification with her preverbal infant; repeatedly, she receives his cues, imagines his inner life, and verbally expresses his desires and intentions, providing meaning and emotional guidance that suit his developmental capacities. We chose to tape the same mother-son pair in order to capture the dramatic physical, motoric, and cognitive changes of the first few months of life and to portray the ways in which these lead to modifications in the dyad's mutual regulation and affective sharing. For example, at 10 months, the mother's presence serves as an emotional base for this baby, who has begun to crawl away from the mother's body and explore exciting items in his surroundings. The mother's gentle verbal admonishments as he determinedly pursues the family's electronic equipment presage the more specific, active superego training characteristic of the toddler phase.

Chapter 3: The Toddler

• **Toddler and Mother (2:39)**

The **"Toddler and Mother"** video should be viewed with Chapter 3 ("The Toddler: Early Sense of Self and Gender, Rapprochement, Libidinal Object Constancy, and Superego Precursors"). This clip illustrates the mother's ongoing, foundational role as her 20-month-old son's base of security even as he achieves a separate sense of self and gains autonomous capability; when she briefly leaves the room, he immediately grows sober and somewhat unfocused. His emerging cognitive and communicative abilities allow the dyad to rely increasingly on language and play as vehicles for sharing affective experience. In addition, their interaction illustrates the mother's early empathic efforts to enforce behavioral standards and foster the seeds of superego development: having mastered motoric resistance and the beloved word "no," this toddler energetically evades her attempts at a diaper change, but her playful demeanor helps soften his negativity and elicits eventual cooperation.

Chapter 4: The Oedipal Phase and Emerging Capacities

- **4-Year-Old Girl** (7:07)

The **"4-Year-Old Girl"** video is designed to accompany Chapter 4 ("The Oedipal Phase and Emerging Capacities: Language, Imagination, Play, Mentalization, and Self-Regulation") and illustrates themes and identifications that are typical of oedipal-phase fantasies through two scenarios of adult-child imaginary play. In the first play episode, a 4-year-old girl eagerly assumes the role of a well-known, beloved fairy tale heroine who embodies such desired qualities as beauty and goodness; as the story unfolds, mostly true to the classical version, her own very personal yearnings for romance, special recognition, and adult-like activities and accoutrements are revealed. In the second play scenario, the child creates an original action-narrative using small dolls and their accessories; this story centers around age-typical, highly moralistic themes, wherein good triumphs over evil and the guilty are severely punished, reflecting the oedipal youngster's ongoing struggle to master angry, possessive, and jealous feelings and impulses. The oedipal child's deep pleasure and absorption in play, the use of pretense to achieve temporary identification with admired adults, and the role of narratives to express and organize intense feelings are portrayed vividly in this video vignette. Moreover, the tape exemplifies the scaffolding function of adult involvement, demonstrating how adults expand the child's play by adding structure and complexity to the preschooler's spontaneous actions and ideas.

Chapter 6: The Latency Phase

- **7-Year-Old Girl** (2:30)
- **7-Year-Old Boy** (5:01)
- **10-Year-Old Male Friends** (4:43)

There are three video clips that illustrate different aspects of the momentous social and cognitive gains of the latency phase, as discussed in Chapter 6 ("The Latency Phase: Cognitive Maturation, Autonomy, Social Development, and Learning"), particularly as these relate to the world of school and friendships. In the first clip, **"7-Year-Old Girl,"** a young child applies her increasing logical and analytic capacities, as well as her emerging self-restraint, to social dilemmas such as peer competition and conflict; she reasons aloud about potential motivations and solutions. In the next video, **"7-Year-Old Boy,"** the latency child's unprecedented capacity for learning and cooperation are emphasized as this child and his father construct a model; in another segment, he describes perceived unfairness at school, reasons about boy-girl differences, and relates his sense of novel academic pressures. The final tape pertaining to this phase, **"10-Year-Old Male Friends,"** presents two lively, highly verbal fifth-grade boys whose anxieties and interests revolve around the daily world of same-sex peer socialization. With obvious excitement and nervous anticipation, they discuss the upcoming shift to middle school, where they will be separated for the first time and called upon to forge new social connections.

Chapter 8: Early and Mid-Adolescence

- **Early Adolescent Girl (4:09)**
- **Mid-Adolescent Boy (10:06)**

The next two videos help the viewer distinguish major features of adolescent subphases and should be viewed with Chapter 8 ("Early and Mid-Adolescence: The Importance of the Body, Sexuality, and Individuation, the Role of Action, and Special Problems of the Teen Years"). In both videos, teens describe the development of their personal attitudes and values and review decisions they have made about friendships and peer pressure in the context of a growing sense of independence and autonomy. In the first video, **"Early Adolescent Girl,"** a pubescent girl (age 13 years) discusses the importance of her peer group and her ongoing connection to her family. In the second video, **"Mid-Adolescent Boy,"** a slightly older teen (age 15 years) defines himself both within and apart from his complex, blended family; he reflects on friendship, describes his romantic involvement with a girl his age, and discusses the pull of risky social behaviors. Both videos illustrate the adolescent's dawning realization of personal freedom and self-responsibility and the growing awareness that decisions and choices now carry consequences.

Chapter 9 (Late Adolescence)

- **Late Adolescent Boy (4:23)**
- **Late Adolescent Girl (7:02)**

The next two videos illustrate later adolescent trends and should be viewed in tandem with Chapter 9 ("Late Adolescence: Identity, Sexuality, Autonomy, and Superego Formation in the Late Teens and Twenties"). These videos exemplify the older teen's increased capacity to reflect on the past and contemplate the future, the concern about establishing a unique personal identity in the wider world, and the pressures of self-definition as the "real world" looms. The first video, **"Late Adolescent Boy,"** portrays an 18-year-old high school senior; on his final day of high school, he ponders the end of his familiar surroundings and looks ahead to college. He wonders aloud about his future identity and how to establish his place in a novel social environment. The second video, **"Late Adolescent Girl,"** features a 20-year-old college student as she reflects over the events of her life, analyzes the impact of family history, and describes the inevitable changes in her close parental relationships. As she looks forward, imagining her adult life, she considers the concrete decisions she will soon face about who and what she will become.

Chapter 10 (Emerging Adulthood)

- **Young Adult Male, Age 25 (6:57)**
- **Young Adult Male, Age 26 (5:55)**

The final two video clips depict young adulthood and should be viewed while reading Chapter 10 ("The Odyssey Years: Emerging Adults on the Path to Adulthood"); both illustrate men in their mid-20s whose lives have taken some unexpected turns, with trajectories shaped by events, losses, or personal revelations. The first video, **"Young Adult Male, Age 25,"** features one individual who needed to rely heavily on his own internal resources after being faced with a series of real-life stressors, including financial pressures and the death of a parent; along the way, a mentor provided guidance. The final video, **"Young Adult Male, Age 26,"** depicts how the expected pathway of college was interrupted by a personal realization; after a period of uncertainty, this young man ultimately found meaning and satisfaction in an unanticipated professional opportunity.

CHAPTER 1

A Psychodynamic
Developmental Orientation

This book is intended for people interested in understanding the minds of others, both children and adults, in a comprehensive, in-depth way. Our approach is based on the premise that every individual at any given moment is a complex product of his or her endowment, developmental history, current circumstances, and relationships with key figures, as well as the relationship unfolding in the here-and-now patient-therapist interaction. In this book we hope to provide a basis for considering the individual in the first three decades of life in developmental context by offering a way of thinking about traditional developmental phases and clarifying the developmental tasks and challenges associated with each phase, many of which are culture specific. From our point of view as psychodynamic thinkers and therapists, this approach offers the most compassionate and informed method for considering a human life and figuring out how best to help it proceed.

Most psychodynamic thinkers subscribe to some theory of development (Michels 1999), because developmental ideas inform their approach to treatment of adults and children alike. Despite their contemporary diversity, psychodynamically oriented psychotherapists can agree that the nature of the personality, the quality of relationships, the regulation of impulses and affects, and attitudes toward work and myriad facets of life are powerfully influenced by an individual's personal history, especially his or her early history. Moreover, these psychotherapists tend to think about the person they are hoping to help by placing the person's conflicts and patterns into a context that considers the developmental surround, the quality of mental organization, and the nature of the cultural expectations and pressures, historically and in the present.

There is considerable disagreement among psychodynamic thinkers, however, about the legitimacy of the traditional developmental phases (Coates 1997), which have unfortunately been associated with prescriptive progression and linear thinking. This is perhaps especially true in regard to the oedipal phase, which was historically viewed as the period of development that determined the future personality and that followed a normative sequence. A modern perspective on development avoids linear concepts and refers instead to hierarchically ordered mental organizations that occur, like attractor states in the terminology of systems theory, in a relatively reliable way across individuals and across cultures (Abrams 1983; Galatzer-Levy 1995, 2004; Gilmore 2008). Thus, each phasic shift is the product of multiple interacting systems, none of which can fully realize the given state independently. Anna Freud was a pioneer in this way of thinking; even though she used the misleading term *developmental lines,* she was actually proposing a highly integrative multisystem approach to considering complex developmental outcomes (Freud 1963; Mayes 1999). This idea of transactional developmental systems obviates the tendency, among developmental thinkers, to assign decisive importance to a singular system, such as genetic endowment, environment, or their interaction, or developmental moment, such as infancy or early childhood. Although we concur that certain basic interpersonal, emotional, and biological needs must be met in infancy for development to proceed, we do not see infancy as the preeminent developmental moment.

In addition, there is some controversy about the end point of development and the presence and power of developmental forces in the adult. The popular Eriksonian approach to development throughout the life cycle, with developmental tasks and challenges extending into old age (Erikson 1951/1959), is, for some psychodynamic developmentalists, insufficiently grounded in the consideration of mental reorganizations and internal maturational pressure characterizing the first two decades of life; it is "psychoanalytic sociology" (Abrams 1983). These critics feel that the term *development* should refer exclusively to a biologically driven progression toward the mature form and should be considered officially completed with the establishment of adult mental structure and the full array of adult capacities—cognitive, emotional, sexual, and so on (Abrams 1983, 1990; Neubauer 1996). Others take a middle ground and suggest that psychological development continues throughout adulthood, albeit at a slower pace, with shifts primarily in the contents of mental organization and minimally in the organization itself. For example, Blatt and Luyten (2009) describe certain dimensions of personality, specifically interpersonal relatedness and self-definition, and document their developmental transformation over the lifespan. Still others embrace a lifespan developmental model of "a never-ending series of transformations [so that] the only difference between infancy—or adolescence, for that matter—and any other period or phase of lifespan is one of degree, that is, rate of internal change and rate of encountering drastically new context" (Stern 1995, p. 192). For these thinkers, adult development assumes a central role, and tasks such as mature love, childbearing and child rearing, mentoring, midlife crisis, climacterium, and death can be considered intrapsychic developmental tasks (Colarusso and Nemiroff 1979; Emde 1985). Such theoretical differences obviously affect ideas about whether adult psychotherapeutic treatment has a development-promoting function or, alternatively, recruits other types of internal processes to effect change.

An interesting phenomenon bearing on the question of the overall trajectory of development is the fact that developmental phases have undergone two significant addenda in social psychology: developmental literature and the popular imagination. Before the turn of the twentieth century, adolescence was not granted the status of a developmental stage with its own challenges in regard to the familiar dimensions of the body, object relations, cognitive function, superego consolidation, values, and goals. This seems patently absurd to the contemporary observer who is steeped in awareness of adolescent culture, adolescent transformation, adolescent-specific developmental tasks, and the gradual maturation of the body in the years following puberty. Moreover, modern neuroscience offers a steady stream of new information about changes in the brain during this period (see, e.g., Tamnes et al. 2010). In the twenty-first century, a new developmental phase has been proposed, roughly corresponding to the decade between ages 20 and 30 and variously called emerging adulthood, the odyssey years, or contestable adulthood (see Chapter 10, "The Odyssey Years"). Clearly, this new phase is a by-product of the interface of the contemporary social structure and the young adult. Some thinkers suggest that statistically significant delays in milestones of adulthood (marriage, childbearing, employment) over the last 50 years reflect the interplay of social forces such as technology, employment opportunities, and improved prevention of unwanted pregnancy. Others believe that these delays have unmasked a legitimate developmental period with physiological underpinnings, just as adolescence was unmasked by the rise of the twentieth-century emphasis on a college education. For those who embrace a lifespan developmental model or, at the very least, extend developmental impact past adolescence, it is self-evident that the 20s are fraught with developmental challenges (Chused 1987; Colarusso 1995).

THE ROLE OF DEVELOPMENT IN PSYCHODYNAMIC TREATMENT

Despite the disagreements about the extent to which development is a life-long process and the question of stability in the conceptualizations of developmental phases, developmental ideas are invariably invoked in describing psychopathology and clinical interventions. Indeed, most psychodynamic thinkers privilege the role of development in determining adult personality and view treatment as an inquiry into personal history. For many psychodynamic clinicians, the unfolding relationship between patient and therapist contains information about the patient's childhood relationships, trauma, and experience. The way the individual personality emerges in psychotherapy is conceptualized as a window into the past of the patient; specifically, transference-countertransference dynamics are understood as an illumination of past relationships (Govrin 2006). As it evolves over the course of treatment, the present patient-therapist relationship provides a system of checks and balances for hypotheses about the patient's history, informing and modifying the patient's and therapist's understanding of both present and past, with the ultimate outcome of a coherent personal narrative and better integrated sense of self.

Developmental ideas are invoked in psychodynamic clinical descriptions in a number of ways in addition to the fundamental notion that the transference recapitulates important childhood relationships and illuminates developmental experience. One is by analogy; the treatment process is conceptualized as a new developmental opportunity. To this way of thinking, the therapeutic relationship is in and of itself "developmental"; the therapist is seen as a "transformational object" (Bollas 1979), like a parent figure, and the process is understood as a corrective to the deficits in the patient's childhood experience. Sigmund Freud (1940/1962) himself observed that both patient and therapist approach treatment with attitudes corresponding to parent-child dynamics and warned that, however eagerly this dynamic might be embraced by the patient, it was the therapist's task to resist the pressure to take on a parental role. Nonetheless, as both metaphor and meaningful analogy, the notion of "restoring the child to the path of normal development" (Neubauer 1990, p. 106) in treatment through the development-promoting functions of the therapist has been revisited repeatedly over the history of the field and remains a key concept of child psychotherapy (Abrams 1978b; Rangell 1992; Sandler 1996). Children's development is frequently described as derailed by conflict, trauma, or constitutional factors, and dynamic treatment is deemed successful when the child returns to age-appropriate developmental tasks unencumbered by pathology. Moreover, because the patient in child treatment is "in process" of development, there has been a sustained interest in differentiating therapeutic functions into those promoting conflict resolution and those facilitating developmental progression. These functions are sometimes synergistic, but often they are at odds because the developmental press forward heightens resistance to looking backward and reviving past relationships (Abrams et al. 1999; Neubauer 1996, 2003).

The role of ongoing development in adult treatment is more controversial, in part because, as noted in the introduction of this chapter, there is some disagreement about whether adults "develop" at all, whether adult psychopathology can be understood as representing a developmental arrest or deformation, and whether the developmental process can be rekindled in the course of therapy. Those who promote the idea of adult development, especially self psychologists, view treatment as an opportunity to reactivate compromised developmental processes to achieve a more adaptive outcome (Settlage 1996); to them, treatment itself is "developmental" in patients of every age. The pioneers of attachment theory have similarly maintained that effective treatment must include the "provision of a secure framework to support the recovery of the patient's mentalizing capacity" (Fonagy et al. 2003, p. 447). Fonagy, Target, and their colleagues, who have systematically sought a convergence between psychodynamic and attachment theories, introduced the idea of *mentalization* as a powerful interpersonal capacity that is established in early childhood in the mother-infant interaction, reverberates in subsequent development on multiple levels, from cortical to self-representation to interpersonal relations, and is essential for managing complex environmental conditions. Interference with its development constitutes a "psychic autoimmune deficiency" (Fonagy et al. 2003, p. 435); treatment creates the opportunity to develop this core foundational component of mental health that was bypassed in early childhood.

Another common and related use of developmental ideas in clinical work is derived from the tradition of psychodynamically informed infant research and observations of mother-infant interactions. Especially among attachment theorists, self psychologists, and some intersubjectivists, mother-infant mutual regulation and attunement serves as a template for the exchanges in the treatment dyad. For example, Beebe and Lachmann derive many of their ideas about the relationship between adult patient and therapist from observations of mother-infant interaction (Beebe and Lachmann 1998; Lachmann and Beebe 1996). Although they caution against any direct correlation of the "dynamic content" of these disparate dyadic situations, they emphasize that the "process of mutual interactive regulation" between therapist and adult patient illuminates and is informed by the early regulatory relationship between the patient as baby and the caregiver.

In contrast to those theorists who believe that understanding development is intrinsic to treatment, theorists representing some "postmodern" schools of psychodynamic therapies, such as other intersubjectivists and relationalists, have challenged the importance of a theory of development from a range of different vantage points (Corbett 2001; Reisner 2001). These schools suggest that all the necessary information is in the here and now. Attempts to sketch a veridical history by extrapolating or reconstructing from the present picture are, for better or worse, myth making and a co-creation of patient and therapist (Michels 2006). Nonetheless, it is our impression that a close look at the clinical work reported by proponents of this viewpoint demonstrates that the therapist approaches the patient with an implicit developmental theory; all dynamically oriented practitioners use their developmental theories as scaffolding to build up their picture of the patient before them, to frame their understanding of his or her "way of being in the world" (Winnicott 1965), and to help the patient make sense of his or her own experience and inner life.

A Contemporary Psychodynamic Approach to Development

This book is intended to provide the framework for the psychodynamic approach to development. Our purpose is to familiarize the reader with the unfolding development of the person from birth to "emerging adulthood" (Arnett 2004). In our view, such knowledge best orients the clinician to consider the idiosyncratic inner world of the patient and is central to the therapeutic task of restoring continuity and a sense of coherence in the here and now.

This version of psychodynamic developmental theory is concerned with certain key dimensions and recognizes that they are embedded in a multiplicity of interacting systems that influence individual development. The course of individual human development can be best understood as the evolving interface of a complex dynamic process in which biological, psychological, familial, and cultural systems all play a role. The process of mental development is profoundly dependent on the reliable presence of a nurturing human environment, interacts with it, and then loops back to further influence its own evolution; the human environment extends beyond the immediate family to the ambient culture, which in turn influences and is influenced by the interplay between subculture and society at large.

Our viewpoint is consistent with contemporary scientific thinking about human development (Sroufe et al. 2005). It embraces a perspective that is by definition complex, infinitely variable, and yet subject to certain psychodynamic organizing principles that remain consistent from individual to individual and result in recognizable patterns, at least within a given culture (Corbett 2001). These fundamentals include the following:

1. *Body:* A focus on the body and the powerful impact of the maturing body on the mental life of the individual. This was Freud's seminal insight: "the ego…is first and foremost a body-ego" (Freud 1923/1962, pp. 26–27); his earliest developmental theory was indeed based on the maturation of bodily drives, called *psychosexual* stage progression. Since that time, the body has been in and out of fashion among psychodynamic theorists; it has lost ground as a fundamental source of mental life in recent contemporary thinking that eschews the importance of sexuality and with it, the role of the body, such as attachment theory and relational theory. However, interest in the body is currently undergoing a renaissance as its central importance in building up the interpersonal world from earliest infancy is now recognized on a neuroscientific basis; mirror neurons and bodily maps that facilitate the baby's imitation of the caretaker in the first days of life are hypothesized to establish the fundamental recognition that "here is something like me" (Beebe et al. 2003; Gallese 2009; Gallese and Sinigaglia 2010; Meltzoff 2007). Moreover, the body has been restored to its rightful position in cognitive psychology, replacing the information-processing computer metaphor with the idea of embodied cognition (Fonagy and Target 2007). The concept of body as bedrock is threaded through contemporary theoretical literature (see also Fonagy 2008; Lemma 2010). It is also central to recent neuroscientific formulations of consciousness (Damasio 1999).

2. *Phases:* A delineation of developmental phases and progression, even while acknowledging that linearity, lockstep progression, and prescribed pathways, often attributed to traditional developmental theories, are unfortunate and erroneous conceptualizations. There are broadly recognizable developmental periods, demonstrable within and across cultures, that rise to the level of recognizable patterns and are associated with recognizable environmental demands and expectations. Nonlinear systems theory would term these "attractor states" that result from the interface of relatively similar progressions of developing systems across individuals. Any given individual's success or failure within these smaller developmental units reverberates throughout that person's developmental trajectory and so becomes another factor that influences its course.

3. *Ego:* A focus on the role of *maturing ego capacities* in the mind while recognizing their ready recruitment into conflict, their fluidity, and their idiosyncrasies. Psychodynamic developmental theory elucidates the

transformations in the organization of the mind, including changes in cognitive capacities and defense mechanisms, in different developmental epochs. The understanding of the kind of mind that characterizes a given developmental period and the individual's idiosyncratic version of it facilitates an appreciation of his or her specific mental experience in previous iterations. This inevitably leads to an interest in the dynamics of memory as early experience is developmentally reconstructed throughout childhood and adolescence (Tuch 1999).

4. *Superego:* Recognition of the crucial role of the *process of internalization,* which builds mental structure via representations of self and others. This process is central to the gradual establishment of self-regulation, and especially of the primary self-regulatory agency, the superego. This agency and its associated affects of shame and guilt are reconfigured and matured over the entire span of development, becoming increasingly self-determined.

5. *Environment:* The central importance of the near environment and the still larger remote environment, including the cognitive, emotional, and social expectations of each developmental epoch as realized in a given culture. Our viewpoint considers how these environmental factors affect the individual child as a product of a particular culture in a particular time.

6. *Family system:* The contribution of the immediate environment and the powerful role that adaptation between mother and infant and the family system play in the individual's unfolding. Our viewpoint recognizes the profoundly important experience of early caretaking and how interpersonal engagement and emotional connectedness in infancy contribute to the origins of thought, the awareness of the self, and the understanding of the minds of others (Hobson 2002).

7. *Inner life:* A focus on certain key areas that are of enduring interest in psychodynamic theorizing and clinical work—the dynamic unconscious, sex and aggression, object relations including the attachment system, ego capacities including defenses, and the subjective self-experience or sense of self. The breadth of focus distinguishes the psychodynamic developmental viewpoint from other forms of developmental inquiry. Thus, while committed to recognition of the environmental influence, this approach considers its purview to be *the world as represented in the inner life* of the individual.

8. *Other sciences:* An open and inquiring posture toward the information obtained from *other neighboring developmental sciences,* because these can only enrich the fund of knowledge about development, offering new insights and contributing new directions to inquiries (Gilmore 2008).

9. *Accrued meaning:* An overarching emphasis on the *meaning* that the developmental trajectory and its events accrue in the mind, because the

individual developmental experience is continuously reinterpreted over the course of life.

Such a psychodynamic approach to development will redress some popular misconceptions that grew out of the partial theories of various psychoanalytic schools. Because psychodynamic developmental thinking was never brought into a unifying theoretical frame, it appears as disparate threads woven through various contributions, some old, some new, some based on outdated thinking, and some entirely contemporary.

For example, Sigmund Freud's earliest developmental sequence of psychosexual stages was based on a singular causality—that is, a biologically driven libidinal progression of erotogenic zones. Today, psychodynamic developmental thinking, even the most classical Freudian theory, takes many more factors into account. Developmental progression into latency, for example, does not depend on a castration threat and the repression of the oedipal constellation, although indeed these events and mental processes can occur. Latency marks the confluence of many interacting dynamic systems, which together move the developing child to a new equilibrium, with a new set of mental capacities, a new relationship to a body significantly altered by maturation, a new range of environmental expectations, new possibilities of object relations, and a new ability to work. Our preference would be not to privilege one system over another in this complex interplay, but rather to recognize that all the elements, including a number of others, both universal and unique, work synergistically to achieve the new organization. Therefore, we reject the idea of any simple linear causality in human development.

Similarly, we do not embrace the notion that the search backward for psychodynamic roots provides a complete explanation for mental phenomena. This type of dated thinking led to the proliferation of theories that equated psychodynamic understanding of psychopathology with assertions of ultimate etiology. For example, because we can trace a particular psychotic fantasy to a childhood experience does not mean that we understand why the patient is psychotic. We may better understand the way that experience has been recruited into the patient's psychosis and how such a fantasy became important. We now know, however, that all complex psychological states, such as autism, schizophrenia, so-called psychosomatic disorders, borderline personality, learning disabilities, homosexuality, and infertility, arise in the infinitely interwoven interplay of biology, genetics, mental life, and environment.

We also caution against a prevalent but unfortunate categorical tendency to consider certain developmental outcomes as "normal" or "healthy" and others as, by definition, pathological (Auchincloss and Vaughan 2001;

Coates 1997; Grossman and Kaplan 1988). This error is by no means exclusive to psychodynamic theory; it is built into the fabric of culture and is clearly the result of the interface of culture and science. For example, contemporary views of women have a huge impact on how female psychological development is conceptualized; previous attitudes toward women's ambition, objectivity, moral depth, or sexuality, for example, were influenced by prevailing sociopolitical conventions and represented as bedrock. Similarly, perspectives on the development of homosexuality have been revolutionized by the contemporary view that homosexuality is at least partially biologically determined; a continuum of homosexual development can be considered, ranging from healthy to disordered.

We believe these historical misconceptions can best be avoided by a degree of humility in regard to the question of "why" a certain outcome occurred in individual dynamics. We cannot necessarily determine ultimate causality, if indeed it exists, but rather seek the more straightforward but nonetheless clarifying answer to "how" the patient became who he or she is. Our conviction is that such an open and inquiring developmental framework helps in work with patients, both children and adults. It orients the clinician in listening to the patient and in the prolonged process of collaborative work that constitutes transformative psychotherapy. Because the past is felt to operate in and shape the present and because distortions based on past experience constrain the degrees of freedom possible for a given individual, an elucidation of the past is not only illuminating but also essential for better adaptation. In turn, the elucidation of the present achieved in a treatment relationship "predicts" the individual's psychological past (Hartmann and Kris 1945) and helps restore meaningful continuity to the autobiographical self. Thus, the therapist's capacities to imagine the child in the adult patient, to appreciate the serial translations of earlier experience, and to link these disparate editions into a narrative thread are essential to the integrative process that occurs in treatment. A cohesive view of human development forms the infrastructure of the evolving picture of the specific individual presentation.

Every practitioner has a more or less coherent picture of human development, of the demands and expectations of contemporary culture, and of phase-specific conflicts and challenges. The degree to which these developmental ideas are grounded in a complex appreciation of the developmental trajectory is surprisingly variable. Areas of ignorance and bias, based on personal psychology or obsolete information, are ubiquitous among clinicians of considerable experience. Better appreciation of development can only clarify such blind spots, enhance the skill of the therapist, and improve the depth and sensitivity of clinical work.

Psychodynamic Organizing Principles

- A focus on the transforming body and its impact on the mind. The ego is "first and foremost a body ego" (Freud 1923/1962, p. 27).

- A delineation of developmental phases and progression, while recognizing infinite variations and the complexity of interacting dynamic systems.

- A focus on maturing ego capacities.

- A focus on the processes of internalization in the formation of mental structure.

- Recognition of the importance of the near (familial) and distal (social) environment.

- Emphasis on subjective meaning

- A concentration on the following key areas:
  — The dynamic unconscious
  — Sex and aggression
  — Object relations (including attachment systems)
  — Ego development, including defenses
  — Subjective sense of self

BASIC PRINCIPLES OF A PSYCHODYNAMIC THEORY OF DEVELOPMENT

Our proposal begins with five fundamental hypotheses of human development (Abrams 1977) that delineate its transactional nature.

1. *Maturational emergence:* There is an expected sequence of emerging functions in the psychic apparatus leading to progressively differentiated structures of hierarchical organization. The sequences, the functions, and the structures are rooted in biological sources.
2. *Milieu:* To materialize and flourish, new structure requires environmental stimulation. The range of stimulation and the timing are important variables influencing outcome.
3. *Experiential interface:* The experiential products of the "outer" and "inner" interaction also codetermine what is to follow.
4. *Transformations of mental organization:* Each step in the sequence involves transformations as well as sequences.
5. *Progression-regression processes:* Development is also effected by intrinsic regressive and progressive processes that influence intensity, duration, and cadence (Abrams 1978, pp. 388–389). This form of developmental

regression should be distinguished from that implied in the notion that certain symptoms represent regression to a previous form in the adult (see next section, "The Genetic Point of View").

In human development, the individual maturational timetable (principle 1) requires the milieu (principle 2)—the environment and the people in it—for stimulation and direction. The interaction (principle 3) is the stuff of personal experience that feeds back into the transaction. In his elaboration of these principles, Abrams (1978) emphasized transformation and hierarchical organizations wherein qualitatively different mental configurations replace each other, by reconfiguration and addition of new elements, as development proceeds (principle 4). This is analogous to what systems theorists call "attractor states," which typify each developmental epoch. Individuals passing through these epochs show roughly comparable levels of cognitive organization, object relationships, moral development, and affective complexity and regulation in roughly comparable time frames, which identify them as being "in" a certain phase. The pace of this progression, the variability of different arenas within the personality, the ease of shifting back and forth, and the pressure to move forward (principle 5) are all intangibles that contribute to the individual trajectory.

Core Psychodynamic Principles of Theory of Development

- Maturational emergence
- Milieu
- Experiential interface
- Transformations of mental organization
- Progressive-regressive trends

THE GENETIC POINT OF VIEW

Abrams (1977) observes that developmental principles are implicit in much early theorizing but never consolidated into a cohesive theory. This may be due to the reality that psychodynamic thinking, to the extent that it is interested in the patient's past, tends to travel backward in search of psychological antecedents and meanings and to be less interested in the recognition of the transformations and potentialities of forward progression (Novick and Novick 1994). Looking backward, or the *genetic viewpoint,* was one of the "minimal assumptions" on which dynamic thinking rests (Rapaport and Gill 1959). Most psychodynamic practitioners, with few exceptions, apply some form of *genetic thinking* in their therapeutic work, meaning that they seek the psychological origins and development of present symptoms; they understand a patient before them as a complex product of an evolving past.

Unfortunately, as noted in the section "A Contemporary Psychodynamic Approach to Development" earlier in this chapter, the search for psychological origins has been confused with the idea that all mental phenomena have psychological *etiology.* This is an important distinction; understanding the psychological history, even if the beginnings can be traced with conviction, is not the same as determining etiology. When we as therapists explore mental origins and evolution over time, we do not claim to be clarifying *why* a given symptom, personality organization, or sexual preference is present but rather *how* it figures into the development of our patient (Gilmore 2008). Although we might figure out when a learning disability first was diagnosed or posed challenges, then consider its impact on the developing mind, examine its recruitment into conflict throughout development, and assess how it is operating in the here and now, we do not presume to know what caused a given person to have a learning disability. We are interested in how this cognitive problem and its history affect the person we are seeing. In a similar fashion, we consider the effects of a special talent, such as prodigious musical gifts, on an individual's development without making claims for a psychological etiology. Also, although we are eager to understand the influence of a given sexual orientation on childhood and adolescent experience, we do not suggest that this clarifies why a person is so oriented.

The genetic viewpoint has more or less importance in different theoretical schools. To the extent that therapeutic benefit relies on the "uncovering" of the forgotten past by the lifting of repression, often through examination of the nature of the relationship unfolding between patient and therapist, genetic reconstruction is a central tool. However, many contemporary thinkers feel that this is a problematic simplification, inconsistent with contemporary understanding of memory. It is conceptually linked to an *archeological metaphor* for personality—that is, the idea that prior mental organizations are buried in historical sequence in the course of development (Dowling 2004). This idea has, for many practitioners, been replaced by the recognition that the past is significant primarily for how it has shaped psychology—the nature of object relations, self-regulation, and the like (Fonagy 1999)—and for how it is reworked throughout development, and reshaped in its present invocation.

The archeological metaphor is connected to a reification and "concretization" of the idea of regression, invoked to explain the emergence of "primitive" fantasies, mental organizations, or defenses, for example, as a result of a backward slide toward more "archaic" forms (Inderbitzen and Levy 2000).

Regression proper is indeed part of the developmental process in childhood, because developmental milestones can be temporarily lost or internalizations reprojected in the process of development. However, even in childhood, there is never pure regression, because the loss of the developmental acquisition or function occurs in an individual who has already moved forward to a more mature organization. In childhood, the time frame is compressed and so this incongruity is not pronounced. In adulthood, however, regression to primitive mental organizations is a misnomer; the past is never available in pure form, like a buried artifact. It is a past that is reconstructed in the moment of remembering or reexperiencing it. (See Freud [1899] for a remarkably modern discussion of memory.) Adults do not regress to earlier forms. Dowling (2004) proposes that the present is continuously constructed from elements of the present moment and the myriad memories—conscious, unconscious, or procedural—from the past. Past forms are "all... present, all variably accessible, all richly contributing to the typical patterns that follow while altering those that have already been." The present "draw[s] upon but [is] distinct from all that preceded it. Now one past pattern contributes more strongly to the unique, age-determined pattern of the moment, now another, and now another" (Dowling 2004, p. 202). Although it is unlikely that the idea of regression as a shorthand for a very complex process will vanish from the literature or even from this volume, it needs to be understood as a signifier of the quality of the current manifestation, and not as a description of a mental process retreating to earlier forms (Inderbitzen and Levy 2000).

Connecting each patient to his or her past is a vital part of facilitating a more integrated and expanded self-experience, but it is not a quest for specific memories or an attempt to reconstruct a veridical narrative. Historical events are important, but it is their effect on the developing mind that counts. We believe that psychodynamic thinking is greatly enhanced by a more nuanced understanding of developmental process. Looking backward carries with it a tendency toward linearity and simple causality, whereas consideration of developmental progression is inherently nonlinear, unpredictable, complex, and full of serendipity and surprise.

The current zeitgeist among psychodynamic developmental thinkers is increasingly informed by nonlinear thinking. Many writers note their debt to the insights and principles of nonlinear systems theory (Galatzer-Levy 1995, 2004; Mayes and Spence 1994; Tyson and Tyson 1990) or second-generation cognitive psychology (Fonagy and Target 2007). These contemporary contributions urge the embrace of a more complex and open-ended theory of dynamic developmental processes and their role in the individual's mental life at the moment of clinical presentation. Our conviction is that genetic reconstructions and appreciation of current dynamics can be greatly enhanced by awareness of development; in fact, that is the premise of this book. It is this complex and dynamic developmental process that we address throughout the text.

Nonlinear Dynamic Systems Principles in Psychodynamic Thinking

- Development is a product of multiple interacting systems, each self-organizing, individually paced, and impacted by its interaction with others.
- Recognizable developmental phases are *attractor states,* which are both universal and infinitely variable.
- Development is nonlinear as each hierarchically emergent mental organization rearranges and recycles old elements.
- In this conceptualization, the classical notion of regression—linear backward movement to old fixation points—is not feasible.

Key Concepts

- Development is the process that integrates endowment, emerging capacities, environment, and experience, and results in nonlinear sequential mental organizations.
- Developmental tasks are the specific challenges to the mind emanating from the following:
  - Environmental expectations
  - Individual maturation
  - Their interaction in personal experience
- Modern psychodynamic developmental thinking utilizes a multisystem approach, recognizing the following:
  - Human development is a transactional process integrating a range of systems into a relatively consistent progression while allowing for infinite variations.
  - Ego capacities, object relations, physical maturation, subjective experience, superego evolution, environmental demand, and the drive to move forward—to name but a few—must all be accounted for in considering an individual mind and the evolving life story.
- Understanding development is relevant to any exploration of the human psyche; most theories concerning mental life are in agreement with Freud's endorsement of the old aphorism "the child is father to the man" (Freud 1913/1962, p. 183).

- Understanding the sequential mental organizations that characterize human development helps the clinician recognize the following in patients:
  - Naïve cognitions
  - Traumatic deformations
  - Distortions of current relationships
  - Deleterious patterns of perception, emotion, and behavior derived from childhood experience that remain in the life of the adult
- Some active memories of the past reflect specific events (episodic memory) and are usually elicited by the present moment. However, most memories are procedural.
  - They are contained nonverbally in the way the individual walks, talks, thinks, relates, fears, and loves.
  - Greater attunement to childhood forms facilitates recognition and clarification of patterns and feelings that were presumably necessary in the past but that are currently the source of conflict and suffering.

REFERENCES

Abrams S: The genetic point of view: historical antecedents and developmental transformations. J Am Psychoanal Assoc 25:417–426, 1977

Abrams S: The teaching and learning of psychoanalytic developmental psychology. J Am Psychoanal Assoc 26:387–406, 1978

Abrams S: Development. Psychoanal Study Child 36:113–139, 1983

Abrams S: The psychoanalytic process: the developmental and the integrative. Psychoanal Q 59:650–677, 1990

Abrams S, Neubauer PB, Solnit AJ: Coordinating the developmental and psychoanalytic processes: three case reports—introduction. Psychoanal Study Child 54:19–24, 1999

Arnett JJ: Emerging Adulthood. New York, Oxford University Press, 2004

Auchincloss EL, Vaughan SC: Psychoanalysis and homosexuality: do we need a new theory? J Am Psychoanal Assoc 49:1157–1186, 2001

Beebe B, Lachmann FM: Co-constructing inner and relational processes: self- and mutual regulation in infant research and adult treatment. Psychoanal Psychol 15:480–516, 1998

Beebe B, Sorter D, Rustin J, et al: A comparison of Meltzoff, Trevarthen, and Stern. Psychoanal Dialogues 13:777–804, 2003

Blatt S, Luyten P: A structural-developmental psychodynamic approach to psychopathology: two polarities of experience across the lifespan. Dev Psychopathol 21:793–814, 2009

Bollas C: The transformational object. Int J Psychoanal 60:97–107, 1979

Chused JF: Idealization of the analyst by the young adult. J Am Psychoanal Assoc 35:839–859, 1987

Coates S: Is it time to jettison the concept of developmental lines? Gender and Psychoanalysis 2:35–53, 1997

Colarusso CA: Traversing young adulthood: the male journey from 20 to 40. Psychoanalytic Inquiry 15:75–91, 1995

Colarusso CA, Nemiroff RA: Some observations and hypotheses about the psychoanalytic theory of adult development. Int J Psychoanal 60:59–71, 1979

Corbett K: More life: centrality and marginality in human development. Psychoanal Dialogues 11:313–335, 2001

Damasio A: The Feeling of What Happens. New York, Harcourt Brace, 1999

Dowling S: A reconsideration of the concept of regression. Psychoanal Study Child 58:191–210, 2004

Emde RN: From adolescence to midlife: remodeling the structure of adult development. J Am Psychoanal Assoc 33(suppl):59–112, 1985

Erikson EH: Growth and crises of the healthy personality (1951), in Identity and the Life Cycle, Psychological Issues Monograph 1. Edited by Erikson E. New York, International Universities Press, 1959, pp 50–100

Fonagy P: Memory and therapeutic action. Int J Psychoanal 80:215–223, 1999

Fonagy P: A genuinely developmental theory of sexual enjoyment and its implications for psychoanalytic technique. J Am Psychoanal Assoc 56:11–36, 2008

Fonagy P, Target M: The rooting of the mind in the body: new links between attachment theory and psychoanalytic thought. J Am Psychoanal Assoc 55:411–456, 2007

Fonagy P, Target M, Gergely G, et al: The developmental roots of borderline personality disorder in early attachment relationships: a theory and some evidence. Psychoanalytic Inquiry 23:412–459, 2003

Freud A: The concept of developmental lines: their diagnostic significance. Psychoanal Study Child 18:245–265, 1963

Freud S: Screen memories (1899), in The Standard Edition of the Complete Psychological Works of Sigmund Freud, Vol 3. Translated and edited by Strachey J. London, Hogarth Press, 1962, pp 299–322

Freud S: The claims of psychoanalysis to scientific interest (1913), in The Standard Edition of the Complete Psychological Works of Sigmund Freud, Vol 13. Translated and edited by Strachey J. London, Hogarth Press, 1962, pp 163–190

Freud S: The ego and the id (1923), in The Standard Edition of the Complete Psychological Works of Sigmund Freud, Vol 19. Translated and edited by Strachey J. London, Hogarth Press, 1962, pp 1–59

Freud S: An outline of psychoanalysis (1940), in The Standard Edition of the Complete Psychological Works of Sigmund Freud, Vol 23. Translated and edited by Strachey J. London, Hogarth Press, 1962, pp 144–208

Galatzer-Levy RM: Psychoanalysis and dynamical systems theory: prediction and self-similarity. J Am Psychoanal Assoc 43:1085–1113, 1995

Galatzer-Levy RM: Chaotic possibilities. Int J Psychoanal 85:419–441, 2004

Gallese V: Mirror neurons, embodied simulations, and the neural basis of social identification. Psychoanal Dialogues 19:519–536, 2009

Gallese V, Sinigaglia C: The bodily self as power for action. Neuropsychologia 28:746–755, 2010

Gilmore K: Psychoanalytic developmental theory; a contemporary reconsideration. J Am Psychoanal Assoc 56:885–907, 2008

Govrin A: The dilemma of contemporary psychoanalysis: toward a "knowing" post-postmodernism. J Am Psychoanal Assoc 54:507–535, 2006

Grossman W, Kaplan D: Three commentaries on gender in Freud's thought: prologue to the psychoanalytic theory of sexuality, in Fantasy, Myth, and Reality: Essays in Honor of Jacob A. Arlow. Edited by Blum H, Kramer Y, Richards AK, et al. New York, International Universities Press, 1988, pp 339–370

Hartmann H, Kris E: The genetic approach in psychoanalysis. Psychoanal Study Child 1:11–30, 1945

Hobson P: The Cradle of Thought: Explorations of the Origins of Thinking. Oxford, UK, Macmillan, 2002

Inderbitzen LB, Levy ST: Regression and psychoanalytic technique: the concretization of a concept. Psychoanal Q 69:195–223, 2000

Lachmann FM, Beebe BA: Three principles of salience in the organization of the patient-analyst interaction. Psychoanal Psychol 13:1–22, 1996

Lemma A: An order of pure decision: growing up in a virtual world and the adolescent's experience of being-in-a-body. J Am Psychoanal Assoc 68:691–714, 2010

Mayes L: Clocks, engines, and quarks—love, dreams, and genes: what makes development happen? Psychoanal Study Child 64:169–192, 1999

Mayes L, Spence D: Understanding therapeutic action in the analytic situation: a second look at the developmental metaphor. J Am Psychoanal Assoc 42:789–817, 1994

Meltzoff AN: "Like me": a foundation for social cognition. Dev Sci 10:126–134, 2007

Michels R: Psychoanalysts' theories, in Psychoanalysis on the Move: The Work of Joseph Sandler. New Library of Psychoanalysis, Vol 35. Edited by Fonagy P, Cooper A, Wallerstein R. London, Hogarth Press, 1999, pp 187–200

Michels R: Unpublished discussion of psychoanalytic developmental theory by Karen Gilmore, MD. Association for Psychoanalytic Medicine Scientific Meeting, New York, NY, June 6, 2006

Neubauer P: First day. Bull Anna Freud Centre 13:79–122, 1990

Neubauer PB: Current issues in psychoanalytic child development. Psychoanal Study Child 51:35–45, 1996

Neubauer PB: Some notes on the role of development in psychoanalytic assistance, differentiation, and regression. Psychoanal Study Child 58:165–171, 2003

Novick KK, Novick J: Postoedipal transformations: latency, adolescence, and pathogenesis. J Am Psychoanal Assoc 42:143–169, 1994

Rangell L: The psychoanalytic theory of change. Int J Psychoanal 73:415–428, 1992

Rapaport D, Gill MM: The points of view and assumptions of metapsychology. Int J Psychoanal 40:153–162, 1959

Reisner S: Freud and developmental theory: a 21st-century look at the origin myth of psychoanalysis. Studies in Gender and Sexuality 2:97–128, 2001

Sandler AM: The psychoanalytic legacy of Anna Freud. Psychoanal Study Child 51:270–284, 1996

Settlage CF: Transcending old age: creativity, development and psychoanalysis. Int J Psychoanal 77:549–564, 1996

Sroufe A, Egeland B, Carlson E, et al: The Development of the Person: The Minnesota Study of Risk and Adaptation From Birth to Adulthood. New York, Guilford, 2005

Stern D: The Motherhood Constellation: A Unified View of Parent-Infant Psychiatry. New York, Basic Books, 1995

Tamnes CK, Ostby Y, Fjell A, et al: Brain maturation in adolescence and young adulthood: regional age-related changes in cortical thickness and white matter volume and microstructure. Cereb Cortex 20:534–548, 2010

Tuch RH: The construction, reconstruction, and deconstruction of memory in the light of social cognition. J Am Psychoanal Assoc 47:153–186, 1999

Tyson P, Tyson R: Psychoanalytic Theories of Development: An Integration. New Haven, CT, Yale University Press, 1990

Winnicott DW: The Maturational Processes and the Facilitating Environment: Studies in the Theory of Emotional Development. London, Hogarth Press and Institute of Psycho-Analysis, 1965

CHAPTER 2

Infancy

Parenthood, the Mother-Infant Relationship, and the Mind of the Infant

INTRODUCTION TO THE INFANT

The mysterious mind of the preverbal infant has captured the imagination of modern psychodynamic thinkers. Fascinating discoveries of the newborn's relational capacities and a deeper grasp of the inherently reciprocal mother-infant bond have powerfully affected and broadened theories on early mental development. A diverse group of psychodynamic and developmental thinkers has clarified the foundational influence of the dyad's *attachment relationship* and its unique contribution to enduring social and emotional patterns; such groundbreaking work has generated novel thinking about the intersubjective nature of relationships throughout the lifespan, including in the therapeutic situation.

Role of the Mother-Infant Relationship

Despite a dazzling array of innate abilities, many of which serve to maintain close contact with the mother, the newborn arrives in a state of considerable dependency and relies heavily on maternal ego resources. The mother's emotional *mirroring* and physical responsiveness—delivered largely through the dyad's bodily contact—are profoundly shaped by identifications with her own parents, her relational history, and her unique responses to the baby's gender and temperament. As the mother repeatedly provides timely and consistent care, the very young infant begins to form mental representations of his or her shifting psychological and somatic states in combination with the mother's comforting presence. Over the course of the first few months, the baby's mind is structured by increasingly complex, organized internalizations

21

of the dyad's bodily and affective interactions; by the conclusion of infancy, these representations serve as templates for lifelong interpersonal and self-regulatory tendencies.

The stunning cognitive, social, and motoric achievements of infancy inevitably transform the dyad's initial intense bodily and emotional connection; less immediate modes of affective communication, such as verbalization and social referencing, begin to substitute for intimate physical contact. Although the mother continues to function as a beacon of emotional orientation, the baby's natural desire for exploration and determined pursuit of motor mastery broadens his or her previous, exclusive focus on the parent. The child's intellectual and motor milestones support a dawning sense of separateness and differentiation, laying the groundwork for entry into the toddler phase of development.

Historical Influences and a Modern Psychodynamic Approach to Infancy

The current widespread interest in preoedipal phases of childhood (i.e., infancy and toddlerhood) developed gradually within psychodynamic theory. An influential and highly original group of writers (e.g., Fairbairn 1954; Klein 1945, 1946) hypothesized about infant mental life; their unprecedented thinking about the lively, relationship-oriented minds of babies—much of which was later validated by empirical study—led to expanding interest in early childhood and mother-infant observation. Although a full review is beyond the scope of this chapter, we consider the following work to be particularly influential: Spitz's (1945, 1946) pioneering studies on institution-reared infants; Winnicott's (1956/1958, 1960) and Bion's (1962) elaborations of the maternal mind; and Mahler's (1972, 1974) depiction of separation-individuation theory, which describes the child's gradual achievement of differentiation and autonomy. These writings elucidated the inextricable link between mothers' and babies' mental lives, the critical role of stable and responsive parental care, and the developmental consequences for infants who are deprived of maternal bonding.

Since the 1970s, there has been a burgeoning literature on infancy (certain key studies are referenced in the current chapter); much of this work was inspired by Bowlby's (1963, 1969, 1973, 1980) seminal writings on *attachment theory*, which postulates the baby's innate need for maternal proximity and the sense of security that the mother's physical presence provides. Enormously influential in both academic and more popular venues, attachment theory and its basic principles have permeated current culture. Such common notions as maternal attunement and responsiveness are derived from the work of Bowlby and his successors. A number of prominent theorists (e.g., Stern 1985, and more recently Fonagy 2001; Gergely 2000; and Slade 2000) have integrated psychodynamic principles with attachment theory and developmental research, heightening scholarly and clinical interest in infancy within the psychodynamic community.

Substantial mutual benefit has resulted from the bridging of psychodynamic and research perspectives on infancy, but each retains unique objectives and illuminates different aspects of the mother-infant dyad (Pine 2004; Shuttleworth 1989). Empirical work tends to emphasize the external, measurable capacities that are manifest when the infant is calm, alert, and available for engagement. At such moments of opportunity, babies display remarkable social abilities and sophisticated knowledge about the world. However, we believe that the infant's subjective experience is not limited to these points in time. Particularly in the first weeks of life, when psychological and somatic states fluctuate rapidly, periods of distress and inaccessibility may dominate. To add to the complexity, the parent's inner life both influences and accommodates the baby's changes. The shifting, mutual, and often unquantifiable mental states of parent and child remain central to what we see as the psychodynamic purview.

PARENTHOOD, PREGNANCY, AND MOTHER-INFANT AFFECTIVE SHARING

Pregnancy and the Maternal Reverie

The psychological life of the baby begins in the parental mind. Expectant parents' fantasies are powerfully shaped by memories and unresolved conflicts from childhood, feelings about their own mothers and fathers, emotional and relational styles, and attitudes toward the baby's gender (whether known or imagined); these multiple conscious and unconscious factors will immediately influence the parents' care of and reactions to the newborn (Blum 2004; Slade and Cohen 1996; Stern 1995; Winnicott 1960).

Although fathers and adoptive parents share many of the biological mother's prenatal anticipations and anxieties, the pregnant woman's dramatic physical and hormonal changes, and the birthing process itself, create distinct psychological and bodily transformations. In the final weeks of pregnancy many women experience an increasingly inward focus, with intensified fantasizing about the baby and a relative withdrawal from the pragmatic concerns of the external world. A unique maternal reverie begins to develop; this "primary maternal preoccupation" (Winnicott 1956/1958) will facilitate the mother's identification with the newborn's shifting affective states as well as her capacity to mirror and contain the baby's feelings of distress and discomfort (Bion 1962; Winnicott 1956/1958). Such availability is particularly crucial during the first weeks of life, when the child requires highly *contingent responsiveness*—that is, timely parental care that is closely geared to the baby's specific signals and needs. Gradually, over the course of the first few months, the mother will regain her normal investment in the world beyond the baby; simultaneously, the infant's expanding interest in people and things outside of the mother-infant dyad develops.

Mother-Infant Affective Communication and the Role of Marked Affect

In the first months of life, the mutual affective processes of mother-infant identification and communication are conveyed primarily through bodily contact. Repeatedly, the mother mentally absorbs the infant's preverbal signals, identifies with his or her shifting affective and somatic states, and experiences her own emotional arousal. Without becoming overwhelmed or distracted by deep empathic feelings and anxieties, she interprets the infant's needs and delivers timely, consistent care. As she feeds, holds, and rocks her newborn, the baby actively takes in the sound, smell, and feel of the mother's body, along with the sense of her comforting presence.

Typical maternal responsiveness, which operates largely outside of conscious awareness, is uniquely suited to the young infant, who distinguishes between real and *marked* (i.e., modified) affective expressions (Gergely 2000). Interacting with a distressed baby, the mother's face and demeanor reflect an empathic but marked version of the child's emotion. She does not concretely mimic the infant's crying and manifest discomfort; such direct replication of negative states would intensify the infant's anxiety. Rather, the mother portrays a recognizable but playfully transformed version of the baby's subjective experience, such as "mock sad" pouting and accompanying verbalizations when the baby cries.

The mother's capacity to identify with the infant's needs reflects a modulated form of emotional arousal and enables her to deliver meaningful care that facilitates the child's gradual awareness, understanding, and tolerance of affective and bodily experience. Mental representations of bodily states, along with the mother's transforming care, begin to structure the infant's mind, forming essential building blocks for autonomous emotional self-regulation (Bion 1962; Gergely 2000; Gergely and Watson 1996; Winnicott 1960). During the infant's first weeks of life, the mother's responsiveness and active ministrations protect the infant from overwhelming distress; soon, however, the baby's mental representations lead to measurably increased tolerance for temporary discomfort and a sense of anticipatory relief. The young infant's diminished crying and distress, and the more frequent and prolonged periods of calm alertness, reassure the mother and strengthen her confidence about the effectiveness and quality of her care.

The sweeping, life-changing potential of parenthood creates a unique opportunity to revisit and rework earlier relationships and unresolved conflicts; many adults report transformations in their sense of self. The depth of these adjustments has led a number of theorists to postulate parenthood as a developmental phase (Benedek 1959; Stern 1995). A newfound closeness and identification with one's own parents, major shifts in values and priorities, a deeper sense of meaning and purpose, and increased intimacy with the child-rearing partner are common experiences.

• **See the video "Pregnant Woman" for an example of one woman's thoughts and feelings about the experience of pregnancy, the impact of motherhood on her relationship with her own mother, and her anticipation of upcoming changes in the family constellation.**

A number of risk factors—such as infant illness, lack of social support, and maternal psychopathology—can impede the experience of parenthood and compromise the mother's mirroring and caretaking capacities. The combined pressures of physical exhaustion, bodily and hormonal changes, and the sudden loss of the unique pregnancy experience create special vulnerabilities during the postpartum period, when the infant's dependency needs and the demand on maternal ego strength are at their most acute. Myriad biological, social, and emotional variables, including the unconscious conflicts that are aroused by motherhood, may contribute to postpartum anxiety and depression (Blum 2004, 2007; Murray and Cooper 1997).

The mother's mental representations of her own attachment history and her capacity for emotional self-reflection are powerful predictors of parent-infant attachment (Fonagy et al. 1993; Main et al. 1985). For the parent with unresolved trauma and deep relational conflicts, the newborn's intense needs and distressed states may evoke "ghosts in the nursery" (Fraiberg et al. 1975); these unwanted feelings and associations, which derive from the mother's distant past, interfere with maternal reverie and responsiveness in the here-and-now mother-infant situation. Moreover, they lead to distorted views and negative fantasies about the baby. For example, one mother who suffered from childhood neglect perceived her own newborn as voraciously demanding and impossible to satisfy; another, who had been raised by an intermittently violent foster parent, experienced her young infant's cries as reproachful critiques of maternal care. Memories of unmet childhood longings and helplessness, rage at the inadequacy of parental figures from the past, and the concomitant urgency to suppress such responses can cause the mother to misinterpret, minimize, or simply "tune out" the baby's affective signals (Slade and Cohen 1996).

The Role of the Maternal Mind in Infancy

- The primary maternal preoccupation is a unique reverie that helps prepare the mother for an emotional identification with her newborn.
- Maternal fantasies and attitudes (about gender, prenatal activity, etc.) immediately attach to the newborn and powerfully influence the baby's mental development.
- The infant relies heavily on maternal ego capacities, particularly the mother's mirroring and empathic responding.
- "Ghosts in the nursery" refers to unresolved memories, feelings, and conflicts from the mother's own childhood that may distort and impede maternal reverie and empathic responsiveness.

NEWBORN PERIOD, EMERGENCE OF SOCIAL SMILING, AND ROLE OF TEMPERAMENT

First Weeks of Life

Newborns are uniquely equipped and motivated to seek and engage their mothers. Their first communicative capacities, such as crying, powerfully affect the parent and help elicit the care they require. The baby's body is the center of experience. As discussed in the previous section, "Introduction to the Infant," the young infant's fluctuating somatic states and the mother's soothing care are gradually internalized, forming early mental structure. Consistent, *contingent* maternal responses (i.e., those that are closely geared to the baby's specific needs), along with the infant's growing social and cognitive capacities, soon lead to better tolerance for brief states of distress; the newborn's initially fleeting and highly intermittent periods of calm alertness and social availability are steadily increased and prolonged in the first weeks of life.

Our modern view of infancy has been greatly enriched by John Bowlby's (1969, 1973) work, which postulates that an innate, biologically based attachment system is activated whenever the baby experiences distress due to loss of the maternal presence; the child's emerging social, cognitive, and motor capacities—crying, smiling, creeping after the mother, vocalizing—are recruited to maintain or reengage the mother's attention and restore her physical closeness. During the first few months of life, based on repeated mother-infant interactions, the baby develops *internal working models*—that is, mental representations of self and other in a relational context. These models, which gain in complexity and organization, begin to create an enduring framework for the child's relational style and social expectations. Within this theory, contingent responsiveness and reliable mothering are seen as highly conducive to infants' immediate sense of efficacy, as well as to their more permanent feelings and beliefs about attachment relationships.

The nature of the baby's subjective preverbal experience is elusive. Copious developmental research has revealed previously unimagined capacities for sociability, affective communication, and perceptual organization in the first weeks of life. For example, a neonate can discern his or her own mother's unique smell, discriminate her voice, and integrate complex sensory information (Gergely and Watson 1996; Grosse et al. 2010; Stern 1985). However, the helplessness and dependency of the newborn are profound, and the gradual development of mental structure requires substantial, stable parental care. We find certain theorists' vivid, evocative descriptions to be particularly helpful for imagining the baby's fluctuating inner states and the comforts of maternal holding; these include the restoration of bodily integration after fragmentation, the sense of being gathered together after falling apart, and a feeling of continuity (Bick 1968; Bion 1962; Shuttleworth 1989; Winnicott 1960).

Mahler's (1972, 1974) theory of separation-individuation postulates that the infant initially experiences the self and the mother as an undifferentiated unit. Mahler suggests that for many months, babies have only limited awareness of their own and their parents' mental and bodily boundaries. In this model, a major task of early development is the gradual achievement of psychological and physical separateness. Mahler's elaborations of the newborn's initial "autistic-like" state have needed revision in light of more recent findings about innate relational capacities (Gergely 2000; Pine 2004). Nonetheless, we find that Mahler's descriptions of the newborn remain relevant; they capture the unfathomable nature of preverbal experience, the baby's intense need for highly contingent responsiveness, and the adults' sense of helplessness and bewilderment when the baby appears acutely distressed or unreachable.

Social Smiling and Its Impact on Mother-Infant Bonding

At around age 2 months, with the emergence of responsive *social smiling,* the infant's overall appearance and behavior shift markedly. The arrival of this uniquely meaningful milestone reflects maturities in the infant's underlying mental organization, including better self-regulation of somatic states, more prolonged periods of alert availability, and increased cognitive and perceptual abilities. These advances immediately impact the mother-infant relationship, deepening the dyad's pleasure in face-to-face interaction and expanding the overall scope of affective communication (Spitz 1965; Stern 1985). As anyone familiar with infants can attest, eliciting their smile is intrinsically rewarding; moreover, a new level of increased social responsiveness makes the 2- or 3-month-old child appear to be a far more recognizable, comprehensible creature than the newborn. After navigating the sleepless and often confusing first weeks of life, many parents feel an enormous sense of relief and a renewed confidence in their capacity to understand and care for their infant.

Temperament and Its Role in Mother-Infant Relations

Unique aspects of infant endowment find expression early in the first year of life. The baby's innate temperament, encompassing such factors as susceptibility to arousal and reactivity, influences his or her availability for social engagement, tolerance for stimulation, and capacity for self-regulation (Kagan 1997). Importantly, infant qualities elicit deep maternal reactions; when combined with the baby's gender, for example, they may arouse the mother's unconscious feelings and associations about perceived passivity or aggression. The mother-baby temperamental "fit" is not necessarily ideal; an active, highly engaging parent may find herself with a slow-to-warm, easily overwhelmed infant. Maternal flexibility and willingness to accommodate the infant's individual needs and vulnerabilities will be key factors in the baby's emerging personality. The complex interaction between infant endowment and maternal responsiveness leads to an emerging "basic core" (Weil 1970) of possibilities that guide future developmental trends.

The following vignette illustrates one mother's adjustment to her baby's unique temperament and relational needs.

> Ruth and her husband, both busy and successful 33-year-old educators, knew that the arrival of their first child would mean dramatic changes in their active, highly scheduled lives. However, Ruth was not prepared for baby Heather's distinct qualities. Although Heather was contented and healthy, and was a good eater and sleeper, the baby was easily overstimulated by avid social interactions, preferring to warm slowly to her mother's overtures. At times, she fussed or averted her gaze when Ruth approached her with characteristic enthusiasm, loud tones, and lively physical handling. Friends commented that Heather appeared to be a "quiet observer," content to spend long periods of time in her infant seat or on a blanket gazing at people or interesting toys; other parents openly envied her pleasant temperament and quick achievement of eating and sleeping routines.

Privately, Ruth wished her daughter were less placid and more aggressive; these were the assertive qualities that Ruth admired and associated with successful, powerful women. She watched as her own mother, who was low-keyed and soft-spoken, patiently elicited Heather's slow but wonderful smile, allowing the infant to sustain a comfortable interaction. Although Ruth had always felt frustrated by her mother's timid, hesitant ways, she was grateful for her quiet grandmotherly presence and began to copy her gentle approach.

Initially, Ruth is surprised that her daughter possesses tendencies so different from her own; she had daydreamed about a zesty, athletic child. The infant's subdued style stirs up confusion, as well as a sense of incompetence, in this active, vivacious mother who was used to being "on top of" her life. However, Ruth is an open, reflective parent, able to acknowledge her rather unrealistic prenatal fantasies about perfect mother-daughter bonding, her mild disappointment, and her sense of inadequacy. Newfound empathy for her own mother, whose interpersonal style is somewhat quiet and reserved, helps her absorb the grandmother's modeling and assistance, and this first-time mother soon learns to accommodate her baby's need for gentler handling.

The following case example describes a less favorable maternal adjustment in a mother-infant dyad buffeted by serious psychological pressures.

Naomi, 24 years old, intensely wished for a boy. She was reassured by active fetal movement, which convinced her that this baby could not possibly be female. She had long-standing private convictions about boys' superior status, power, and capacity for happiness. Her own mother, divorced when Naomi was young, kept the household going but derived little pleasure from life. Naomi's sense of her mother's endurance and forbearance had dominated her childhood. Her father, meanwhile, was a distant, rather exciting character, more vivid in fantasy than in his real contributions to her upbringing. At 19, Naomi married a steady, kind, and undemanding boyfriend; she sometimes doubted her respect for him, but she was certain of and grateful for his devotion.

When baby Michael was born, she was delighted by his alert, active demeanor; to friends, she proudly described him as "strong." She speculated that as a boy, he would surely not be victimized and vulnerable; on the other hand, she began to anticipate that he would undoubtedly strike out on his own sooner than a female child; indeed, her own brother had, in her perception, "fled" home in late adolescence, leaving her alone with her depressed and needy mother. Her own baby's first signs of self-soothing—such as sucking his fingers and quieting at 3 months—filled her with ambivalence; she was gratified by his "strength," but felt her own role in his life to be diminished. When alone with Michael, Naomi sometimes—but not always—postponed responding to his cries, rationalizing that she was teaching him "self-reliance." Inevitably, after a few minutes of self-sucking, he would gradually grow more distressed and frantic. At these moments, she felt he truly needed her, but she was simultaneously enraged by the intensity of his helplessness and needs.

This mother's capacity for empathic responsiveness is impeded by her underlying abandonment fears and unresolved rage at male figures from the past, as well as her largely negative sense of her own mother's parenting. Fears of rejection, memories of her own helplessness, and intense, angry feelings are stirred up as she confronts her infant's normal neediness and efforts at self-regulation. These "ghosts" from an unhappy childhood place enormous psychological pressures on the dyad and create an unresolvable bind for Naomi and the infant: she can neither tolerate Michael's dependency nor accept his self-reliance. Her unpredictable, occasionally negligent behavior threatens to disrupt the baby's sense of security and stability, making it far more challenging for him to develop internal emotional controls.

Face-to-Face Interaction and the Process of "Hatching"

Ages 3–6 Months and Dyadic Interaction

The 3- to 6-month-old infant is intensely social, showing immense interest and unmistakable pleasure in face-to-face interaction. His or her entire body responds; smiling, cooing, intent gazing, and bicycling limbs all convey the baby's total engagement in dyadic exchanges. Key components of human socializing, such as vocal turn-taking and reciprocity, can already be recognized in these early face-to-face encounters. Close inspection of mother-infant interaction reveals ongoing processes of affective communication and mutual regulation, conducted through minute, unconscious shifts and adjustments in behavior (Beebe 2000; Stern 1985). In contrast to newborns, older infants are less dependent on immediate, contingent responsiveness; they are now interested in slightly novel experiences and can wait brief periods before their bodily states receive attention.

• See the video "3-Month-Old Infant and Mother" for an example of face-to-face interaction and an illustration of how the mother's ongoing conversation reflects her attempts to imagine the child's experience.

Mahler's (1972, 1974) depiction of mother-infant "symbiosis" captures the dyad's deep affective connection and mutual dependency; the powerful reactions and sense of exclusion that third parties, from family members to infancy researchers, experience when they are in the presence of the dyad attests to the pair's intense mutual absorption (Rustin 1989). By the fourth month of life, infants have internalized a sense of familiar, unfolding dyadic interactions and are disturbed by changes in maternal behavior. This awareness is demonstrated in the "still face" experiment (Tronick 1989; Tronick et al. 1978). In this paradigm, mothers are initially instructed to engage in typical responsive face-to-face exchanges with their babies; then, they are asked to shift to an impassive expression. In response to the mother's still face, many infants redouble their efforts at engagement by increasing vocalizations and motor activity. When these attempts fail to restore normal interaction, most babies manifest apparent distress and avoidance via crying, gaze aversion, or sudden drowsiness.

Age 6 Months, the Process of "Hatching," and the Transitional Object

Halfway through infants' first year of life, their intense absorption in face-to-face interaction begins to shift. Increasingly, they direct their attention beyond the mother's face, actively pushing away to examine her body, clothing, and accessories. In addition, they begin to show greater awareness of and interest in objects and the surrounding environment. Mahler (1972, 1974) describes this as the process of *hatching*, a dawning sense of separateness from the mother fueled by the infant's enhanced cognitive and sensorimotor apparatus. Better able to sit and manipulate interesting items, and even to creep a short distance away from the mother, the baby achieves a new view of the world and an increasing desire for exploration. *Orality* is a dominant mode of learning; throughout the first year of life, infants take in the social and inanimate world through their sensory organs and attempt to bring all objects, including parts of their own and their mothers' bodies, to their mouths for sucking and exploration.

During this phase of emerging separateness, while infants' awareness of objective reality is still dim, they often become attached to a special *transitional object*; typically, this item is a soft, familiar toy or blanket that provides comfort as the baby experiences the gradual loss of mother-child bodily intimacy and security. The value of such an object, which is the child's "first not-me" possession (Winnicott 1953), is intuitively grasped by mothers, who tend to allow their child to retain the item despite its inevitable dirtiness and decrepit condition. Over time, the object loses its meaning and desirability; older children's play and imaginative activities are natural continuations of transitional phenomena, giving them access to fantasies and creative ideas that are not bound by the world of objective reality.

Affective Sharing in Late Infancy and the Attachment Relationship

Emergence of Joint Attention and Social Referencing

The last quarter of the infant year marks a period of momentous change in the mother-child relationship. Cognitive, social-emotional, and motoric advances equip the baby for a far more active role within the dyad. Expressive babbling, responses to familiar words and phrases, increasingly sustained attention and interest in shared activities, and improved motoric coordination (crawling, cruising, and manipulation of objects) all contribute to the infant's drive toward exploration and motor mastery while allowing for more distal modes of mother-infant communication. As the baby ventures beyond the immediacy of the mother's body, he or she now possesses an array of capacities that serve to maintain affective sharing and connection.

A greater awareness of mother-child separateness and a growing ability to differentiate the mother from other adults leads to the emergence of *stranger anxiety* and *separation anxiety.* Even familiar, previously accepted substitute caregivers, such as grandparents and babysitters, may suddenly find themselves rejected. Moreover, babies begin to expect and protest the mother's departures, linking the loss of her presence with specific behaviors, such as mother putting on her shoes. The infant does not yet fully grasp the mother's permanence or mentally anticipate her return, and is therefore susceptible to acute distress over temporary separations.

Despite these novel vulnerabilities, however, the older infant's discovery that mental states and affects can be shared with the mother is a transformative development that deepens the parent-infant bond and provides vastly enhanced self-regulatory possibilities. The emergence of *joint attention,* wherein babies shift their gaze between the mother's face and an object of mutual interest, is a subtle but crucial sign of new, social-emotional reciprocity. During ambiguous or stressful situations, older infants begin to engage in the process of *social referencing,* whereby they seek the mother's emotional signals and then use those signals to gauge their own affective reactions (Emde 1983; Stern 1985). This process is vividly demonstrated in the "visual cliff" experiment, in which babies are subjected to a perceived threatening situation and their mothers are instructed to provide either negative or positive affective feedback (Sorce and Emde 1981). In this experiment, an infant is placed on a structure with a transparent surface over a checkerboard pattern, which creates the illusion of a sharp drop-off. The mother stands in front of the baby, who begins to crawl toward her. As babies approach the apparent "cliff," they tend to hesitate, show apprehension, and look toward the parent for emotional guidance. In conditions where the mother beckons and encourages, babies cross the cliff; however, when the mother's behavior reflects negative or frightened affect, the babies refuse to move.

Emotional Refueling and Mother-Infant Attachment

The older infant is increasingly motivated for mobility and exploration but remains affectively anchored in the dyadic relationship; the mother functions as a "beacon of emotional orientation" (Mahler 1952). Repeatedly, after the baby crawls a short distance away or becomes engrossed in interesting objects, he or she looks back at the mother in order to share pleasurable feelings and receive reassurance; frequently, the child returns to the mother's lap for brief emotional refueling before setting out once again to play and explore. If made anxious by an unexpected noise or the arrival of a stranger, the infant quickly seeks the mother's facial expression or moves closer to her body for comfort. Such tangible behaviors were famously recruited in the "strange situation" experiment (Ainsworth et al. 1978), a widely used assessment of mother-infant interaction that reveals distinct patterns of attachment by age 12 months. In this paradigm, babies and their mothers initially acclimate to a laboratory environment; after a series of brief but stressful separations, designed to elicit the infants' attachment and proximity-seeking behaviors, researchers evaluate the babies' reactions to reunion with their mothers. Judgments about the infants' quality of attachment are based largely on their effective use of the mother as a "secure base"—that is, as a source of security and comfort after distress—and as a facilitating presence for return to exploratory play.

The studies by Ainsworth et al. (1978) yielded three attachment classifications: *Secure* infants play and explore in the mother's presence and manifest ongoing affective sharing and reciprocity; despite considerable distress during the separation conditions, these infants are soon reassured by the mother's return. *Avoidant* infants appear emotionally detached from their mothers and behave as if they are impervious to the experimental conditions; such children have learned to minimize their affective reactions, despite physical evidence of heightened anxiety during separation (e.g., increased heart rate). *Ambivalent/resistant* infants are highly aroused and distressed throughout the assessment, unable to make use of the maternal presence for exploration or self-regulation either before or after separation. An additional insecure group, *disorganized/disoriented* infants, was later identified. These babies manifest inconsistent, incoherent reactions to separation conditions; their failure to develop an organized strategy for managing distress, which is believed to derive from the mother's own unresolved trauma history and her tendency toward confusing, alternately frightened or frightening behaviors, places them at risk for later mood and self-regulatory disorders (Hesse and Main 2000; Main and Hesse 1990). The American "standard" distribution for typical dyads is considered to fall at around 70% secure, 20% avoidant, and 10% resistant; a meta-review of attachment studies, which includes data on disorganized dyads, reveals the following frequencies: securely attached (62%), avoidant (15%), resistant (9%), and disorganized (15%) (van IJzendoorn et al. 1999). In populations under pressure from social, psychological, or environmental stress, the proportions of dyads with insecure attachment are substantially higher.

The categorization of attachment soon gave rise to a burgeoning collection of studies in which links between the quality of early mother-infant relationships and broad areas of later social and emotional development were postulated. When compared to their insecure counterparts, securely attached babies are found to demonstrate enhanced functioning in such developmental domains as peer relations, emotional self-regulation, cooperative behavior, and adjustment to school (see Sroufe et al. 2005 for an extensive review of these findings). In later chapters, we more fully elaborate the consequences of secure early attachment as they apply to the specific phases and age-salient tasks of childhood.

Moreover, corresponding classifications of maternal attachment styles, as measured by narratives and relational descriptions on the Adult Attachment Interview (George et al. 1985), yielded the following categories: *secure–autonomous* mothers (like secure infants) value personal bonds and are open to emotional signals; *dismissive* mothers (similar to avoidant infants) deny the importance of their own and others' relational and emotional experience; *preoccupied* mothers (like ambivalent-resistant infants) tend to become overwhelmed by personal feelings and memories; and *unresolved* mothers (like disorganized-disoriented infants) manifest chaotic, poorly organized strategies for coping with emotional distress and frequently report a history of early loss and trauma (Hesse and Main 2000; Main 2000). Distributions for typical U.S. and Canadian mothers are as follows: autonomous (58%), dismissive (23%), and preoccupied (19%); 18% are further classified as unresolved (Bakermans-Kranenburg and van IJzendoorn 2009; van IJzendoorn and Bakermans-Kranenburg 1996).

Research into the intergenerational transmission of attachment yields complex findings. Results suggest very high (approximately 75%) continuity, from mother to baby, for the nondifferentiated categories of secure and insecure patterns (van IJzendoorn 1995). However, the powerful influence of the maternal mind—her tolerance for affect, fantasies about parenthood, and memories and representations of her own childhood bonds—does not necessarily result in an exact replication of the mother's relational style. Continuity is quite robust between "autonomous" mothers and secure children; emotionally flexible, self-reflective mothers discern, accept, and interpret their infants' emotional signals and needs, ultimately fostering secure attachments (Fonagy 2001; Slade 2000; van IJzendoorn 1995). On the other hand, transmission between subcategories of insecure attachment (i.e., dismissive parent to avoidant infant, preoccupied to resistant, unresolved to disorganized) is less predictable; although insecure mothers tend to foster insecure babies, intervening factors such as specific maternal traumas or fantasies, or children's use of multiple behavioral strategies in coping with a distant or overwhelming parent, contribute to greater variability (Shah et al. 2010; Slade and Cohen 1996). Intergenerational pathways, even in the first year of life, are remarkably diverse and will continue to accrue unique features as the child's range of reactions and defenses gains in scope.

Although his work predates by many years the studies described previously in this section, we find Winnicott's (1960) notion of the *false self* to be especially useful and rich; indeed, many of his ideas about the mother-infant relationship were validated by later research. Winnicott poses a universal infant (and, more broadly, human) dilemma: how to maintain intimate connection with the mother (or any intimate other) while achieving unique and individual selfhood. In his theory, failures of maternal mirroring, such as persistent overstimulation or nonresponsiveness, severely curtail the baby's potential resolutions, leading to the gradual suppression of his or her true needs and natural tendencies. To preserve closeness to the mother, the poorly mirrored infant must adopt a false self and identify with the mother's defensive reactions, such as denial of the baby's dependency and hunger for attention. The infant prematurely accommodates the mother's emotional requirements, such as for a more subdued, less demanding, or less needy baby. In essence, the infant's *true self* is sacrificed, and he or she becomes the child required by the mother. This vivid description of dyadic process is highly consistent with the avoidant infant of attachment theory, who adapts to the mother's poor affect tolerance via the minimization of needs and emotions. In both theories, the infant makes substantial internal adjustments in order to maintain proximity and security.

The Mother-Infant Relationship and Mental Structure

- The baby begins to form mental representations of bodily feelings and sensations in combination with the mother's emotional and physical responsiveness.

- By age 2–3 months, the infant has an internalized sense of mother-infant affective interactions.

- The infant's internal working models of self, mother, and their relationship form building blocks for later, more enduring patterns of relating and emotional self-regulation.

- By the end of the first year, stable patterns of attachment can be discerned in the infant.

- These secure and insecure patterns are assessed by measuring the infant's use of the mother as an emotional base for exploration and self-regulation.

PHYSICAL DEVELOPMENT, MOTORIC PRACTICING, AND THE TRANSITION TO TODDLER PHASE

The infancy period is one of unparalleled physical growth and central nervous system maturation, including rapid gains in weight and length (nearly tripling and doubling, respectively, in the first 12 months of life); evolutions in muscle mass, tone, coordination, and strength; and changes in bodily proportions (Thelen et al. 1984). Momentous advances in motoric capacities, from the normative "fidgety movements" of the first few months to the milestones of grasping, sitting, crawling, and ultimately walking, further contribute to the transformations of this phase (Hempel 1993).

As the first year comes to a close, infants' preoccupation with standing and walking becomes all-absorbing; their persistent, determined pursuit of upright mobility is aptly described as part of the "practicing phase" (Mahler 1972, 1974). Previous intense focus on the mother is noticeably diminished as infants' physical and mental energies turn to the mastery of motor skills, and as they increasingly derive pleasure and excitement from their own movement and autonomous exploration. Moreover, now that their bodily connection to the mother is slightly diminished, older infants are more aware of their fathers and siblings, who in turn find them more responsive and engaging. Although the infant's emotional life is still anchored in the mother-child relationship, separate attachments to the other parent, siblings, and important caregivers are established. The almost-toddler begins to notice and imitate the actions of others, and shows enhanced interest in their possessions.

◆ **See the video "10-Month-Old Infant and Mother" for an example of an older infant who is increasingly engrossed in exploration and motor accomplishments.**

The following two vignettes depict typical behaviors for mobile infants.

Eliza, age 12 months, is devoted to the task of walking, which she has not yet quite mastered. Rising at dawn, she cruises around her crib. Once her mother sets her on the floor, Eliza uses whatever furniture or surfaces she can find for assisted movement, or walks along while holding onto her older sister's toy shopping cart. On a number of occasions, this sibling resentfully pulls the cart away, causing Eliza to tumble; however, the 1-year-old barely reacts to these minor setbacks and soon finds a way to regain upright mobility. One day at the playground, Eliza grabs hold of another infant's push toy and begins to toddle along, never looking back as she approaches the border of the park. Her mother follows at a slight distance, repeatedly calling her name, but eventually she is forced to corral Eliza and return the toy to its rightful owner. Eliza wails piteously until she is set down on the ground again, and then she quickly begins to cruise along the park benches.

Jay, age 11 months, is rapidly crawling toward the family's entertainment center; his mother calls him and cautions him to stop, but he seems not to hear her as he focuses on the temptation of attractive knobs and lights. As she begins to pursue him, Jay squeals excitedly and makes an attempt at wobbly acceleration; he tumbles onto his face, momentarily stops, but then recovers and continues on his way. When his mother scoops him up right before he reaches the television, he momentarily cries and protests; very soon, however, he is redirected to a new activity and location. This entire sequence of actions will be repeated many times in a day.

The practicing infant continues to return to the mother's side for emotional refueling, but the exhilaration of independent movement and exploration is powerfully motivating; the baby appears engaged in a "love affair with the world" (Greenacre 1957). Newfound symbolic abilities, such as the beginnings of imitative play and first words, allow for more distal forms of dyadic sharing and relating, further allowing the infant's horizons to expand beyond the immediate mother-baby orbit. The physical act of walking and the infant's dawning sense of control over mother-child distance are essential to the development of autonomy. Olesker (1990) notes that gender differences may impact the baby's awareness of separateness. She suggests that girls tend toward a greater overall focus on and sensitivity to their mothers' emotional states and are more precociously aware of differentiation than boys. Moreover, she reports that mothers are more straightforward and active in their efforts to promote independence in male infants, whereas their reactions to their daughters' self-reliance are often more ambivalent. In Olesker's view, girls' more mature sense of separateness, heightened awareness of maternal affect, and exposure to the mother's conflictual feelings can interfere with exuberance during the practicing phase and dispose female infants to increased anxiety during the achievement of motor milestones.

As a number of writers (e.g., Mahler 1974; Stern 1985) have poignantly noted, the new capacities and enlarged perspectives of late infancy inevitably lead to losses for both mother and child. Emerging motoric and symbolic abilities usher in the toddler period, which is characterized by a growing sense of separation from the mother. Affective sharing and communication continue, but the walking baby's fascination with the world beyond the mother's body and increasing capacity to represent experience through words and play transform the dyadic relationship, permanently altering the physical intimacy of the mother-infant bond.

Summary of Infant Milestones

- At birth, an innate attachment system equips the newborn with capacities to seek maternal proximity.
- Social smiling begins to emerge at around age 2 months; the infant then enters an intensely social period of development and actively seeks face-to-face interaction.
- By around age 3 months, distinctions of temperament are discernible and a basic core of developmental trends is formed.
- Halfway through the first year, the infant enters a period of "hatching," marked by increasing awareness of mother-infant differentiation.
- When the child is between 8 and 10 months of age, awareness of the mother as a distinct person intensifies, resulting in stranger and separation anxieties.
- At around the same time, social referencing and joint attention emerge, representing the baby's increased capacity for sharing affects and other mental states.
- As the infant gains motor skills, the mother functions as a secure base or beacon of emotional orientation.
- Stable secure and insecure (avoidant, resistant, and disorganized) patterns of attachment are discernible by the end of the first year.
- Intense focus on the mother shifts during the practicing phase as preoccupation with upright mobility dominates and the infant appears to enter a love affair with the world.

Key Concepts

The mother-infant relationship forms the context for the baby's mental development. An innate attachment system motivates the newborn to seek maternal proximity and equips the baby with uniquely social capacities. From the earliest weeks of life, the newborn creates mental representations of feelings and bodily states along with the mother's physical and emotional care; initially, he or she relies heavily on maternal ego capacities, especially the mother's empathic identifications and responsiveness. The baby's constitutional factors, such as temperament, and the mother's particular fantasies, associations to the past, and here-and-now care yield a basic core of trends that serve to guide future development.

As the infant receives consistent relief from physical distress and emotionally reciprocal attention, internal working models of the self, the mother, and their ongoing relationship are consolidated; these form the building blocks for later, more enduring patterns of relating. The process of differentiation, in which the infant increasingly grasps a sense of self as separate from the mother, begins to unfold by around age 6 months. Cognitive and motoric capacities expand, and the infant is an increasingly active participant in the dyad's affective sharing, seeking the mother's joint attention and her emotional information in order to inform the infant's own reactions (*social referencing*). By the end of the first year of life, distinct styles of secure or insecure mother-infant attachment can be discerned. A preoccupation with achieving upright mobility dominates the final weeks of infancy, as the child approaches the toddler phase.

- The *primary maternal preoccupation* is a unique reverie that begins to prepare the mother for an intense, empathic identification with the baby.
  - The mother's capacity for *affective mirroring* and *contingent responsiveness* is essential during the initial weeks of infancy, when babies have few resources to manage their fluctuating states.
  - Maternal reverie can be impeded by "ghosts in the nursery"; these are unwanted, disavowed feelings and memories from the mother's own childhood, which may stem from traumatic events or highly conflictual relationships with her own parents.
- The body is the center of infant experience.
  - Early mental structure begins to develop as the child internalizes bodily states and feelings in combination with the mother's repeated feeding and holding.
  - Orality is a dominant mode of learning and relating to the world.
- By the end of the first 3 months, the infant's unique temperamental qualities can be discerned. A *basic core* of develop-

mental trends, which comprise innate characteristics and maternal influences, begins to emerge.

- The young infant is intensely social.

- *Attachment theory* posits a biologically based predisposition to seek maternal proximity and felt security.

  - After social smiling emerges, at 2–3 months, the infant enters a period of focused interest in face-to-face interaction with the mother.

  - Internalizations of ongoing, repeated mother-infant interactions become increasingly organized and integrated over the course of the first months; such mental structures form the basis for later, more enduring relational patterns and self-regulatory capacities.

- At around age 9 months, the infant begins to assume a more active role in the mother-child relationship.

  - Joint attention and social referencing are major signposts of increased capacity to initiate and make use of affective sharing.

  - The infant is more aware of the mother's distinct features and may experience separation and stranger anxiety.

- As the infant acquires greater motoric abilities, the mother functions as a beacon of orientation; the baby repeatedly leaves the mother's side, briefly explores, and returns for emotional refueling.

- By the end of the child's first year, attachment theorists can identify both secure and insecure patterns of mother-child relating.

- An increasing preoccupation with upright mobility diminishes older infants' previous intense focus on the mother. Babies' horizons expand and they experience a "love affair with the world."

References

Ainsworth MDS, Blehar MC, Waters E, et al: Patterns of Attachment: A Psychological Study of the Strange Situation. Hillsdale, NJ, Erlbaum, 1978

Bakermans-Kranenburg MJ, van IJzendoorn MH: The first 10,000 Adult Attachment Interviews: distributions of adult attachment representations in clinical and non-clinical groups. Attach Hum Dev 11:223–263, 2009

Beebe B: Co-constructing mother-infant distress: the microsynchrony of maternal impingement and infant avoidance in the face-to-face encounter. Psychoanalytic Inquiry 20:421–440, 2000

Benedek T: Parenthood as a developmental phase. J Am Psychoanal Assoc 7:389–417, 1959

Bick E: The experience of skin in early object relations. Int J Psychoanal 49:484–486, 1968

Bion WR: The psychoanalytic study of thinking. Int J Psychoanal 43:306–310, 1962

Blum HP: Separation-individuation theory and attachment theory. J Am Psychoanal Assoc 52:535–553, 2004

Blum LD: Psychodynamics of post-partum depression. Psychoanal Psychol 24:45–62, 2007

Bowlby J: Pathological mourning and childhood mourning. J Am Psychoanal Assoc 11:500–541, 1963

Bowlby J: Attachment and Loss: Volume 1. New York, Basic Books, 1969

Bowlby J: Attachment and Loss: Volume 2. New York, Basic Books, 1973

Bowlby J: Attachment and Loss: Volume 3. London, Hogarth Press, 1980

Emde RN: The pre-representational self and its affective core. Psychoanal Study Child 38:165–192, 1983

Fairbairn W: An Object Relations Theory of the Personality. New York, Basic Books, 1954

Fonagy P: Attachment Theory and Psychoanalysis. New York, Other Press, 2001

Fonagy P, Steele M, Moran G, et al: Measuring the ghost in the nursery: an empirical study of the relation between parents' mental representations of childhood experience and their infants' security of attachment. J Am Psychoanal Assoc 41:957–989, 1993

Fraiberg S, Adelson E, Shapiro V: Ghosts in the nursery: a psychoanalytic approach to the problem of impaired infant-mother relationships. J Am Acad Child Psychiatry 14:387–421, 1975

George C, Kaplan N, Main M: Adult Attachment Interview. Berkeley, Department of Psychology, University of California, Berkeley, 1985

Gergely G: Reapproaching Mahler: New perspectives on normal autism, symbiosis, splitting and libidinal object constancy from cognitive developmental theory. J Am Psychoanal Assoc 48:1197–1228, 2000

Gergely G, Watson JS: The social biofeedback theory of parental affect mirroring. Int J Psychoanal 77:1181–1212, 1996

Greenacre P: The childhood of the artist: libidinal phase development and giftedness. Psychoanal Study Child 12:47–72, 1957

Grosse G, Behne T, Carpenter M, et al: Infants communicate in order to be understood. Dev Psychol 46:1710–1722, 2010

Hempel MS: Neurological development during toddling age in normal children and children at risk of developmental disorder. Early Hum Dev 34:47–57, 1993

Hesse E, Main M: Disorganized infant, child and adult attachment: collapse in behavioral and attentional strategies. J Am Psychoanal Assoc 48:1097–1127, 2000

Kagan J: In the beginning: the contribution of temperament to personality development. Modern Psychoanalyst 22:145–155, 1997

Klein M: The Oedipus complex in the light of early anxieties. Int J Psychoanal 26:11–33, 1945

Klein M: Notes on some schizoid mechanisms. Int J Psychoanal 27:99–110, 1946

Mahler MS: On childhood psychosis and schizophrenia—autistic and symbiotic infants. Psychoanal Study Child 7:286–305, 1952

Mahler MS: On the first 3 subphases of the separation-individuation process. Int J Psychoanal 53:333–338, 1972

Mahler MS: Symbiosis and individuation: the psychological birth of the human infant. Psychoanal Study Child 29:89–106, 1974

Main M: The original category of infant, child and adult attachment: flexible versus inflexible attention under attachment-related stress. J Am Psychoanal Assoc 48:1055–1095, 2000

Main M, Hesse E: Parents' unresolved traumatic experiences are related to infant disorganized attachment status: is frightened and/or frightening behavior the linking mechanism? in Attachment in the Preschool Years. Edited by Greenberg MT, Cicchetti D, Cummings EM. Chicago, IL, University of Chicago Press, 1990, pp 161–182

Main M, Kaplan N, Cassidy J: Security in infancy, childhood and adulthood: a move to the level of representation. Monographs of the Society Research Child Development 50:66–106, 1985

Murray L, Cooper PJ: Postpartum Depression and Child Development. New York, Guilford, 1997

Olesker W: Sex differences during the early separation-individuation process: implications for gender identity formation. J Am Psychoanal Assoc 38:325–346, 1990

Pine F: Mahler's concept of symbiosis and separation-individuation: revisited, reevaluated, refined. J Am Psychoanal Assoc 52:511–533, 2004

Rustin M: Encountering primitive anxieties, in Closely Observed Infants. Edited by Miller L, Rustin ME, Rustin MJ, et al. London, Duckworth, 1989, pp 7–22

Shah PE, Fonagy P, Strathearn L: Is attachment transmitted across generations? The plot thickens. Clin Child Psychol Psychiatry 15:329–345, 2010

Shuttleworth J: Psychoanalytic theory and infant development, in Closely Observed Infants. Edited by Miller L, Ruskin ME, Ruskin MJ, et al. London, Duckworth, 1989, pp 22–51

Slade A: The development and organization of attachment: implications for psychoanalysis. J Am Psychoanal Assoc 48:1147–1174, 2000

Slade A, Cohen L: Parenting and the remembrance of things past. Infant Ment Health J 17:217–239, 1996

Sorce J, Emde R: Mothers' presence is not enough: effect of emotional availability on infant exploration. Dev Psychol 17:737–745, 1981

Spitz RA: Hospitalism—an inquiry into the genesis of psychiatric conditions in early childhood. Psychoanal Study Child 1:53–74, 1945

Spitz RA: Hospitalism—a follow-up report on an investigation described in Volume I. Psychoanal Study Child 2:113–117, 1946

Spitz RA: The First Year of Life. New York, International Universities Press, 1965

Sroufe LA, Egeland B, Carlson EA, et al: The Development of the Person: The Minnesota Study of Risk and Adaptation From Birth to Adulthood. New York, Guilford, 2005

Stern DN: The Interpersonal World of the Infant: A View From Psychoanalysis and Developmental Psychology. New York, Basic Books, 1985

Stern DN: The Motherhood Constellation: A Unified View of Parent-Infant Psycho-therapy. New York, Basic Books, 1995

Thelen E, Fisher DM, Ridley-Johnson R: The relationship between physical growth and a newborn reflex. Infant Behav Dev 7:479–493, 1984

Tronick EZ: Emotions and emotional communication in infants. Am Psychol 44:112–119, 1989

Tronick EZ, Als H, Adamson L, et al: The infant's response to entrapment between contradictory messages in face-to-face interaction. J Am Acad Child Psychiatry 17:1–13, 1978

Van IJzendoorn MH: Adult attachment representations, parental responsiveness and infant attachment: a meta-analysis on the predictive validity of the AAI. Psychol Bull 117:387–403, 1995

Van IJzendoorn MH, Bakermans-Kranenburg MJ: Attachment representations in mothers, fathers, adolescents, and clinical groups: a meta-analytic search for normative data. J Consult Clin Psychol 64:8–21, 1996

Van IJzendoorn MH, Schuengel MH, Bakermans-Kranenburg MJ: Disorganized attachment in early childhood: meta-analysis of precursors, concomitants, and sequelae. Dev Psychopathol 11:225–249, 1999

Weil A: The basic core. Psychoanal Study Child 25:442–460, 1970

Winnicott DW: Transitional objects and transitional phenomena: a study of the first not-me possession. Int J Psychoanal 34:89–97, 1953

Winnicott DW: Primary maternal preoccupation (1956), in Collected Papers: Through Paediatrics to Psychoanalysis. New York, Basic Books, 1958, pp 300–305

Winnicott DW: The theory of the parent-infant relationship. Int J Psychoanal 41:585–595, 1960

CHAPTER 3

The Toddler

Early Sense of Self and Gender, Rapprochement, Libidinal Object Constancy, and Superego Precursors

INTRODUCTION TO THE TODDLER

The toddler is both motorically and developmentally on the move. In the exciting months between the first and third birthdays, the young child's upright mobility and expanding mental capacities transform his or her sense of self and relationship with the mother. A series of momentous and highly visible evolutions—from wobbly initial steps to competent movement, non-verbal gestures to elaborate language-based communication, and imitation to creative symbolic play—expands the toddler's world beyond people and things in the immediate environment. At the same time, more hidden but crucial internal changes, such as growing self-regulatory abilities and increased self-awareness, help the toddler begin to achieve mastery over bodily functions and emotional urges, laying the groundwork for superego development.

By the middle of the second year, the toddler's interior life is already far more complex and nuanced than during infancy. As noted by a number of theorists (Bergman and Harpaz-Rotem 2004; Mahler et al. 1975; Stern 1985), the acquisition of myriad new physical and psychological capacities creates unfamiliar challenges and vulnerabilities for the walking, talking toddler. An increasingly objective and differentiated *sense of self* leads to intensified anxiety about the mother's presence. Once the elation of the practicing phase has diminished, the toddler enters a period of dawning self-awareness—recognizing his or her real limits, helplessness, and smallness—and becomes acutely conscious of the new physical and psychic separateness from the mother; moreover, the emergence of *self-aware emotions*,

45

such as pride and shame, brings a capacity for self-evaluation. The development of language enriches and expands the mother-child relationship but contributes to the gradual loss of bodily intimacy that characterized the dyad's preverbal bond (Stern 1985). Discrepancies between the toddler's urges and the mother's desires, as well as between the wished-for state of things and reality, become part of the child's conscious awareness. The baby's earlier sense of "the world as his oyster" (Mahler 1972) has begun to fade.

We find Mahler's (1972) descriptions of the *rapprochement phase,* marked by the toddler's entry into a period of increased anxiety and resurgent need for maternal comfort, to be especially meaningful. For the first time, the small child experiences the inner pressure of conflicting urges, such as the inward push toward newfound independence and autonomy versus the equally intense wish to refuel emotionally in the mother's lap (Blum and Blum 1990; Erikson 1968; Mahler et al. 1975). The toddler is not yet emotionally equipped to manage or resolve ambivalent feelings; the parent's consistent empathy and patience will be needed as the child gradually gains tolerance for internal tensions. Moreover, as toddlers develop awareness of their own and their mothers' separate and distinct bodies and minds, they must simultaneously grapple with a new set of cultural requirements. In infancy, the baby's limited motor, cognitive, and communicative capacities necessitated nearly total dependence on parents; during this period of time, parental demands and expectations were minimal. However, as the child acquires language and rudimentary self-restraint, societal standards—largely transmitted through the mother—begin to enter the parent-child relationship; the 2- or 3-year-old child is expected to wait and share, manage aggressive impulses, and begin controlling bowel and bladder urges. Inevitably, these behavioral limits clash with the child's natural inclinations and lead the toddler into conflict, both with the parents and with his or her own desires. Such inner turmoil contributes to the familiar scenario of the overwrought, negativistic, tantrum-throwing toddler who is no longer as easily distracted and redirected as the same child in infancy.

Despite the inevitable struggles of the toddler phase, young children are highly motivated to learn and to develop self-control. Longing to acquire the perceived strength and skill of parents, the toddler watches, mimics, and practices adults' actions; imitation of parents and internalization of their behaviors form the *superego precursors* that presage later, more autonomous self-regulatory and moral developments. Moreover, the toddler is driven by loving feelings for the mother and actively seeks maternal affirmation of behavior. Unlike the infant, the toddler fears not only the loss of the mother's physical presence but also the loss of her love and approval (Mahler et al.

1975). As awareness of parental injunctions and expectations sharpens, the child can no longer pursue private aims and pleasures without internal stress.

The body is central to the toddler's experience and emerging self-awareness (Damasio 2003; Fonagy and Target 2007). Maternal involvement with the young child's physical care remains an important feature of their relationship, but responsibility for eating and toileting is slowly shifted toward the toddler (Freud 1963). Bodily urges and *anal phase conflicts*, such as competing desires for messing and cleanliness, are powerful forces during the toddler period and affect mothers' reactions as well as children's behavior (Furman 1992). The accomplishment of sphincter control and the evolving capacity to control impulses and resist immediate pleasures are fundamental to the toddler's sense of independence and mastery (Blum and Blum 1990; Yorke 1990). In addition, increasing awareness of anatomical boy-girl differences begins to shape the toddler's feelings about the self.

EMERGING SENSE OF SELF, SEPARATION, AND GENDER

Self-Awareness and Mother-Child Separation

The emergence of an increasingly complex, differentiated sense of self is a profound and transformative toddler development. Although psychodynamic definitions of the self are highly varied, many theorists view the self as a relatively stable set of structures or mental representations that are the center of subjective experience. The self has a pivotal role in organizing and regulating relatedness, continuity and coherence, agency and mastery, emotionality and morality (Emde 1983; Emde et al. 1991; Stern 1985; Tyson and Tyson 1990). During the toddler phase, the emerging sense of a separate, self-conscious, and gendered self begins to create a foundation for enduring self-experience.

By the middle of the second year, most toddlers acquire a fundamental concept of an objective self. Within the research literature, mirror self-recognition has been used as a signpost for the achievement of this internalized self-representation. In a well-known experiment, 15- to 18-month-olds' noses are surreptitiously marked with rouge; when these toddlers view their reflection in a mirror and perceive the red mark, they respond by touching their noses, demonstrating a basic notion of the self as an empirical entity (Lewis and Brooks-Gunn 1979). In contrast, younger babies respond by patting the mirror image. Importantly, the affect that accompanies this test of self-recognition is deeply influenced by the quality of mother-child attachment; whereas most children react to their reflections with pleasure, the self-recognition performance of maltreated toddlers is accompanied by neutral or unhappy emotion (Schneider-Rosen and Cicchetti 1984). These findings strongly suggest that the toddler's earliest self-aware feelings reflect the history of mother-infant relational experience.

The young child's newly acquired symbolic skills contribute to the increasing awareness of a separate physical and mental self, differentiated from the mother (Lewis and Ramsay 2004; Meissner 2008; Tyson and Tyson 1990). Early language development, particularly initial use of self- and other-referential pronouns and the toddler's affinity for the beloved word *no*, helps delineate mother-child separateness. In addition, early forms of mother-directed pretend play (e.g., the toddler's feeding the mother a spoonful from an empty bowl) further signify and reinforce the toddler's sense of self-other boundaries. Moreover, toddlers increasingly distinguish between their own and their mother's less tangible features, such as private intentions and wishes; a growing realization that the self and others may possess different and at times opposing desires and plans is foundational to the child's developing social understanding and self-regulation capacities (Fonagy 1995; Sugarman 2003).

As toddlers achieve a sense of physical and psychological separation, moving further from the sheltered dependency of the infant situation, both children and parents experience a sense of loss. Furman (1996)observes that during the gradual shift from the exclusive "mother-child bodily unit" of infancy, the dyad "gropes its way uneasily toward bodily differentiation and new body and ego boundaries" (p. 442). The toddler's dawning sense of self leads to more realistic awareness of personal vulnerability, smallness, and powerlessness. Simultaneously, the parent's limits are more keenly understood; the toddler grapples with inevitable disappointment as he or she increasingly realizes that the mother is not always able to restore his or her sense of happiness or alter reality-based conditions. One 2-year-old boy, whose plans to visit the zoo were thwarted by rain, insisted that his mother "make the sun come"; he erupted angrily and inconsolably as she explained that she could not.

The Self and Gender

Most current psychodynamic theorists view gender as a fundamental aspect of identity that begins to develop in the first months of life. As the young child's sense of a gendered self evolves, it is deeply affected by parental attitudes and feelings; moreover, like all aspects of the self, it is integrated and reorganized with increasing complexity as cognitive and emotional capacities mature (Kulish 2010; Yanof 2000). At around age 2 years, most toddlers achieve a beginning grasp of gender; they can label themselves as a boy or girl, and they possess a rudimentary, concrete idea of gender differences. Toddlers' understanding of boy-girl distinctions is limited, however, by their thinking and reasoning capacities; concepts of male and female are associated with familiar, perceptual characteristics, such as long hair or blue-colored clothing, or with specific behaviors. The deeper meanings of gender and the permanence of sexual differences are not yet grasped; the concept of gender is not yet associated with the genitals (de Marneffe 1997). Coates (1997) provides a revealing example of toddler thinking: when a 2-year-old boy is presented with unclad, anatomically correct male and female dolls and asked to identify them by gender, he protests, "I don't know, they don't have their clothes on" (p. 39).

Given the opportunity to observe sexual differences, toddlers express interest and curiosity as well as pride in their own gender (de Marneffe 1997). However, psychodynamic theorists emphasize the inevitable, deeper anxieties that attach to early perceptions of anatomical distinctions, particularly during a time when children's thinking is highly concrete. These include girls' envy of penises (described as "fancy" by one 3-year-old girl, and as "fun for squirting" by another) and their concomitant sense of something missing, and boys' worries that girls have somehow lost their penises and that such potential losses have implications for their own bodies. Many clinicians view these wishes, fears, and fantasies as significant developmental influences that are easily discernible in the clinical material of both children and adults. In her observational study of toddlers, Olesker (1998) describes a 27-month-old girl who begs for a penis at Christmas time and is bitterly disappointed when she receives toys; another toddler insists that her parents refer to her genitals as they do her brother's (i.e., as a penis).

Toddlerhood and the Sense of Self

- Between 15 and 18 months, most children manifest awareness of the self as a separate, empirical entity.

- Self-conscious emotions, such as shame and pride, appear along with the sense of self.

- Enhanced awareness of the physical and mental self as differentiated from the mother leads to unprecedented feelings of vulnerability.

- Toddlers label themselves as boy or girl, but do not yet grasp the link between gender and genitals; they view sex assignment as based on concrete characteristics such as hair and clothing.

- Although toddlers manifest positive feelings about their own sex, their concrete thinking can lead to genital envy and anxiety.

Maternal reactions to toddlers' unrestrained curiosity about gender differences and to their children's early genital self-exploration are often intense (Furman 1992). These responses are communicated in myriad, often nonverbal ways and internalized by watchful young children. During the anxieties of the toddler phase, the child makes frequent use of social referencing to ascertain the mother's emotional state; such emotional information is integrated into the overall sense of self and feelings about gender. Multiple daily diaper changes, wherein the pre–toilet trained child is supine and observing the maternal visage, offer an important opportunity to glean information about the parent's reaction to bodily products and hygiene. Girls may be particularly attuned to maternal attitudes, making their self-esteem and body image more vulnerable to the perceived sense that the genital area is regarded as dirty and distasteful (e.g., Gilmore 1998; Olesker 1990, 1998)

THE RAPPROCHEMENT PHASE, INNER CONFLICT, AND EARLY SUPEREGO DEVELOPMENT

The Rapprochement Crisis and Internal Conflict

The elation of the newly walking 1-year-old is short-lived. Achieving upright mobility permits the child to control distance from the mother, reinforcing a dawning sense of separateness and autonomy (Mahler 1972; Mahler et al. 1975). As toddlers increasingly grasp mother-child bodily and psychological differentiation, confront their own and their parent's limitations, and encounter the ordinary frustrations of daily life, their previous sense of imperviousness gives way to a more anxious, sober realization of personal vulnerability. This shift of mood and enhanced feeling of insecurity, often evident by age 15–18 months, leads to renewed desire for maternal proximity and ushers in the period that Mahler referred to as the rapprochement phase. Many toddlers exhibit an increase in separation anxiety, reverting to earlier habits of protesting the mother's absences and seeking her body for constant reassurance and refueling.

A hallmark of rapprochement is the toddler's contradictory gestures and feelings. He or she vividly displays frustration, aggression, and mounting *ambivalence* toward the mother, often demanding and simultaneously rejecting maternal contact. The child's disrupted interior states are transformed into outward struggles with the mother, frequently taking the form of age-typical whining and tantrums. Toddlers' behavior often engenders parallel confusion in the mother; for example, the child may shadow her insistently, only to dart away, or may beg to be lifted and then immediately clamor to be set down. The peak period of the toddler's inner stress and tumultuous behavior signals a "rapprochement crisis" (Mahler 1972), which gradually recedes as the child learns to tolerate strong emotions and inner tensions (see section "Libidinal Object Constancy" later in this chapter, for a fuller discussion of this process). Within psychodynamic theory, the shift away from the rapprochement crisis and the child's increasing tolerance for internal conflict are viewed as foundational steps in the slow, arduous progression of emotional self-regulation and superego formation. Such developments depend heavily on the parent's ongoing availability and stable, nonretaliatory reactions in the face of the toddler's fluctuating moods and behaviors.

An alternative model to psychodynamic theory is attachment theory (e.g., Lyons-Ruth 1991), wherein the toddler's conflicted states are seen neither as inevitable nor as growth promoting, but rather as a reaction to problematic mother-child relating. Within this perspective, insecure attachment and low maternal affect tolerance are the underlying conditions that contribute to toddlers' noncompliant and poorly regulated behaviors, such as tantrums. Both psychodynamic and attachment theories concur that the toddler's emerging tolerance for internal turmoil and beginning self-regulatory capacities are inherently linked to the ongoing mother-child relationship. Well-established dyadic capacities for shared pleasure and affective communication provide a solid foundation as the pair enters the natural challenges of the toddler years. Social referencing behavior continues to be prominently manifested in the second year of life, as toddlers repeatedly seek and imitate maternal reactions (Emde et al. 1991).

We adhere, however, to the basic psychodynamic concept of *ubiquitous conflict* and believe that Mahler's (1972) notion of rapprochement captures the child's inevitable and ultimately growth-promoting interior struggles. Moreover, even a secure, well-functioning mother-infant dyad may encounter novel challenges as the toddler begins to demand greater autonomy or as the mother's own unresolved struggles over authority and control are revived in the context of developmental tasks of the 2- to 3-year-old (e.g., toilet training). Furthermore, we suggest that highly attuned mothers cannot ever completely shield their toddlers from frustration or fully compensate for the necessary loss of the infant experience of gratification.

• **See the video "Toddler and Mother" for an illustration of a toddler's separation reaction and ambivalent behavior.**

Internalization of Parental Standards, Morality, and Feared Loss of Maternal Approval

The gradual maturation of superego capacities is a lengthy process, beginning with the preverbal baby's internalization of parental holding and affective reactions in the first months of life. During the toddler phase, the child's rapidly increasing verbal comprehension, motoric control, and self-awareness facilitate a period of socialization in which both child and parent actively participate; superego precursors, such as imitation of parental behavior, emerge and form the building blocks for later, more complex and autonomous self-regulation and moral functioning. Parental injunctions and approvals are gradually absorbed and retained by the toddler, giving rise to mental *introjects* (i.e., inner representations of the parental voice and function). Once these internalized images are established, externalized mother-child struggles over good versus bad behavior are transformed into interior conflicts between inner wishes and self-prohibitions (McDevitt 1983). Indeed, empirical findings suggest that children demonstrably associate affective discomfort with wrongdoing, attach positive feelings to prosocial actions, and attempt intentional control of their impulses by early in the third year of life (Kochanska 1993; Kochanska et al. 2010); increasingly, moral feelings and reactions are integrated into the sense of self (Emde et al. 1991; Vaish et al. 2011). Although some recent research attributes a moral "compass" to preverbal infants, most writers agree that the child's awareness of morality and conscious feelings about moral transgressions originate during the toddler phase, beginning in the second year of life (Dunn 2006; Smetana et al. 2012).

The toddler encounters an array of cultural pressures and standards, many of which are initially experienced as sudden, unfamiliar impediments to pleasurable pursuits. Although crawling infants are subjected to and appear to comprehend the parental "No," adults begin to impose far more elaborate restrictions and demand cooperation from their increasingly verbal and mobile toddlers; often, aggressive behavior and bodily functions are the first targeted areas of socialization. The toddler of the rapprochement phase, while highly motivated to seek mastery and parental approval, simultaneously resists passive compliance and adult control (Mahler 1972); familiar negative and oppositional behaviors, such as tantrums, help define and consolidate the child's sense of self-other boundaries but also create tension within the dyad.

Many psychodynamic and developmental theorists view inevitable toddler-parent clashes as normative, growth-promoting opportunities, particularly when they are accompanied by the parent's verbal communication (e.g., Blum and Blum 1990; Laible et al. 2008); indeed, age-appropriate parental admonishments over moral transgressions (e.g., "Look, you made him cry") encourage the young child to think about others' perspectives (Smetana et al. 2012). As the process of cultural transmission unfolds, via the parent's limit setting and guidance, parental disappointment and irritation are inevitably evoked. Such maternal reactions have enhanced meaning for the toddler, who is increasingly conscious of self-other distinctions and shame versus pride reactions, and therefore is newly vulnerable to parental dissatisfaction; moreover, the pressures of the rapprochement phase, with its increased fears of maternal loss and separation, further sensitize the child to the mother's emotional state. In infancy, loss of physical proximity to the mother leads to anxiety; in toddlerhood, feared loss of maternal approval and love begins to emerge as a major danger, threatening the young child with diminished self-esteem and feelings of abandonment. These various developments—the toddler's increasing awareness of others' needs and perspectives, realization that maternal approval is connected to child actions and can be withheld, and desire to share positive feelings with the mother— begin to create substantial inner discomfort when the child pursues forbidden behaviors.

The Role of Parental Self-Regulation

When parents handle their toddler's behavioral training and resistances with tact and sensitivity, eschewing the use of physical power and angry outbursts, they facilitate the child's internalization of critical self-regulatory capacities, including self-control during emotional arousal, verbal (rather than action-based) expression of negative affect, management of interpersonal conflict, and social perspective taking. Moreover, the toddler's freedom from acute anxiety about maternal overreaction and rejection frees up internal resources for new developmental tasks, such as social learning (Kochanska et al. 2004). The mother's ability to manage her own aggressive feelings and handle the toddler's "violent swings between love and hate" (Freud 1963, p. 253) is essential for the child's sense of stability and his or her gradually increased tolerance for and understanding of inner feelings and tensions (Blum and Blum 1990; Furman 1992; Sugarman 2003; Winnicott 1965).

Such maternal capacities are frequently put to the test during the toddler phase, when possessiveness, negativism, and stubborn reactions—often manifested by the young child's love affair with the words *no* and *mine*—are natural expressions of internal discomfort and of the ongoing struggle for self-definition and autonomy. Battles for control of the toddler's body may emerge as the balance of mother-child power and responsibility slowly shifts and the child assumes greater involvement in toileting and self-feeding. Teasing, withholding, and controlling behaviors are common, particularly during toilet training, when mother-child clashes can evoke high emotion (Furman 1992); similarly, the toddler may refuse food or manifest increased pickiness and fussing over eating. The mother's capacity to resist embroilment in such struggles and avoid unnecessary intrusion in the child's bodily self-management ultimately facilitates the development of autonomy.

The following vignette depicts a mother and toddler who are caught in a typical rapprochement dilemma. The mother's considerable self-awareness, playful attitude, and empathy allow her to manage the child's confusing, erratic behavior without undue anger or retaliatory urges; because the mother remains relatively constant and composed, her toddler, Rachel, is eventually able to return for comfort and achieve a restored sense of security. Over time, Rachel's repeated experiences of inner turmoil, within the context of the mother's constancy, will move her toward greater affect tolerance and a more integrated sense of her own and her mother's complex emotional lives.

> Rachel, age 18 months, had been an active, alert, and sunny-tempered infant, but her mother, Miriam, discerned a recent sobering of the toddler's mood; in addition, there were occasional unpredictable eruptions into crying, whining, and clinging. For the past few weeks, Rachel protested her familiar sitter's arrival and cried piteously as Miriam prepared to leave for work. Even on days when her mother was home, it became impossible to anticipate what would set Rachel off; often, it seemed as if the impetus for a meltdown stemmed from mysterious internal tensions and had little to do with her mother's behavior. Miriam began to feel cross, tentative, and controlled, waiting for Rachel's next scene. She was initially thrilled by Rachel's new walking and talking skills, but now she guiltily confessed to her husband that the "terrible twos" were worse than anything she had expected. Ruefully, she joked that Rachel's newfound willfulness was their punishment for having bragged to friends about her easy infancy.
>
> During a trip to a familiar ice cream parlor, part of their weekend routine all summer, a tantrum began. After Miriam handed Rachel the usual treat, which Rachel had always eaten with obvious pleasure, the child refused it and began to whine and fuss. Even as she looked longingly at the cup of ice cream, the toddler belligerently asserted, "No! No!" Bewildered, her mother masked her own mounting frustration and embarrassment. Miriam offered Rachel an alternative flavor, which was also rejected, and then tried to pick her up in an attempt to soothe. Rachel struggled, pushing and protesting, as Miriam, now mortified, carried her out of the store. Finally, Rachel collapsed into a damp exhausted heap in her mother's arms and accepted comfort, insisting on being carried all the way home. Once there, Rachel recovered fairly quickly; she and her mother then played with puzzles and looked at picture books, as they always did on Miriam's days at home.

The following vignette, by contrast, presages a potential derailment of a 2-year-old child's fragile self-esteem and self-regulatory capacities, due to his mother's unresolved conflicts around autonomy and control and her fears of male dominance. Sam's age-typical possessiveness and negativity evoke the mother's associations to an aggressive, authoritarian older brother who caused her to feel helpless and enraged for much of her childhood; when she encounters her son's age-typical grabbing and spilling, she responds angrily and attributes to him her brother's perceived narcissism and self-interest.

> Deborah has found 2-year-old Sam's pleasure in messiness, both in and out of the bathroom, hard to tolerate; often, she has reacted with open disgust, much preferring her older daughter's fastidious, even compulsive adherence to neatness and order. Sam and Deborah managed the first year relatively well. Deborah enjoyed her male infant's dependency and responsiveness. However, his newfound willfulness and oppositional behaviors are stirring up Deborah's unwanted feelings from the past, causing her to respond in ways that frustrate and confuse the toddler. The pair is increasingly enmeshed in sadomasochistic exchanges, wherein the level of emotionality intensifies and conflicts are ratcheted up into real, consequential situations.
>
> Deborah has just prepared lunch for herself, her 5-year-old daughter, and Sam. There is a bowl of chips, his favorite snack. He eagerly grabs one, spilling a few out of the dish while asserting, "Mine!" Deborah fixes him with an annoyed look and retorts, "They aren't just for you." His sister primly asks for a chip, which Deborah passes to her approvingly. "He thinks everything is his; he's selfish," she comments to her daughter. Sam looks away; he cannot understand his mother's words but he recognizes her familiar angry voice. He begins to crumble his chip in his hand and then suddenly sweeps it onto the floor. Coldly, Deborah removes the bowl from his reach and then roughly carries him away from the lunch table. She says, "Now you're punished. No dessert for you." Sam begins to cry and throw the toys nearest him. Deborah ignores him; she and her daughter continue their lunch while Sam works himself into a full-blown tantrum.

The Rapprochement Phase

- When the toddler is between 15 and 18 months old, motoric achievements and sense of a separate self lead to intensified separation anxiety and renewed concern about maternal proximity (rapprochement).

- The child experiences ambivalence toward the mother and displays contradictory behaviors (e.g., shadowing the mother and then darting away).

- The development of libidinal object constancy (stable, internalized representation of the self and other) helps resolve the anxiety and mood instability of the rapprochement phase.

- Maternal self-regulatory capacities are instrumental in toddler's increasing tolerance for inner discomfort and conflict.

Superego Precursors: The Wished-For Self-Image and the Role of Shame in Toddler Socialization

As toddlers becomes increasingly aware of self-other differentiation, they perceive more clearly the disparity between their own and their parents' tangible features and capacities; their growing realization that they cannot do what adults do creates a threat to their fragile self-esteem and engenders feelings of frustration and longing. We find Jacobson's (1964) and Milrod's (1982) elaboration of "the wished-for self-image" to be particularly relevant to the plight of the newly self-conscious toddler; this term refers to fantasied self-representations—such as notions of being big or strong—that emerge at the height of young children's narcissistic vulnerability, as they begin to grasp their own smallness and helplessness. These self-images, which derive largely from observed and admired parental behaviors, are fueled and reinforced by the toddler's playful imitations of adult actions. Early parental identifications and wishful self-images serve as superego precursors and are important vehicles for social learning and identification; indeed, empirical studies draw links between early imitation of parental behavior and later development of conscience (Forman et al. 2004; Lewis and Ramsay 2004). Through action-based pretend replications of what they see and hear, toddlers seek to acquire highly visible, concrete adult characteristics. The parents' ordinary activities, such as pushing a stroller, watering the garden, or using the toilet, are repeatedly mimicked and practiced.

The gap between the toddler's wishful self-image and what he or she can actually attain creates tension and discomfort, motivating the child toward growth and development. One 20-month-old boy, momentarily saddened because he could not lift a heavy watering can as he had seen his father do the day before, persisted until he had edged the can closer to the flowers; eventually, he accepted his parent's tactful offer of a slightly smaller, lighter substitute that he could more easily manipulate and happily engaged in garden care for an extended period. Although temporary feelings of shame and inadequacy can serve as necessary motivators for learning and persistence, it is essential that the young child not be overwhelmed by defeat and mortification. Shame, in particular, functions as an intense, highly averse social anxiety that is a painful but necessary tool in the gradual process of toddler socialization; shame predates guilt, an anxiety that has more to do with concerns about moral deficiencies and does not fully emerge until oedipal development (Yorke 1990). However, an abundance of shameful experience can overwhelm the toddler's fragile self-esteem, which is easily boosted or deflated by immediate conditions, such as parental praise or disapproval. A sense of pride, confidence in the mother's admiration, and the expectation that perceived disparities with adults can be narrowed are central to the toddler's maintenance of positive self-regard and hopefulness (Blum and Blum 1990; Milrod 1982).

As toddlers gradually copy and absorb adult behaviors and prohibitions, they remain highly dependent on the reinforcing physical presence of the parent; certain familiar parental commands ("no hitting," "share with your sister") may be partially internalized, but they are not yet automatic and consistent. Increasingly, the mother's disciplinary and praising voice is evoked and remembered. However, once the parent is no longer in the room, the toddler is an unreliable standard bearer. The following vignette illustrates a toddler who has begun to develop self-control, but cannot resist aggressive impulses directed toward his little sister when left to his own devices.

> Joshua, age 2 years 5 months, has been momentarily left alone with his 3-month-old baby sister, Sarah. His mother has been working hard to help Joshua feel proud and included in the infant's care; often she models gentle behavior, such as caressing Sarah, and praises him when he mimics this, verbally appealing to his newfound identity as the "big brother." Although this momentarily makes him feel proud and grown up, Joshua is not always so sure he wants to be a big brother, particularly when his mother is holding and nursing Sarah. Occasionally, he demands a bottle himself or tries to take the baby's blanket. From time to time, he good-naturedly suggests to his parents that they "throw Sari away"; both adults respond without anger, patiently explaining that the baby is now part of the family.
>
> After his mother briefly leaves the room to answer the front door, Joshua draws close to Sarah's cradle and begins to mimic his mother's stroking and crooning. In his mother's tones he repeats, "We love our Sari" while carefully stroking her arm as he has seen and heard their mother do so many times. He continues this mantra as he strokes more and more roughly, growing curious as she soon begins to fuss. Less than a minute later, his mother returns to find Sarah wailing with a red mark on her arm. Joshua, averting his face, quickly asserts, "Sarah hit me," and he begins to cry as well.

Inner Conflict and Early Superego Development

- Toilet training is a major context for toddler socialization, self-control, and increased autonomy.
- The toddler's language and cognitive capacities facilitate internalization of the parental voice of authority.
- As the toddler's awareness of parental prohibitions and approvals sharpens, he or she can no longer pursue pleasurable aims without experiencing inner conflict.
- Internal discomforts are expressed via action and conflict with the parent.

- Feared loss of maternal approval becomes a major source of anxiety.
- Early superego precursors, such as the wished-for self-image, help the toddler internalize parental limit-setting.

This scenario depicts the toddler's typical struggle for self-regulation and self-control, even in the face of empathic parents who are sensitive to their young child's interior struggles. Left momentarily to his own resources, Joshua is able to evoke his mother's voice and behavior as a model for his own actions. However, in the absence of her reassuring and restraining presence, his feelings of jealousy and resentment become overwhelming. Moreover, he does not fully grasp the effect of his behavior on the baby's body and mind. At first, he is curious as she begins to fuss, responding to the increasing pressure of his hand. Afterward, when his mother returns and reacts with consternation, he is aware of behaving badly and feels ashamed. By externalizing blame onto the baby, he tries to rid himself of his uncomfortable feelings, which include his diminished self-regard, concerns about maternal disapproval, and sense that he has done real harm to the infant.

The Anal Phase of Toddlerhood and the Role of Toilet Training in Early Development

Sigmund Freud's (1923/1962) assertion that "the ego is first and foremost a bodily ego" (p. 26) is brought to life vividly by toddlers, particularly when toilet training is under way. The accomplishment of sphincter control is a complex psychological and bodily task, requiring parent and toddler capacities for mutual communication and self-control. As the child acquires toileting habits, he or she develops and strengthens important defenses (i.e., identification with the aggressor and reaction formation, both described later in this section) and self-regulatory processes (e.g., a heightened awareness of inner and outer body boundaries, identification and compliance with adult standards for behavior, a sense of responsibility for self and bodily control, and the capacity to relinquish natural pleasures in order to achieve shared pride, self-esteem, and mastery). Such crucial mind-body connections and advances make toilet training a key growth-promoting task with major implications for social, emotional, and superego development.

Toddlers and their mothers acclimate slowly to the shift away from exclusive maternal responsibility for the baby's body (Freud 1963; Furman 1992); this profound change in the dyadic relationship stirs up deep fears, losses, and conflicts. On the surface, mothers may welcome the end of their diapering days and experience a sense of real pride in their toddler's toileting accomplishments; unconsciously, however, many fear a loss of control over the child and feel bereft of the special physical relationship they shared with the baby. Power struggles fought on the ground of the toddler's body may emerge, particularly if parents are internally pressured by unresolved conflicts from their own childhood battles for autonomy. Moreover, mothers are not impervious to societal judgments and may react with shame if their toddlers do not achieve toilet mastery within expected time frames; their own sense of inadequacy and embarrassment impacts their feelings toward the toilet training process.

The anal-sadistic trends of the toddler period evoke strong reactions from the mother; immersed in the child's daily care and hygiene, she is buffeted by strong regressive pulls and inevitable frustrations. Toddlers' controlling behaviors, negativism, tendencies toward withholding and expulsion, and often teasing and provocative demeanor make for a highly stimulating and challenging maternal experience. Furman (1992) comments that "mothers' true feelings about their toddlers' anality run deep" (p. 150); these intense reactions are rarely and reluctantly divulged. Mothers may respond with unexpected anger and retaliatory urges toward their toddlers' provocations, disgust over their unrestrained messiness, and envy of their open pursuit of instinctual gratification. As they attempt to manage the unwanted and overwhelming feelings stirred up by a child's scatological fascinations and pleasures, mothers themselves may begin to manifest increased messiness or compulsive neatness.

For the toddler, the demands of toileting are similarly daunting, requiring an unprecedented level of self-control and increased awareness of the inner body and its signals. Early in the toilet training process, toddlers tend to overlook bodily cues or mistake one urge or sensation for another; when bowel or bladder pressures are experienced, young children may erroneously conclude that they are hungry or thirsty, or they may respond to such urges by increasing their level of activity. Moreover, the child soon discovers that strong maternal reactions can be elicited by toileting mishaps, refusals, and teasing; the toddler's accompanying sense of power, pleasure in controlling the mother, and desire for independence all foster an emotional excitement and satisfaction in oppositional and provocative behaviors. The toddler's ambivalent participation in toileting is influenced by both negative and positive motivations. Loving feelings for the mother, a strong desire for her positive regard, the joys of mastering new tasks, and the pleasure in identification with adults are major impetuses for accomplishing this developmental task. At the same time, the looming threat of maternal disapproval and the concomitant fear of shame shape the young child's behavior.

Left to their own devices, toddlers manifest considerable pleasure in messing and spilling, as well as in bodily products and odors; such affinities must be gradually renounced in favor of more socially acceptable hygiene and orderliness. *Reaction formation,* a process that transforms the child's interest, excitement, and pleasure into the opposite feeling (in this case disgust), and *identification with the aggressor* (i.e., with the parent's prohibitions and disapproving attitudes) evolve as major tools for self-control. These unconscious defense mechanisms, along with the loving aspects of the parent-child bond and the toddler's own pride and shame reactions, help the young child gain mastery over primitive wishes and begin to repudiate them with adultlike repugnance. As such defense mechanisms develop, the child may begin to feel uncomfortable with sloppy activities that were previously enjoyed, such as paints or mud; some toddlers manifest intense concern with neatness, compulsively avoiding messes and overreacting to small stains or drips. Despite this, identifications and defensive disavowals are crucial in the toddler's socialization, far beyond the toilet training situation. For example, similar mechanisms help convert envy and aggression toward a new baby sibling into more acceptable, loving big brother or sister feelings.

THE TODDLER'S THINKING AND ADVANCES IN SELF-REGULATION

Preoperational Thinking and the Toddler's Naïve Cognition

At around age 2 years, toddlers transition to the *preoperational* period of cognitive development. *Deferred imitation* (i.e., mimicking of actions that have been observed, without the immediate presence of a model) is an early hallmark of this phase, signaling the toddler's increasing capacity for stable mental representations and laying the groundwork for more complex pretend play and parental identifications. In addition, the acquisition of early language and fundamental concepts about the animate and inanimate world (e.g., object permanence and the sense of a separate self) transforms the child's mental life and brings the action-oriented, *sensorimotor* phase of infancy to a close (Piaget 1926, 1962). Toddlers begin to think and talk about important people and events in their lives, even when these are not immediately perceived. With greater mental freedom from the tangible world, the young child can engage in thought rather than action and draw on internal images for emotional self-regulation (Blum 2004). For example, the mother's comforting presence can now be evoked through memories, words, images, and simple pretend games.

Toddlers' relatively concrete thinking affects their social, emotional, and cognitive life. Judgments are heavily influenced by tangible properties and intuitive, rather than logical, problem solving; for example, a preoperational child will typically determine that three large stones are "more" than five small ones, based on the conspicuous size of the latter. The toddler's perspective is *egocentric;* he or she cannot fully comprehend other people's viewpoints or consider multiple dimensions of a situation. Such immaturities in social understanding limit toddlers' awareness of their own behavioral impact; for example, they do not fully grasp the effect of their own grabbing, hitting, or biting on another child's physical or mental experience. Abstract concepts, such as generosity and kindness, are not yet socially meaningful unless the parent links them to specific, tangible behaviors and indicates their desirability. Toddlers manifest early empathic responses, but these tend to be guided by their own feelings and preferences; for example, one girl, age 2½ years, troubled by her mother's sadness after the death of a relative, rushed to offer her own beloved "blanky" for comfort.

Importantly, the toddler does not fully differentiate internal thoughts and feelings from external reality. Within this mental framework of *psychic equivalence,* inner life is materialized; wishes and fantasies are felt to be consequential, potentially causing events in the real world (Fonagy et al. 2002; Target and Fonagy 1996). Dreams are similarly confused with actual occurrences and may feel "real" to the toddler. Such thinking creates unique vulnerabilities for young children, who may believe that their own jealousy and resentment of a new sibling engenders a baby's sudden illness or injury, or that anger at a parent leads to a divorce. Unclear reality-fantasy and inner-outer boundaries make the child susceptible to multiple fears and phobias; for example, creatures from books or from the child's imagination are not simply pretend. The toddler's naïve cognition leads to intense bodily anxieties. For example, 2-year-olds often perceive feces as precious body parts that may be lost in the toilet, making the toddlers reluctant or even frightened to allow stools to be flushed. Similarly, they may develop new fears of the bathtub, frightened that the self will be swept down the drain. Such fearful fantasies extend to perceived boy-girl anatomical differences; for example, girls' lack of a penis may "mean" to toddlers that an organ has been or can potentially be lost or removed.

Moreover, the toddler's inner resourcefulness for managing intense angry and aggressive feelings is limited. Often, these feelings are externalized, attributed to the mother or other people and objects in the environment, and then felt to originate outside of the self. The combination of the child's externalized affects and the permeable boundary between mind and reality can magnify ordinary experience; mild maternal irritation, the barking of a benign family pet, or familiar dark spaces may suddenly appear unduly threatening. "Reasoning" with a frightened toddler—that is, attempting to use logic and explain the realities of the situation—may have little impact. The toddler's internalized images are similarly affected, so that representations of parental prohibitions and punishments are distorted and misinterpreted, taking on an augmented sense of danger and threat (Blum and Blum 1990). The result is a frightening, exaggerated version of reality; toddlers may fear that even minor mischief will meet with real retribution, such as being abandoned or devoured.

The following examples illustrate typical toddler thinking, age-expected confusion between fantasy and reality, and externalization of feelings.

> Aaron, age 2 years 6 months, is a well-developed, securely attached toddler who suddenly refuses to fetch toys from a dark closet in his room, runs from the vacuum cleaner, and cries when he hears dogs bark in the neighborhood. Chief among his new fears are clowns, whose exaggerated faces and antics cause him to cry and hide. After a trip to the circus and a cousin's birthday party where clown entertainment was hired, he becomes inconsolable when he even thinks he might see one of these creatures. He no longer wants to attend the birthday parties of children in his playgroup, due to possible encounters. In addition, Aaron has begun to have bad dreams and to awaken crying at night. When his mother attempted to comfort him on one occasion, he tearfully described a dream in which she and his father "turned into clowns." Reproachfully, he demanded to know "Why you do that, Mommy?" Momentarily taken aback, his mother attempted to explain that it was "just a dream," but Aaron was unmoved by her remonstrations and continued to be sullen, although he was no longer afraid. She assumed that he was tired and confused, but in the morning he once again approached her in an accusatory manner. Later in the week, he told his day care teacher that "Mommy and Daddy were mean" and repeated his version of events. For the next few weeks, he retold the story multiple times and could not be convinced that this nighttime experience was a product of his mental life.

> Lucy, age 2 years 4 months, has been struggling to master riding her toddler trike. Her 6-year-old brother helps her settle on the seat and stands nearby, murmuring encouragements. Lucy soon becomes distracted and slips off; she is not hurt, but looks crestfallen. Their mother enters the room just as she is pouting, pointing accusingly, and exclaiming, "Tommy pushed me!" Tommy, bewildered, accurately protests that he has just been helping and was nowhere near her when she fell; he attempts to explain to Lucy that she just has to learn how to maintain her balance and cannot look away while she is steering. Lucy cries even harder, continues to blame him for the fall, and insists that she is big enough to ride. Regaining her composure, she threatens that she will no longer play house with Tommy. Now annoyed, Tommy reminds her that he hates playing house and only does so to amuse her.

Libidinal Object Constancy

Toddlers' grasp of *object permanence*—that is, the concept that things and people have an existence outside of immediate action and perception—

helps them anticipate the physical return of the mother after a familiar, reasonable absence. However, this cognitive achievement is not sufficient to maintain an ongoing, enduring sense of the dyad's loving relationship in the face of normal emotional vicissitudes and upheavals. Initially, the toddler does not fully integrate diverse affective states; when one member of the dyad is angry or frustrated, positive memories and feelings are not available for comfort and self-soothing. During the child's own angry spells or when the mother is temporarily punitive or distant, the toddler's sense of loss and abandonment can be intense. For the toddler, it is as if the good, comforting mother has been lost or even destroyed by the child's aggression. The attainment of *libidinal object constancy*—that is, the internalization of a stable, coherent representation of self and mother—is a gradual, complex cognitive-emotional-social development that enables the child to withstand ephemeral, ordinary shifts in affect and mood (Mahler 1974).

When the mother repeatedly demonstrates tolerance for the toddler's mood swings and remains relatively constant in the face of tantrums and provocations, she facilitates the gradual integration of positive with negatively tinged mental representations (Sugarman 2003; Winnicott 1965); ultimately, by the end of the toddler period, these more stable, nuanced images are available for self-regulation during moments of anger and distress. The child can more reliably draw on the mental representation of a soothing maternal presence and experience a sense of emotional connection even when the mother is physically absent (Winnicott 1958). Libidinal object constancy helps bring about a resolution of the rapprochement phase; as the young child begins to feel less internal disruption from uncomfortable feelings, the fragility and mercurial nature of toddler moods begins to subside (Mahler 1974; Mahler et al. 1975). Moreover, the mother's interest in the child's interior life, her increasingly verbal elaborations of the toddler's feelings and intentions, and her constancy during the shifting moods of the rapprochement phase allow the toddler to begin linking his or her own and the mother's external behaviors with psychological states. No longer simply swept up in feelings and impulses, the young child can begin to use language and reflection to mediate affective reactions. Ultimately, such connections help the child make sense and meaning of behavior, strengthen the distinction between psychic experience (or *psychic reality*) and external reality, and regulate the intensity of feelings and impulses (Fonagy et al. 2002; Sugarman 2003).

The resolution of rapprochement phase conflicts and the consolidation of object constancy may be seen as lifelong tasks, rather than as achievements of a particular developmental phase. Throughout older childhood and adulthood, desires for intimacy vie with the individual's need for autonomy and freedom; in addition, ongoing emotional work is required to retain loving, positive feelings toward important others in the moments when strong negative reactions are evoked. Within Mahler's (1972) theory of separation-individuation, these inevitable struggles originate during the toddler period of development but remain part of the human condition for life.

Early Symbolic Functions and Their Role in Self-Regulation

When the child is an infant, the mother performs the tasks of discerning, reflecting, and elucidating the baby's inner states and affects; the dyad's prelinguistic reciprocity and turn-taking form the foundation for the more verbally laden communications of the toddler phase (Beebe et al. 2003; Bruschweiler-Stern et al. 2007). Once language is available, the toddler actively uses words to initiate contact with the mother by labeling and sharing interests and needs. Increasingly, the self is experienced as verbal; the toddler's ability to convey meaningful information across distal modes, share affective experience, and mutually regulate emotional states with the mother becomes inextricably linked to language (Meissner 2008; Stern 1985). In Bloom's (1993) view, the toddler is highly motivated toward language in order to share progressively more sophisticated knowledge and more nuanced emotional reactions with the mother; nonverbal gestures are no longer adequate.

Wide variety is demonstrated in the timing and rate of children's language acquisition. However, by the end of the first year, most infants babble expressively and respond to certain meaningful verbal referents, such as their own and family members' names and labels for familiar routines and games ("bath time," "peek-a-boo," "clap hands"). By the first birthday, the average infant's expressive vocabulary includes a few highly relevant single-word utterances, such as names for self and caretakers; often, first utterances are rooted in the child's immediate perceptual and action-based experience (e.g., "up" while extending arms to be lifted by the parent).

When the child is between 18 and 24 months, development of language is accelerated. Vocabulary increases dramatically and two-word combinations emerge, allowing the toddler to begin communicating more creatively about the basic relationships among important people, objects, and events (Bloom 1993; Nelson 1996). During the same period of time, the emergence of pronouns for self and others reflects a new level of representational thinking and self-other awareness. Indeed, Spitz (1957) theorizes that the toddler's emphatic use of the word *no* represents an important underlying achievement; more than simple imitation of the mother (who must often say "no" to a climbing, grabbing 2-year-old), verbal use of negative words suggests a growing ability to think about things, make judgments, and differentiate between self and other. As the older toddler acquires the use of past and future tense, talking becomes a powerful tool for developing and sharing a sense of self based on autobiographical continuity (Nelson 1996).

Language is also an essential building block in the acquisition of early superego functioning. The toddler's gradual internalization of parental speech, such as maternal praise and prohibitions, enhances the absorption of adult standards and augments the process of socialization. In their initial, shaky attempts at self-control, toddlers often employ literal repetition of maternal restrictions and use these as verbal self-directives. One 2-year-old girl, spooning a whipped cream dessert onto the floor while her mother answered the phone, somberly repeated "No, Becca," over and over again, mimicking the words and intonation her mother had vocalized during similar mishaps. Moreover, as the toddler's linguistic capacities expand, the mother's comforting words and the dyad's verbal exchanges can be evoked for self-soothing and emotional self-regulation to deal with challenging situations. A study of a highly verbal toddler's bedtime monologues (Nelson 1989) demonstrated her use of language to manage the anxiety of nightly separation; in the solitary minutes before falling asleep, this child regularly repeated snippets of conversation with her parents, narrated events from the day, and referenced anticipated activities.

Early language emerges in tandem with pretend play; together, these symbolic functions begin to vastly expand the toddler's potential to internalize adult roles and attitudes, practice social identifications, and engage in emotional self-regulation (Fonagy et al. 2002). Although symbolic play reaches its peak of complexity later in development, during the preschool years, older toddlers begin to add their own imaginary elaboration to everyday events, helping them make meaning of emotionally complex and anxiety-producing situations. Even very young toddlers distinguish between real and playful conditions, as manifested by smiling and exaggerated gestures during pretense (Emde et al. 1997; McCune 1995). Deferred imitation, self-directed pretend play (e.g., "feeding" oneself cereal from an empty bowl), and mother-directed pretense emerge between the first and second birthdays; gradually, when a child is between ages 2 and 3 years, the scope of playful activities is expanded to include more complex, diverse scenarios derived from real-life interactions and events (McCune 1995).

The following vignette illustrates a 2-year-old child's use of pretend play. In this instance, a simple game and narrative derive from real-life events, but the toddler adds his own creative elements to cope with mother-child separation.

David, age 2 years 6 months, struggled with his mother's daily departure for her afternoon job; this event was often anticipated with crying and clingy behavior. In the morning, before she left, he began to develop the following game: He filled a play shopping cart with various items (a combination of real and play food, stuffed animals, his beloved blanket) that he collected from all over the house. Once he filled it to his satisfaction, he gestured for his mother to sit on the sofa and confidently asserted, "Bye-bye, Mommy," explaining that "David go bye-bye now." He then pushed the cart into the next room and out of sight. A few silent moments passed, after which he reappeared and happily greeted his mother. This game was repeatedly enacted and gradually extended by the mother's participation; at times, she would suggest different destinations for his "trip"—a familiar store or his older sister's school. Joining in with playful emotion, she sometimes begged to accompany him on his journey or complained about his absence, to which he kindly but firmly responded, "No, no, I be back later."

As this vignette suggests, maternal involvement in the child's early symbolic play is usually natural and unquestioning; she accepts the toddler's investment in pretense, goes along with the game, and does not articulate the distinction between the child's fantasies and real events (Emde et al. 1997). Secure mother-toddler relationships provide a foundation for the child's imaginary explorations (Cicchetti and Beeghley 1997). Moreover, the mother's participation augments the child's cognitive and imaginative capacities and adds shared enjoyment to an intrinsically pleasurable activity. The narrative extension in this example, wherein the mother plays out David's own inner states, occurs spontaneously and serves a vital function as she enacts his distress and lets him be the "grown-up" in charge, and he achieves a sense of active mastery over a potentially stressful situation.

The Toddler's Physical and Motoric Development

Along with the proliferation of symbolic functions, attainment of upright mobility reorganizes the toddler's relationship to the physical and relational world, immediately impacting the sense of the self as separate and autonomous; moreover, the walking child quickly attracts a proliferation of parental prohibitions. Although the bulk of momentous fine- and gross-motor achievements (grasping, sitting, standing, walking) emerges by the end of infancy, substantial sensorimotor refinement and underlying neural maturation continue throughout the toddler period (Hempel 1993). These qualitative changes, such as greater accuracy and efficiency in motor strategies, vastly enhance the child's range of perceptual experience and contribute to the ongoing development of self-other differentiation as well as to expanding interest in the world beyond the mother-child dyad.

Key Concepts

The toddler phase, between ages 1 and 3 years, is marked by transformative psychological achievements, most notably an emerging *sense of self* and the development of *superego precursors.* A dawning realization of separateness and vulnerability creates an inner crisis for the toddler, who grapples with competing urges toward autonomy and renewed dyadic intimacy. Substantial maternal support is required during the period of *rapprochement,* when the young child demonstrates characteristic ambivalent, negativistic, and moody behavior; the achievement of stable images of self and others—that is, *libidinal object constancy*—contributes to the resolution of this phase, equipping the child with substantially enhanced self-regulatory resources. Expanded symbolic functions, such as imitation, language, and early forms of symbolic play, further contribute to emotional regulation and to the internalization of parental prohibitions.

As the child's cognitive, linguistic, and motoric abilities mature, parents begin the lengthy process of socialization, including toilet training. *Anal phase conflicts* may stress the mother-child relationship but yield important new defense mechanisms and opportunities for self-regulation and bodily autonomy. The child's increased awareness of parental dissatisfactions and the emergence of *self-aware emotions* (e.g., pride and shame) exert a shaping influence on behavior; *feared loss of maternal approval* arises as a major toddler anxiety.

- In the second year of life, an internalized, objective, and gendered sense of a separate self develops.
  - Self-aware emotions, such as pride and shame, begin to emerge and to have a shaping effect on the toddler's self-esteem and capacity for socialization.
  - Boy-girl differences are noted and may elicit anxious reactions.

- The sense of exhilaration and grandiosity that accompanies early walking is diminished as the toddler increasingly comes to terms with reality, including personal vulnerability and the limits of the parents' powers.
  - In the rapprochement phase, a dawning sense of fragility and separateness leads to renewed desire for maternal contact.
  - The toddler displays contradictory, ambivalent, and sometimes aggressive behavior toward the mother.

- The mother's personal self-regulatory capacities are an essential resource for toddler development.
  - Her consistent, empathic, and nonretaliatory reactions help the toddler establish stable and secure internal images of the self and others (libidinal object constancy) which can be evoked when the child is distressed and when the mother is absent.
  - Maternal stability helps increase the child's tolerance for inner conflict.
- Through toileting and other forms of socialization, adults begin to transmit cultural expectations and demands for bodily and impulse control.
  - Anal phase conflicts—withholding, teasing, and negativism—emerge as the toddler struggles to acquire responsibility for bowel and bladder control; these may evoke strong reactions in the mother.
  - Reaction formation, a defense mechanism that helps transform a feeling or attitude into its opposite, helps the toddler renounce messy pleasures, identify with adult standards of cleanliness, and accomplish sphincter control.
- Toddlerhood is a critical period for the emergence of superego precursors.
  - The *wished-for self-image* comprises a set of internal representations of the toddler's desired qualities, such as size and strength.
  - A balance between 1) positive identifications and feelings and 2) more negative experience—such as the toddler's fear of maternal disapproval and concomitant feelings of shame—provides motivation for social learning.
  - The toddler's increased awareness of parental prohibitions makes it impossible to pursue pleasurable but forbidden behaviors without a sense of inner conflict.
- The toddler's thinking is characterized by a *preoperational* (prelogical) approach to problem solving and social-emotional situations.
  - The capacity for deferred imitation is a hallmark of this cognitive period.
  - An egocentric, concrete approach to complex situations limits social understanding and predisposes the toddler to bodily fears.

- The distinction between inner life and reality is not yet clear.

- The toddler's emerging symbolic capacities—language and early play—transform mental life, allowing increasing freedom from the immediate perceptual world.

REFERENCES

Beebe B, Rustin J, Sorter D, et al: Symposium on intersubjectivity in infant research and its implications for adult treatment, III: an expanded view of forms of inter-subjectivity in infancy and its application for psychoanalysis. Psychoanal Dialogues 14:1–51, 2003

Bergman A, Harpaz-Rotem I: Revisiting rapprochement in the light of contemporary developmental theories. J Am Psychoanal Assoc 52:555–570, 2004

Bloom L: The Transition From Infancy to Language: Acquiring the Power of Expression. New York, Cambridge University Press, 1993

Blum EJ, Blum HP: The development of autonomy and superego precursors. Int J Psychoanal 71:585–595, 1990

Blum HP: Separation-individuation theory and attachment theory. J Am Psychoanal Assoc 52:535–553, 2004

Bruschweiler-Stern N, Lyons-Ruth K, Morgan AC, et al: The foundational level of psychodynamic meaning: implicit process in relation to conflict, defense and the dynamic unconscious. Int J Psychoanal 88:843–860, 2007

Cicchetti D, Beeghley M: Symbolic development in maltreated youngsters: an organizational perspective, in Symbolic Development in Atypical Children. Edited by Cicchetti D, Beeghley M. San Francisco, Jossey-Bass, 1997, pp 47–68

Coates SW: Is it time to jettison the concept of developmental lines? Comment on de Marneffe's paper "Bodies and words." Gender and Psychoanalysis 2:35–53, 1997

Damasio AR: Looking for Spinoza: Joy, Sorrow and the Feeling Brain. New York, Harvest Books, 2003

de Marneffe D: Bodies and words: a study of young children's genital and gender knowledge. Gender and Psychoanalysis 2:3–33, 1997

Dunn J: Moral development in early childhood and social interaction in the family, in Handbook of Moral Development. Edited by Killen M, Smetana J. Mahwah, NJ, Erlbaum, 2006, pp 329–350

Emde RN: The prerepresentational self and its affective core. Psychoanal Study Child 38:165–192, 1983

Emde RN, Biringen Z, Clyman RB, et al: The moral self of infancy: affective core and procedural knowledge. Dev Rev 11:251–270, 1991

Emde R, Kubicek L, Oppenheim D: Imaginative reality observed during early language. Int J Psychoanal 78:115–133, 1997

Erikson EH: Identity, Youth and Crisis. London, Faber & Faber, 1968

Fonagy P: Playing with reality: the development of psychic reality and its malfunction in borderline personalities. Int J Psychoanal 76:39–44, 1995

Fonagy P, Target M: The rooting of the mind in the body. J Am Psychoanal Assoc 55:411–456, 2007

Fonagy P, Gergely G, Jurist E, et al: Affect Regulation and Mentalization: Developmental, Clinical and Theoretical Perspectives. New York, Other Press, 2002

Forman DR, Aksan N, Kochanska G: Toddlers' responsive imitation predicts preschool-age conscience. Psychol Sci 15:699–704, 2004

Freud A: The concept of developmental lines. Psychoanal Study Child 18:245–265, 1963

Freud S: The ego and the id (1923), in The Standard Edition of the Complete Psychological Works of Sigmund Freud, Vol 19. Translated and edited by Strachey J. London, Hogarth Press, 1962, pp 1–66

Furman E: Toddlers and Their Mothers: A Study in Early Personality Development. Madison, CT, International Universities Press, 1992

Furman E: On motherhood. J Am Psychoanal Assoc 44(suppl):429–447, 1996

Gilmore K: Cloacal anxiety in female development. J Am Psychoanal Assoc 46:443–470, 1998

Hempel MS: Neurological development during toddling age in normal children and children at risk of developmental disorders. Early Hum Dev 34:47–57, 1993

Jacobson E: The Self and the Object World. New York, International Universities Press, 1964

Kochanska G: Toward a synthesis of parental socialization and child temperament in early development of conscience. Child Dev 64:325–342, 1993

Kochanska G, Aksan N, Knaack A, et al: Maternal parenting and children's conscience: early security as moderator. Child Dev 75:1229–1242, 2004

Kochanska G, Koenig JL, Barry RA, et al: Children's conscience during toddler and preschool years, moral self, and a competent, adaptive developmental trajectory. Dev Psychol 46:1320–1332, 2010

Kulish N: Clinical implications of contemporary gender theory. J Am Psychoanal Assoc 58:231–258, 2010

Laible D, Panfile T, Makariev D: The quality and frequency of mother-toddler conflict: links with attachment and temperament. Child Dev 79:426–443, 2008

Lewis M, Brooks-Gunn J: Theory of social cognition: the development of the self. New Dir Child Dev 4:1–20, 1979

Lewis M, Ramsay D: Development of self-recognition, personal pronoun use and pretend play during the second year. Child Dev 75:1821–1831, 2004

Lyons-Ruth K: Rapprochement or approchement: Mahler's theory reconsidered from the vantage point of recent research on attachment relationships. Psychoanal Psychol 8:1–23, 1991

Mahler MS: Rapprochement subphase of the separation-individuation process. Psychoanal Q 41:487–506, 1972

Mahler MS: On the first three subphases of the separation-individuation process. Psychoanalysis and Contemporary Science 3:295–306, 1974

Mahler MS, Pine F, Bergman A: The Psychological Birth of the Human Infant. New York, Basic Books, 1975

McCune L: A normative study of representational play at the transition to language. Dev Psychol 31:198–206, 1995

McDevitt JB: The emergence of hostile aggression and its defensive and adaptive modifications during the separation-individuation process. J Am Psychoanal Assoc 31:273–300, 1983

Meissner WW: The role of language in the development of the self, I: Language acquisition. Psychoanal Psychol 25:26–46, 2008

Milrod D: The wished-for self image. Psychoanal Study Child 37:95–120, 1982

Nelson K: Narratives From the Crib. Cambridge, MA, Harvard University Press, 1989

Nelson K: Language in Cognitive Development: The Emergence of the Mediated Mind. New York, Cambridge University Press, 1996

Olesker W: Sex differences during the early separation-individuation process. J Am Psychoanal Assoc 38:325–346, 1990

Olesker W: Female genital anxieties: views from the nursery and the couch. Psychoanal Q 61:331–351, 1998

Piaget J: The Language and Thought of the Child. New York, Harcourt Brace, 1926

Piaget J: Play, Dreams and Imitation in Childhood. New York, Norton, 1962

Schneider-Rosen K, Cicchetti D: The relationship between affect and cognition in maltreated infants: quality of attachment and the development of self-recognition. Child Dev 55:648–658, 1984

Smetana JG, Jambon M, Conry-Murray C, et al: Reciprocal associations between young children's developing moral judgments and theory of mind. Dev Psychol 48:1144–1155, 2012

Spitz RA: No and Yes: On the Genesis of Human Communication. New York, International Universities Press, 1957

Stern DN: The Interpersonal World of the Infant: A View From Psychoanalysis and Developmental Psychology. New York, Basic Books, 1985

Sugarman A: Dimensions of the child analyst's role as a developmental object: affect regulation and limit setting. Psychoanal Study Child 58:189–218, 2003

Target M, Fonagy P: Playing with reality, II: the development of psychic reality from a theoretical perspective. Int J Psychoanal 77:459–479, 1996

Tyson P, Tyson R: Psychoanalytic Theories of Development: An Integration. New Haven, CT, Yale University Press, 1990

Vaish A, Missana M, Tomasello M: Three-year-old children intervene in third-party moral transgressions. Br J Dev Psychol 29:124–130, 2011

Winnicott DW: The capacity to be alone. Int J Psychoanal 39:411–420, 1958

Winnicott DW: The Maturational Process and the Facilitating Environment: Studies in the Theory of Emotional Development. The International Psychoanalytic Library 64:1–276. London, Hogarth Press, 1965

Yanof JA: Barbie and the tree of life: the multiple functions of gender in development. J Am Psychoanal Assoc 48:1439–1465, 2000

Yorke C: The development and functioning of the sense of shame. Psychoanal Study Child 45:377–409, 1990

CHAPTER 4

The Oedipal Phase and Emerging Capacities

Language, Imagination, Play, Mentalization, and Self-Regulation

INTRODUCTION TO THE OEDIPAL PHASE

Between the third and sixth birthdays, the young child traverses a unique stage of human development. In psychodynamic theory, the reference to this period as the *oedipal phase,* after the Greek figure Oedipus's fateful embroilment in incest and parricide, captures the child's internal struggle over sexual and aggressive impulses toward the parents. The oedipal young-ster's passionate interest in the mysteries of the adult world, enhanced awareness of anatomical and generational differences, and beginning grasp of the parents' private relationship leads to novel vulnerabilities, such as keen feelings of jealousy and exclusion. The mother-child dyad is irrevoca-bly changed as children develop complex, triadic relationships and fantasies (Blum 1979); moreover, the emergence of guilt feelings intensifies inner con-flict over potential wrongdoing, even in the absence of the adult. A major developmental task of this phase is the integration of aggressive, competitive urges with the child's ongoing love for and dependency upon the parents.

Bodily experience continues to dominate the young child's mental life, as it did during the infant and toddler years. Although toilet training may not be fully mastered at age 3 years, the intense conflicts and preoccupations of the anal phase recede as the child's bodily interests shift to the sexual organs; intensified genital excitement, heightened awareness of boy-girl differences, and avid curiosity about adult sexuality contribute to a period of *genital pri-macy* (Freud 1905/1962; Loewald 1985). Specific anxieties and disappoint-ments arise, including the small child's sense of physical inadequacy and

73

elaborate fears about genital loss and damage. Major challenges of the oedipal phase include making meaning of anatomical distinctions, linking genital features with the sense of a gendered self, and accepting the need to defer wishes for adultlike sexual capacities (Loewald 1985; Mahon 1991; Senet 2004; Yanof 2000).

An explosion of symbolic abilities transforms the oedipal child's cognitive, emotional, and relational world. With a vastly expanded repertoire for language and fantasy, the 3-year-old begins to grasp verbal ideas, engage in elaborate pretend play, contemplate past and future events, and comprehend fictional stories. Children's ardent engagement in make-believe games and fairy stories—highly familiar to parents, therapists, and educators alike—assuages their intense longings for parental qualities and roles; fictional narratives and imaginative play help the child express and organize conflictual feelings, aggressive urges, and age-salient anxieties while deepening their identifications with adults. The capacity for *mentalization*—that is, the ability to interpret behavior based on people's unique feelings and beliefs (Target and Fonagy 1996)—transforms social understanding and emotional self-regulation. The oedipal child's awareness of more nuanced mental aspects of self-other differentiation reinforces a more stable sense of self and others (i.e., *object constancy*) that withstands inevitable shifts in mood and affect. These hugely expanded interior resources, along with the novel presence of guilty reactions and the parents' ongoing empathy and support, facilitate *superego formation.* As the oedipal phase draws to a close, and the child embarks on the grade-school years, the superego serves as an increasingly reliable foundation for independent behavioral and emotional self-control.

In this chapter, we elaborate on the oedipal child's new capacities, all of which are central to the unfolding human drama of the oedipal phase, which is further discussed in Chapter 5, "The Oedipal Phase: Psychosexual Development, Oedipal Complex, Configuration and Constellation, and Legacy in Mental Life." The profound psychological shift, the evolution of an enduring template for relationships, and the internalization of self-regulatory function produce a child who has achieved a fundamental step toward an autonomous self (Loewald 1979).

THE ROLE OF LANGUAGE IN OEDIPAL DEVELOPMENT

As we have described in Chapter 3, "The Toddler," the acquisition of words immediately provides new tools for the toddler's sense of separateness and self-definition, as well as for relational and self-regulatory functioning. The oedipal child's linguistic repertoire is significantly expanded, enabling far more extensive use of language for shared mother-child experience as well as for problem solving and self-control. Transformative changes in the 3-year-old's symbolic capacities lead to vastly more complex and creative mental resources; the emergence of imaginary fantasy, pretend play, and mentalization is inextricably linked to a proliferation of verbal skills. Moreover, the child's growing narrative capability deepens a sense of autobiographical continuity and strengthens emotional self-regulation; the imaginary events of make-believe play, as well as the literary stories that are beloved by the young children, contextualize oedipal themes (romance, adventure, danger) while providing safe, pleasurable outlets for the intense affective upheavals of this developmental phase.

Private Speech and Self-Regulation

Young children's *private speech* is a ubiquitous accompaniment to their play and problem-solving activities. These self-directed, nonsocial, often fragmentary comments reflect children's early attempts at verbally planning and guiding personal behavior. Self-speech peaks during the preschool years and then gradually diminishes; such language is partially internalized by age 4 years (marked by inaudible comments and mutterings) and then largely replaced by silent, inner processes during middle childhood (Winsler et al. 2003). Whereas Piaget (1926) viewed private (egocentric) speech largely as a reflection of the young child's immature cognition, Vygotsky (1962) stressed the intrinsic self-regulatory functions of self-directed talk. In the latter theorist's view, verbal thought originates in social communication and follows an inward trajectory; egocentric speech is a crucial step in the child's gradual internalization of language and self-regulation. The common practice of adults to "talk themselves through" a cognitive challenge or social-emotional dilemma makes it clear that some form of self-directed speech retains usefulness far beyond its ascendancy in early childhood.

Like Vygotsky, psychodynamic theorists view early mental and communicative capacities as arising within the context of mother-child interactions. During the late toddler and early oedipal period, private speech plays an integral function in the child's ongoing internalization of the parental voice. Private, verbal self-directives often mimic maternal praise and prohibitions. A vivid example is provided in Fraiberg's (1996) amusing description of Julia, whose mother momentarily leaves her alone with raw eggs (thereby eliciting the anal-phase temptations of plopping and gooey substances). While energetically dumping this mess on the floor, the small child repeatedly intones the maternal voice: "No No No. Mustn't dood it" (p. 135).

Private speech helps to reinforce parental standards, inhibit impulses, and guide personal behavior (Loewald 1960; Migden 1998); indeed, under experimental conditions, preschool children manifest increased self-speech when tasks are difficult or when their self-restraint capacities are stressed (Winsler et al. 2003). As adult-derived self-directives are continually practiced and internalized, along with more abstract identifications and standards of behavior—for example, ideals such as sharing or being helpful—the physical presence of the parent is no longer essential for reliable self-control. Concerns about punishment, anticipatory anxiety, and guilt serve as further inducements for the child to avoid forbidden actions. Over time, little Julia's desire to dump eggs will yield to stable, inner principles of cooperation and cleanliness, and acceptable outlets, such as baking and painting, can serve as substitutes for her messier urges.

Narrative Capacities

The emergence of narrative capacities transforms the oedipal child's mental life, vastly expanding the potential for communication and self-understanding as well as for creative fantasy. Story-telling activities support social-cognitive development, providing necessary practice for the child's growing ability to shift social perspectives and grasp other points of view. Moreover, narratives promote self-regulation through self-expression and organization of complex feelings and conflicts (Knight 2003; Nelson 1996). The imaginative stories that children use to plan and direct their play allow for the safe exploration of age-typical dilemmas and anxieties; intense feelings and fears are contextualized and modified when they are attached to meaningful events and characters, and when the child can experiment with a variety of emotions and outcomes in a playful, nonconsequential setting.

When the child is between ages 3 and 4 years, enhanced memory and developing narrative skills lead to an increased capacity for and interest in autobiographical storytelling (Nelson 1996). Personal narratives help children interpret complex events and impose meaning on topics of intense curiosity, such as where babies come from. As child and parent share and co-construct autobiographical memories and narratives, the child's sense of self is expanded. He or she experiences a greater awareness of individuated self-history and a deepened sense of continuity. Increasingly, the child's mental life becomes organized around unique, private, and recurrent self-narratives (Abrams 1999; Ginot 2012), which may reflect reality-based events but are heavily influenced by the interpretations, distortions, and fantasies of developmental phases and by emotional experiences with important figures.

As the oedipal child's narrative capacities mature, fictional stories acquire deeper meaning. Tales with romantic and moralistic themes, such as well-known legends about courageous heroes, beautiful princesses, and evil witches, are especially appealing and relevant; such stories offer safe, imaginative outlets for the child's own heightened sexual and aggressive urges, while simultaneously assuaging intense desires for adultlike roles. Forbidden incestuous and parricidal fantasies are easily identifiable in fairy tales that feature guileless but heroic young boys who slay dragons, or motherless girls who triumph over wicked mother substitutes. Cautionary tales of talion or "eye-for-an-eye" justice serve as displaced expressions of both powerfully hostile wishes and equally intense fears of punishment. Such themes appear in many beloved stories, such as "Sleeping Beauty," "Cinderella", "Rumpelstiltskin," "Aladdin," "Puss in Boots," and "The Little Mermaid." As Bettelheim (1975) discusses, many of the classic fairy tales preserve the child's loving feelings for the real parents (e.g., a mother who is idealized in death, or an all-good, all-providing fairy godmother), while offering evil parent substitutes or symbols (e.g., a wicked stepmother or a father-dragon) who can be freely hated and over whom the protagonist (and child listener) can guiltlessly triumph.

The Role of Mother-Child Discourse in Emotional Development

Despite the oedipal child's increasing awareness of and investment in the world beyond the mother, the quality of maternal-child discourse plays a highly significant role not only in the child's language development but in the mentalization capacities described in the next section of this chapter. The dyad's spontaneous dialogues and co-construction of narratives, as mother and child plan or recall daily activities or special outings, promote linguistic competence as well as affective sharing. Adult conversation scaffolds the child's initially shaky narrative coherence and stimulates his or her memory for autobiographical events; moreover, joint storytelling helps the young child learn to consider and incorporate others' unique recollections and views (Nelson 1996). When mothers provide rich, interactive conversation—for example, verbal elaboration of the child's experience and liberal use of mental state expressions, such as "I feel," "I want," or "do you think"—the child's narrative capacities and social-emotional understanding are augmented (Nelson 1996; Ruffman et al. 2002).

As the child acquires more sophisticated language, key maternal ego functions—such as identification, reflection, and modulation of emotional experience—are increasingly performed through shared dialogues; the mother expands and enriches the child's verbalizations, adds to imaginative fantasies, labels feelings, asks simple but relevant questions, and gently stretches the child's awareness of other individuals. Their mutual enjoyment and playfulness contribute to the youngster's deep pleasure in verbal communication and to the sense that words have meaning, can convey important information about the self, and can help achieve mutual validation.

The following mother-child interaction illustrates the way in which typical, ordinary verbal exchanges support the child's emerging cognitive and social development. In this case, a 3-year-old boy and his mother engage in mutually pleasurable conversation about a favorite playmate. The mother's comments and questions are geared to her son's current level of comprehension but also serve to gently pull him beyond and encourage him to think about his friend as a separate individual.

Jeremy, age 3½ years, often requests visits with his preschool friend Isabella, whom he has known since age 2. Recently, he has begun thinking and talking about Isabella between their frequent playdates. As he and his mother engage in daily errands, Jeremy repeatedly initiates dialogues such as the following:

JEREMY: Mommy, what's Isabella doing?
MOTHER: You mean right now? I don't know. What do you think?
JEREMY: I don't know, Mommy. What's she doing?
MOTHER: Maybe she's doing errands with her mommy, like we're doing.
JEREMY: Maybe. Maybe Isabella and her mommy are buying a cupcake like us. Isabella likes cupcakes.
MOTHER: You and Isabella like lots of the same things. That's why you are such good friends.

As they leave the bakery, mother and son playfully speculate about Isabella's other activities, preferred snacks, and desire for another playdate at Jeremy's home.

Language and Self-Regulatory Development

- The child's private speech guides personal behavior and reinforces parental limit setting.
- The parental "voice" is internalized during the process of superego formation.
- Narrative capability allows the child to use oedipal-themed stories and imaginative play in order to express and organize complex, conflictual feelings and impulses.
- Self-narratives are central to the developing personality.
- Stories and classic fairy tales provide safe, displaced outlets for forbidden urges and wishes and allow vicarious enjoyment of moralistic resolutions.
- Mother-child discourse and mothers' use of mental state language contribute to the child's use of language for emotional self-regulation.

MENTALIZATION CAPACITIES AND THE
OEDIPAL CHILD'S RELATIONAL WORLD

Mentalization and Object Constancy

The child's increasingly complex and differentiated understanding of mental states is a major achievement of the oedipal phase. The *egocentric* quality of thinking shifts; objective reality is no longer confused with subjective experience (such as dreaming and wishing), the child's own thoughts and feelings are distinguished from those of other people, and individuals' unique perspectives are increasingly grasped. People's behavior acquires new meaning based on its connection to mental states, such as desires and beliefs; in other words, the child begins to discover what makes people "tick." Within the psychodynamic literature, this developmental attainment is usually referred to as *mentalization,* a concept that has come to be viewed (largely through the work of Peter Fonagy and his colleagues) as central to the regulation and organization of emotional life; indeed, the inability to imagine mental states has been linked to emotional dysregulation, commonly observed in adults with borderline personality disorder (Fisher-Kern et al. 2010; Fonagy and Target 1996). The child's ability to reflect on mental life, connect interpersonal events with inner states, and predict people's actions is highly correlated with a history of secure mother-infant attachment and with the mother's ability to imagine and interpret her child's internal experience (Fonagy and Target 1997).

Within the empirical literature, this truly foundational cognitive-emotional-social milestone is often referred to as the acquisition of a *theory of mind,* which generally manifests at age 4 years; similarly, this concept marks the child's capacity to make meaningful links between people's interior states and their manifest behavior (Mayes and Cohen 1996). As interpersonal behavior becomes intelligible to the child and as he or she is better able to anticipate others' responses, complex social interactions make sense and are less confusing. The child experiences people as more interesting, and the child's curiosity increases (as in the example of Jeremy, above, who begins to ponder and ask questions about Isabella's activities and preferences). More nuanced, less concrete interpretation of the social-emotional world promotes a sense of object constancy, which allows the child to sustain a unified, internal representation of self and significant others, even during moments of emotional upheaval (Mahler et al. 1975). Increasingly, the oedipal child perceives people, personal qualities, and relationships as stable and enduring. Previous fears common during the toddler period, such as the notion that the mother's goodness and love are lost when she is angry, gradually recede. As a result, inner conflicts and ambivalent feelings are better tolerated, and a sense of one's own and others' continuity is strengthened.

Theory of Mind, Chronology, and "False-Belief" Tasks

A substantial body of research suggests that children's acquisition of a theory of mind occurs at individualized rates but tends to follow an orderly and predictable progression. By age 3 years, the oedipal child begins to distinguish between subjective mental experience and external events; however, some young 3-year-olds continue to display trouble differentiating between imaginary contents and factual knowledge, assuming that both reflect real life (Woolley and Wellman 1993). The notion that private beliefs determine behavior is not reliably grasped until later, usually by age 4 years (Woolley and Wellman 1993); the idea that beliefs influence feelings comes slightly later still, at around 5–6 years (Harris et al. 2005; Woolley and Wellman 1993). Very complicated social-emotional concepts, such as the potential for one individual to experience competing feelings, are not fully understood until well into middle childhood.

Much of the developmental research on theory of mind utilizes *false-belief tasks* to measure young children's accuracy in predicting another person's behavior based on that individual's unique point of view (Wellman et al. 2001). To perform such tasks correctly, children must grasp that everyone possesses a subjective (possibly incorrect) view of the world; mastery of mental state words such as *think* and *know* appear to parallel this achievement (Lohmann and Tomasello 2003). Typical false-belief studies present the young child with a scenario such as the following:

> Little Jenny comes home from school. While Mother folds laundry in the living room, Jenny sits down at the kitchen table to play with her new stickers. After a while, she interrupts her play to go to the bathroom, leaving the stickers on the table. While she is gone, Mother enters the kitchen, sees the stickers, and moves them to a drawer, so that she can set the table for dinner. When Jenny comes back to the kitchen, where will she look for the stickers, in the drawer or on the table?

A correct prediction of Jenny's behavior would suggest the capacity to distinguish between the contents of one's own mind, others' mental states, and the exterior world of events. The bulk of research concludes that 4-year-old children consistently pass false-belief tests; they grasp the fundamental notion that people may possess a faulty view of reality, but that their mistaken beliefs may nonetheless guide their behavior (Harris et al. 2005). As one study (Woolley and Wellman 1993) aptly explains, the 4-year-old child has realized "that people have internal mental states, such as beliefs, which represent or misrepresent the world, and that human action stems from a person's representation of the world rather than from objective reality directly" (p. 1). When presented with the Jenny story, 4-year-olds differentiate their own omniscient perspective from the protagonist's. They correctly respond that she will first look on the table, because that is where she left the stickers; they understand that Jenny, unlike the listener, has no knowledge of those maternal actions that took place while she was absent. By contrast, 3-year-old children tend to fail false-belief scenarios. They predict that Jenny will look in the drawer, based on their personal knowledge of where the stickers are currently located. The younger child cannot reliably distinguish between his or her own base of knowledge and another individual's fund of information; egocentric thinking is dominant, limiting the child's ability to hold multiple points of view in mind or to differentiate fully between external events and private mental beliefs.

The Oedipal Child's Expanding Social Life and the Emergence of Triadic Relationships

Their emerging mentalization capacities allow 4-year-old children to imagine the contents of others' minds, giving rise to new levels of empathic reactions; the child can think outside the limits of his or her own needs, preferences, and responses, and contemplate another person's experience. One mother, who had uncharacteristically spent the weekend lying on the sofa because of a mild fever, described the following behaviors of her 3- and 5-year-old daughters, both of whom evinced a concerned and solicitous attitude: the younger child tenderly offered her hugs and a favorite teddy, a personal source of comfort since infancy, while the older girl suggested that they play quietly in another room so that Mommy could rest. Similarly, when faced with the shifting demands of complex social situations, older children are capable of behavioral adjustment based upon the perceived needs of others. For example, when asked to explain a story to a younger child, 4-year-olds are likely to simplify their syntax and vocabulary in order to accommodate the listener's limited verbal skills; 3-year-old children, by contrast, fail to take the younger child's comprehension needs into consideration (Shatz and Gelman 1973).

The acquisition of a theory of mind has far-reaching implications for the oedipal child's emotional and interpersonal life, both in and beyond the family environment. Empirical studies demonstrate links between mental state knowledge and major age-salient developments, such as social competence and self-regulation; As will be elaborated in later chapters, these are foundational areas of inner and relational life which profoundly influence the older child's sense of connection to peers and successful adjustment to learning environments. The capacity to reflect on and interpret mental states correlates with flexible, mature self-regulatory and social functioning: children who display theory of mind knowledge tend to engage in positive friendships, demonstrate prosocial behaviors, and receive high teacher ratings for social skills and classroom adjustment (Denham et al. 2003; Fonagy and Target 2000).

The oedipal child's knowledge of others' minds, more vivid fantasy life, and overall physical and cognitive maturity contribute to an expanding engagement with those outside of the parent-child dyad. Complex, triadic relationships are newly grasped and become an evolving permanent source of emotional and imaginative stimulation. Other people's special bonds, feelings, and activities, from which the child is potentially omitted, elicit intense desire, wishful fantasies, and jealousy. In particular, the private life of the parents (including their mystifying conversations and imagined sexual activities) inspires powerful feelings of curiosity, inadequacy, and exclusion.

Although the parents are major targets of the oedipal child's aggressive and wishful fantasies, siblings are of great importance, and the peer group begins to come sharply into focus. Oedipal children are acutely conscious of sibling-parent bonds; moreover, peer connections and potential exclusion from friendships emerge as a source of growing concern. Such concepts as "best friends" acquire meaning and create new social desires and anxieties. In the context of the child's heightened empathic capacities, deeper grasp of others' needs, and awareness of parental standards, however, angry and jealous reactions give rise to unprecedented conflicts and guilt feelings. A fuller discussion of early triadic relationships, the accompanying feelings and fantasies, and the way in which these contribute to enduring emotional and interpersonal patterns is provided in Chapter 5.

The following examples illustrate differences between the social interactions of children ages 3 and 5 years, as revealed by their verbal exchanges. In the first example, a 3-year-old girl, Jessica, demonstrates her difficulty grasping the distinction between her own and her teacher's mental knowledge. She assumes that Mr. King knows what she knows, and she initiates a conversation about a third party without regard to his perspective. Jessica cannot contemplate the disparity between her own relationship with another child and Mr. King's. When prompted by her teacher to provide additional information, she attempts to clarify but becomes frustrated.

On a Monday morning, 3-year-old Jessica, who was fond of chatting with adults, entered her prekindergarten classroom and approached the teacher with enthusiasm, displaying a tiny bandage on her knee. Eager to discuss the weekend's events, she immediately launched into an explanation of the injury: "Becky did it. She made me fall down. She pushes." Mr. King, who did not know a child named Becky, inquired who she was; in fact, Becky was a cousin who had never had contact with anyone at Jessica's school. Jessica looked annoyed by this question and insisted, "You know Becky, Mr. King."

He responded, "I don't think I've met her, Jess. Is she your friend?"

Jessica briefly considered this request for clarification, and responded, "You know her. She pushed me and she pushed Sandy" (another child unknown to Mr. King).

The following conversation, between two 5-year-old classmates, demonstrates their far greater facility with social understanding and their easy grasp of complex, triadic situations. These girls accommodate each other's perspective; they ask appropriate questions to establish a shared base of knowledge for social exchange, and each spontaneously provides information that the other requires. They understand that each has private relations with other parties, and they attempt to resolve their feelings of empathy and guilt when they make a plan that may affect a younger brother. Moreover, peer relationships are clearly central to the older girls' interests and plans. In contrast to Jessica, whose major focus in the previous vignette was on sharing an experience with her teacher, these girls are intent on securing each other's company, and competently predict adults' thinking and reactions in order to plan for the necessary permissions.

Katie and Abby, 5-year-old classmates who often play together at preschool and attend the same swimming class, but who have never visited each other's homes, are enjoying fantasy play at the school's dollhouse. The school day is about to come to an end, and they are eager to continue their game.

KATIE: I have a really good dollhouse in my room. Do you wanna have a playdate today? Do you wanna come to my house? My mom is picking me up today.

ABBY: I have a dollhouse, too. We can play at your house this time and my house next time. I think my babysitter, Kelly, picks me up today. I have to ask her about playdates. You know my babysitter?

KATIE: She's the one who picks you up from swimming? I know her.

ABBY: She picks me up from swimming and dance.

KATIE: I don't go to dance.

ABBY: Oh. You just see her at swimming?

KATIE: She has red hair and she brings your little brother?

ABBY: Yeah. She doesn't always let me have playdates.

KATIE: Why not?

ABBY: I don't know. Sometimes she has to bring my brother somewhere.

KATIE (*after a thoughtful pause*): My mom always says yes. Let's ask my mom to ask Kelly about the playdate.

ABBY: Kelly will say yes if your mom asks her (*pauses*). But what if my brother wants a playdate too?

KATIE: Then Mom'll bring us to my house, and Kelly can take your brother.

Mentalization and Social-Emotional Development

- Knowledge about the meaningful link between people's internal states and outward behavior is a major cognitive-emotional-social milestone achieved by age 4 years.

- Mentalization is correlated with secure mother-infant attachment and with the child's development of emotional self-regulation.

- In research, false-belief tasks are used to demonstrate theory-of-mind acquisition.

- Mentalization facilitates empathy and moral development, helps the child establish a stable sense of self and other (object constancy), supports behavioral and emotional self-regulation, and contributes to a grasp of triadic relationships.

- Increased awareness of others' minds and relationships (especially the parents' private bond) leads to novel feelings of jealousy and exclusion.

THE DEVELOPMENT OF PRETEND PLAY AND THE ROLE OF IMAGINATION IN THE OEDIPAL CHILD'S LIFE

Transitional Phenomena and the Role of Play in the Child's Mental Life

Beginning with Sigmund Freud's (1920/1962) depiction of a toddler's string game, psychodynamic theorists have privileged play as a unique, development-promoting activity and a window into the young child's internal world. During imaginary play, age-salient conflicts and anxieties are safely expressed without consequence, and passively experienced events are brought under the child's control. The transformations of make-believe allow children to experiment with multiple roles and to participate in complex situations. Reality is temporarily suspended; unlike fantasizing and daydreaming, however, pretend play is both a mental and a physical activity in which action has a central role (Solnit 1987).

According to some theorists (e.g., A. Freud 1963), play represents a circumscribed activity that belongs to the early phases of development and is gradually replaced with reality-bound interests and work. Piaget (1962) expresses similar views; he describes symbolic play as reflecting the prelogical child's attempt to assimilate complex, reality-based experience to his or her immature ego capacities. Like many psychodynamic thinkers, however, Winnicott (1953) suggests that playfulness and imaginary functions are vital across the lifespan. In his theory, play emerges in infancy with the appearance of *transitional phenomena* (as described in Chapter 2, "Infancy," these are typically soft toys or bits of blanket to which babies become attached as they begin the process of self-other differentiation); transitional objects are gradually supplanted by the child's pretend play, and later by the adult's participation in artistic and cultural activities, all of which arise in the potential, creative space between external reality and internal subjectivity. Within the empirical literature, transitional phenomena—which may take the form of sounds and movements, as well as of tangible items—are similarly viewed as normative; up to 60% of toddlers and preschoolers are reported to manifest attachment to blankets or soft objects (Donate-Bartfield and Passman 2004; Passman 1987). However, conclusions differ as to whether these phenomena are related to the quality of the mother-child relationship and whether their presence serves developmental functions, such as self-regulation (e.g., allowing the child to enter an unfamiliar situation without crying).

A number of child clinicians and researchers have elaborated a broad view of imaginative play, emphasizing its importance as a normative, integrative symbolic function that fosters a wide range of intellectual, relational, and self-regulatory capacities and expands the young child's internal representations of self and others (Birch 1997; Gilmore 2005; Lyons-Ruth 2006; Marans et al. 1991; Mayes and Cohen 1992). While playing, children "try on" various roles and identifications and practice perspective taking; during social-dramatic play, with peer or adult partners, a child engages in complex interpersonal exchanges through shared meaning making and narrative building. Indeed, during the state of playing, young children manifest a grasp of other characters' desires and intentions that exceeds their usual, nonplaying capacities (Fonagy and Target 1996; Mayes and Cohen 1996; Vygotsky 1978). Moreover, pretend play allows for the safe expression and exploration of intense, conflictual feelings and anxieties; when these are organized around and attached to creative stories, their sharpness and immediacy is diminished. As the child plays, he or she reintegrates more modulated versions of initial wishes, fears, and impulses.

The development-promoting, self-regulatory functions of play are reminiscent of the mother's role in interpreting and ameliorating the younger child's emotional experience. Indeed, the quality of the early mother-child relationship affects the oedipal child's capacity for play. Children with a history of secure attachment tend to manifest richer, more complex make-believe scenarios; in particular, children with disorganized styles of attachment have difficulty maintaining coherent narratives when affective contents are involved (Hesse and Main 2000; Slade 1987). Moreover, a history of in-secure attachment and early parental abuse and neglect are correlated with poor development of social-dramatic play skills (Alessandri 1991).

Chronology of Pretend Play

Imaginary play attains prominence during the oedipal phase; it gradually recedes as the child enters the next (latency) period of development and begins to seek more structured, rule-bound games. Early forms of pretend play emerge in the second year of life and follow a well-documented progression to-ward increasing levels of cognitive and social-emotional complexity (Born-stein et al. 1996; Fein 1981; McCune 1995; Piaget 1962). However, even in the first months of infancy, the child differentiates between the mother's real and playful affects, suggesting that pretense is grasped in a relational context well before it is manifested in the child's playing behaviors (Gergely 2000). During infancy, the baby's actions are largely presymbolic, involving sensorimotor ac-tivity and exploration; objects, parts of bodies, and toys are observed, mouthed, and manipulated. Around the time of the first birthday, the toddler begins to demonstrate simple self- and other-directed imitations of familiar actions (e.g., "feeding" self or mother from a bowl); the child's smiling and playfully exagger-ated behaviors suggest that the distinction between real and pretense is fully grasped. Soon, he or she also begins to enact simple play sequences that recre-ate scenes of daily life, such as giving a doll a bath (Bornstein et al. 1996).

When a child is around age 2 years, symbolic substitutions emerge. For example, the toddler recruits a block to serve as a pretend phone, or places beads in a dish to be used as imaginary food. Such advances in the level of ab-straction begin to expand the child's play possibilities and stretch the tod-dler's concrete, perceptual, and action-bound thinking. However, the 2-year-old child's play tends to reflect simplistic, familiar themes and situations drawn from everyday experience: a stuffed animal is pushed about in a toy stroller, or a baby doll is put to sleep.

During the oedipal phase of development, an explosion in abstract, narra-tive, and imaginary capacities contributes to increasingly complex and cre-ative pretense. Internal access to fantasy opens up vast possibilities for the contents of play; the child may draw from familiar stories or events, but can also create unique narratives and characters that are imbued with meaningful qualities and wished-for abilities. Ordinary themes, such as playing school or house, are interspersed with more fanciful ones; the adventures of magical creatures, superheroes, and fairy princesses enter the child's repertoire.

As pretend scenarios grow more intricate, involving multiple roles and complex events, the child increasingly seeks and benefits from the participation of peers. Social-dramatic play functions as a major source of interpersonal and emotional learning, requiring that children verbally construct shared meanings and that they agree on the transformative uses of objects. The younger, 3-year-old oedipal child finds it difficult to accommodate the preferences and ideas of others. By around age 4 years, however, most children have acquired the necessary skills for shared fantasy play; these include the capacity to incorporate other players' plans and desires, jointly create and revise complex story lines, and negotiate the assignment of roles. Empirical studies suggest that engagement in shared pretense is linked to higher levels of social cognition (e.g., Howe et al. 2005).

• **See the video "4-Year-Old Girl" for an example of jointly constructed adult-child play narratives with oedipal themes.**

The following vignette illustrates a 3-year-old girl's use of mother-child pretend play to manage the daily task of separation at her preschool classroom. By enacting the role of the mother, this young child engages in a temporary identification with her parent and transforms a passive, negative experience into one in which she possesses mastery and control. Her mother's sensitive role-playing extends the game and elaborates the child's disavowed, unwanted feelings of anxiety and helplessness. The nonconsequential atmosphere of pretense makes it possible for Ginny to evince pleasure over the mother's feigned distress and to relish the role of powerful parent.

> Three-year-old Ginny had recently begun to attend a preschool class and was struggling with the morning separation; often, she cried and clung to her mother, resisting the teacher's attempts to absorb her in various activities. At home, Ginny initiated a new game, called "school drop-off." Ginny drew her mother into the play and enthusiastically suggested, "I'll be the mommy, and you be the big girl." Her mother played along, tactfully avoiding any reference to the obvious link with her daughter's morning struggles; she followed Ginny's lead, accepting her assigned position as the anxious child who was repeatedly abandoned at the classroom doorway. The living room was arranged as the classroom; a large stuffed animal was recruited to be the teacher, "Miss Susan," and smaller animals and dolls were scattered about to represent the various children.
>
> Then, Ginny and her mother solemnly withdrew to the kitchen, clasped hands, and approached the living room entrance. Ginny whispered to her mother sympathetically, "It's okay, sweetie, I'll be back at pick-up time," and gave her a kiss. Her mother evinced mild but persistent protests, insightfully remarking, "I just hate it when you leave, Mommy. I miss you, and the day is so long without you." Ginny offered familiar maternal comfort, such as pats and hugs, and a few suggestions like, "Look, sweetie, Mommy's picture is in your cubby," or reminders about activities they would do together later in the

day. At times, Ginny's portrayal of the mother was more impatient and less compassionate; she resolutely marched off to "work," only briefly looking back and smiling as her mother playfully pouted. This game was often repeated, with slight alterations, and was ultimately abandoned as Ginny gained confidence at school.

Play, the Oedipal Phase, and the Therapeutic Use of Play

The timely emergence of fantasy play during the preschool years is uniquely suited to the internal upheaval caused by oedipal phase conflicts and anxieties: The painful longings, intense ambivalent feelings and potential mortifications of the oedipal child are expressed, modulated, and integrated via creative imagery, story-telling, and character creation (Gilmore 2011). Formidable age-salient tasks, such as self-management of sexual excitement and aggressive urges, are more successfully navigated when the child has access to imaginary outlets. In the secure, nonconsequential world of make-believe, he or she can temporarily acquire coveted qualities and enjoy triumph over rivals; simultaneously, unwanted feelings and vulnerabilities are disavowed and safely displaced onto others.

Such vivid depictions of valued and unwanted aspects of self and other are well known to child clinicians, whose participation in the youngster's imaginary world—via shared play and verbal fantasies—involves accepting assignment to diminished, despised roles which the child is eager to externalize; more desirable, powerful positions are generally reserved for him- or herself. One 5-year-old girl, after setting up an elaborate scene of tiny dolls and furniture, insisted that her therapist play all the naughty children who were severely punished (by having their heads chopped off); she herself assumed the role of the good and beautiful child, who was ultimately chosen to go live in the castle and wed the prince who would one day rule the land. The clinician's playful embellishment of helpless, frightened, or impulsive characters serves to elaborate and clarify the child's own unwelcome feelings and limitations, and soften the sense of danger about forbidden wishes and impulses. Ultimately, these co-created imaginative activities help the child organize and reintegrate complex feelings and conflicts.

The following description of typical 5-year-old girls' sociodramatic play illustrates the way in which children's complex imaginary scenarios allow them to incorporate elements from familiar stories as well as their own fantasies. Playing together requires that these girls accommodate each other's preferences and perspectives, share narratives and meanings, and engage in joint planning. Oedipal themes are apparent: the storyline is magical and romantic, they are working to understand boy-girl differences, and concerns with adult-like status and power are prominent. Moreover, an evil, jealous female figure looms in the background, threatening to take away the girls' dimly defined husbands and force them to return to a less glamorous life, without magic and beauty:

> Anne and Jill, who had both just turned 5, were engaged in sober discussion in a corner of their kindergarten classroom. They had agreed on a basic scenario for a game of mermaids, inspired by a story they both knew well, but each had distinct ideas about additional elements.
>
> ANNE: Who are we gonna marry? Boys can't be mermaids.
>
> JILL: They can too. We'll marry boy mermaids and live in the water.
>
> ANNE: No, no, you're wrong. My cousin June told me. Only girls can be mermaids.
>
> JILL: Who's June?
>
> ANNE: She's nine. She knows.
>
> JILL: Okay. We don't marry other mermaids. We get husbands at the castle.
>
> ANNE: Sometimes we'll be in the water, sometimes in the castle.
>
> JILL (*gesturing toward the housekeeping corner*): Pretend this is the castle and we're living here and we're married and the witch doesn't know (*grabs a dress-up tiara and wand*). And I'm a princess.
>
> ANNE: Wait, that's not fair.
>
> JILL: It's fair. You be the princess next.
>
> ANNE: No, one of us has the tiara, and one of us has the wand.
>
> JILL: Okay, we're both mermaid-princesses (*hands the tiara to Anne*), and I have magic in my wand and you have magic in your tiara (*waves her wand*).
>
> ANNE (*settles the tiara on her head*): To get the power, I just have to touch my tiara (*demonstrates*). And let's pretend the witch doesn't know we have magic, so she comes to the ball and tries to make us not married and go back to the water.
>
> JILL: We're at the ball! (*Both begin to twirl and dance.*) Yikes, the witch is coming, run! (*They both run about the classroom.*)
>
> ANNE: Stop! (*waving her wand at the imaginary witch*). Now you can never get our princes and drag us back to the ocean!
>
> JILL (*touches her tiara, then points to the witch*): Now you're dead!

This pretend game captures the essential elements of play and illustrates how the child's imaginary capacities serve to modulate the inevitable, powerful longings and disappointments of the oedipal phase. Through the safe outlet of fantasy and the metaphors of play, these girls enact and work through central conflicts, such as the dual presence of loving and aggressive feelings toward adults and the competing desires to satisfy urgent wishes and avoid guilty feelings. Experimentation and identifications with perceived adult and gender roles and with idealized standards of behaviors are talked through and then playfully explored in action. The immediacy of intense wishes, urges, and fears is softened; by attaching their romantic desires and their curiosity to a storyline, Jill and Anne achieve a sense of control over their bodies and impulses. In addition, their play is a forum for social learning; they negotiate, invoke esteemed others (in this case, a 9-year-old cousin) to gain power, and ultimately compromise in the service of maintaining their friendship and avoiding disruption of their beloved, shared pastime.

Imaginary Companions

Another familiar phenomenon, the *imaginary companion*—often a benign human or animal "friend"—serves similar functions. Often, these fanciful creatures appear during the oedipal period but may extend into latency, where they tend to assume slightly different forms; they decline sharply in prevalence as children approach puberty. When imaginary friends are defined broadly (i.e., inclusive of invisible companions; those that are based on imagined activities of the child's toys and possessions; and those that take a more abstract form, such as an imaginary friend who is the recipient of the child's diary letters), studies document that between 46% and 65% of school-age children acknowledge a current or past imaginary friend (Taylor et al. 2004; Trionfi and Reese 2009). Although the benefits to older children are less clear, preschoolers with imaginary companions manifest the following characteristics compared to peers without them: richer fantasy and play narratives, better developed communication skills, and higher levels of social-emotional knowledge and competence, including theory of mind acquisition (Roby and Kidd 2008; Taylor et al. 2010). Parents tend to be very aware of the oedipal child's imaginary friends; however, the older child's more subtle creations often elude parental notice.

Imaginary companions of the oedipal phase emerge as the child is struggling to gain mastery over powerful wishes and urges; the particular qualities and behavioral tendencies with which their creator imbues them reveal the child's fears and ongoing battles to achieve self-control. Moreover, these companions arise during a period of novel loneliness, as the child is coming to terms with his or her exclusion from important relationships between parents or peers. Instinctively appreciating their importance to the child, parents tend to accommodate these companions, who are alternately fussed over and ordered about by the child. One lively 3-year-old boy who suffered from intense fear of dogs and was often admonished for poor table manners and general impatience created a nonthreatening canine friend; after a frightening encounter with a large but harmless dog, the child announced the arrival of "Bouncy Doggy," a meek male pet who accompanied the family on trips outside of the home. On many occasions, when the creature was allowed his own seat at a local restaurant, Bouncy Doggy's owner reprimanded him for slurping, refusing new foods, and kicking under the table. This faithful, undemanding companion served multiple functions: assuaging the child's specific bodily anxieties (including castration fears about biting and injury) by transforming a threatening, large-toothed dog into a benign creature within the child's total control; providing a constant friend, with no potential for jealous or excluded feelings; and serving as a repository for the child's own impulsive urges and unwanted behaviors, while the child was free to embody the adultlike role of disciplinarian.

The Role of Imagination in Oedipal Development

- Pretend play and its accompanying creative stories serve as an outlet and organizer for oedipal wishes, anxieties, and conflicts.

- Play allows the child to achieve mastery over passively experienced events, such as mother-child separation.

- During play, children practice perspective taking, try on a variety of identifications, and satisfy their desire for adult roles.

- Social-dramatic play with parents or peers serves as a learning experience wherein children jointly create meaning and accommodate another's plans and preferences.

- Imaginary companions are a normative creation that provides the child with companionship and a sense of mastery over his or her own fears and impulses.

PREOPERATIONAL THINKING AND THE OEDIPAL PHASE

Although oedipal children have vastly increased verbal capacities and mental state knowledge, their inner life is deeply influenced by *preoperational thinking* (Piaget and Inhelder 1969); this prelogical and impressionistic approach to solving problems and evaluating complex, emotionally laden events makes these children highly susceptible to idiosyncratic, magical interpretations. Particularly in those under age 4 years, some continuing confusion between products of the imagination and reality-based events persists (Woolley and Wellman 1993). Even the 4-year-old child's social and emotional comprehension may be overwhelmed by complicated actions and exciting feelings. For example, one group of researchers (Harris et al. 2005) employed the widely known "Little Red Riding Hood" story to test preschoolers' ability to comprehend multiple perspectives; despite 4-year-olds' well-documented mentalization capacities, these writers concluded that many in that age group expect Little Red to be frightened when she knocks on Grandma's door, even though the story makes clear that she could have no knowledge of the earlier, calamitous events (i.e., that the wolf had already intruded in Grandma's house and is now dressed up in her clothing).

Moreover, concrete and perceptually bound thinking tends to dominate the oedipal child's understanding of problems and situations; often, a single conspicuous dimension, such as size, governs the child's judgments. As a result, "bigger is better" becomes a guiding principle for oedipal values. For example, a nickel may be perceived as more valuable than a dime, because it is larger and therefore impressionistically experienced as more desirable. When given a choice, the young child will select objects that are larger, shinier, or fancier. These various limitations and immature interpretations are brought to bear when the child contemplates matters of keen oedipal phase importance, such as bodies and sexuality.

The Oedipal Child's Reproductive Theories and the Primal Scene

The oedipal child's thoughts and feelings about highly relevant and complex topics, such as generational and anatomical distinctions, are acutely affected by naïve cognition. Perception, action, and bodily experience dominate the child's sense of self; self-definitions and self-understanding are expressed in action-based language, rather than through proffering abstract beliefs and opinions (Auerbach and Blatt 1996). Enhanced abilities to compare and contrast their own small physical endowments with their parents' bodily equipment, as well as intense oedipal-phase curiosity about genitals, are experienced in the context of children's naïve cognition. Concrete reproductive theories and mortification over perceived inferiorities, vis-à-vis adults' larger, more complex sexual equipment, can engender deep anxieties and feelings of inadequacy.

The oedipal child's avid interest in the body and its functions and in settling the question of "where babies come from" can lead to active investigation. Young children may engage in mutual bodily exploration with peers or devote considerable energy and ingenuity to the task of viewing their parents' unclad bodies, including intrusions into the adult bedroom. One especially enthusiastic 3½-year-old girl proposed that her parents "make a baby right now so I can *see how it gets maked.*" Young children are vocal about their biological theories; commonplace beliefs revolve around oral and anal cavities, such as the notion that babies get into the body via the mouth, like food, and are excreted through the anus. Making meaning of the body, anatomical differences, and gender distinctions is a central developmental task for the oedipal child (Yanof 2000) and absorbs considerable intellectual and emotional effort.

Although children begin to grasp the link between gender and genitals around age 3 years, they remain quite confused about adult sexuality (Senet

2004). Within psychodynamic theory, the oedipal-age child's perception of parental sexual activity—referred to as the *primal scene*—is viewed as a formative, universal fantasy. As Blum (1979) describes, "the confused child wonders, 'who does what, how, why, and to whom?'" (p. 30). Primal scene fantasies may or may not be based on actual, visual observation of the parents but are always subject to the young child's distortions and concrete thinking. Interpretations of the sexual act as aggressive, misperceptions about the mechanics of intercourse, and oversimplified notions about internal organs are common.

The following clinical example illustrates the way in which developmental achievements—in this case, toilet training—can be derailed by oedipal-phase thinking and anxieties. This 4-year-old girl, whose very fine verbal and play capacities cause her to appear precociously sophisticated, is relentless in her pursuit of anatomical and reproductive information. Often, she trails her father into the bathroom to try (unsuccessfully) to convince him to let her view and touch his penis; on a number of occasions, she walks in on the parents embracing in bed or when they are unclothed. Inspired by the pregnant mother of her best friend, she begs her parents for information about anatomy and childbirth, which they attempt to provide. Her comprehension of such material, however, is limited by 4-year-old logic and reasoning capacities and is highly influenced by her own fears and fantasies.

> Four-year-old Natalie was described by her parents as "always an intense, high-strung child, even as a baby." In response to fervent questions, her mild-mannered parents had given her basic biological facts, such as labels for female anatomy and simple information about human reproduction. Nonetheless, she adhered to her personal theories about the origins of life, which centered around a vague notion that eggs, which she imagined resembled those she and her mother cracked for baking, and some sort of swimming seed collided within the female abdomen; she "knew" that the egg was a girl, and the seed a boy.
>
> During the pregnancy of her best friend's mother, Natalie suddenly rejected her favorite breakfast, consisting of hard-boiled eggs and tomatoes, and assiduously avoided this combination of these foods. Natalie explained that eggs and tomato seeds would "mix up in my tummy." After her friend's baby brother was born, Natalie's anxiety about foods expanded; she began to refuse many former staples, particularly seeded fruits. In addition, her successful bowel training suffered a setback and she began to have accidents and demand diapers. Her concerned parents contacted a child therapist and play therapy was initiated.
>
> Through pretend play with dolls and her accompanying narratives, Natalie soon revealed the multiple ideas, anxieties, and conflicts behind her food and toilet phobias. These included her firm belief that ingesting seeds and eggs could lead to her own pregnancy, jealousy of the friend's new baby

brother, desires to be grown up and have a baby of her own, and worries that a newborn could grow in her body and then be eliminated in the toilet. Play therapy and parent counseling led to a gradual return of normal eating and age-appropriate toileting.

Bodily Anxieties and Fears of Punishment

The preschool child's naïve cognition affects the capacity to manage intense, conflict-laden feelings and impulses. Typical oedipal wishes—such as desirous, possessive, or hostile inclinations toward a parent—may be invested with the magical potential to control objects and events in the real world; such beliefs cause the child to fear real-life consequences for private emotions and fantasies. A parent's illness, a sibling's injury, or a marital separation during this phase of development can elicit intense anxiety in the child, because such events appear to validate his or her mental powers and reinforce the sense that forbidden thoughts and feelings have catastrophic potential.

The young child's sense of justice and fears of punishment are similarly concrete and simplistic, often taking the form of bodily consequences. Fantasies of talion-like retribution for prohibited desires make the oedipal child especially vulnerable to worries about physical loss and injury, such as castration. The following vignette of a typically developing 3-year-old boy who is exposed to sexual differences, via a newborn female cousin, illustrates the way in which such thinking can engender deep anxiety and briefly interfere with daily life. In this instance, Daniel's verbal capacities and his parents' reassuring attitude help make his sudden phobic reactions fleeting and manageable.

> Daniel, age 3½ years, had achieved toilet training with little difficulty, taking pride in his accomplishment of bodily self-control. He enjoyed urinating like his father into the grown-up toilet, rather than the potty, and then pressing the handle for flushing. After a visit to the home of a newborn female cousin, where he witnessed frequent diapering and dressing activities with great interest, he asked persistent questions about boy-girl bodily differences; his parents responded naturally and comfortably to his queries as to why the infant had no penis, where her penis had gone, and so on. He seemed satisfied, and his parents assumed that he had accepted their simple explanations.
>
> Several days later, Daniel refused to walk past a familiar dog on his way to preschool, insisting "That dog wants to bite my penis" while pointing to the animal's open mouth and large teeth. Soon he began to refuse to urinate in the downstairs toilet, insisting that the bowl looked like "a mouth that wants to eat my penis." His parents were surprised at the sudden emergence of fearful reactions; their reassurances were somewhat comforting, but he was not fully convinced that the dog and toilet were safe. His parents offered to carry him as they walked past the dog's home and were casual about Daniel's avoidance of the first-floor bathroom. After several months, these avoidant behaviors subsided.

Superego Formation

Morality and Guilt

From around age 3 years, the young child's sense of self is increasingly connected to an internal self-monitoring system that helps regulate emotionality and guide behavior. Variously referred to as the *superego* (in psychodynamic literature) or *conscience* (in empirical studies), this set of inner standards and controls gives rise to moral emotions, such as guilt and empathy, that are integrated into the self-representation (Kochanska 1994; Kochanska et al. 2010). Within the empirical literature, *guilt* is defined as a complex social emotion involving feelings of contrition and responsibility toward another, clearly evident by around age 4 years but not fully developed until the grade school years. The young child's acquisition of a theory of mind, and concomitant grasp of others' needs and feelings, is a critical underpinning for mature empathy and moral functioning. However, complex social concepts and the meanings behind emotional interactions are only partially grasped by the preschooler; for example, at age 4 years, children recognize that "saying sorry" represents a form of conciliation, but they do not fully understand the implied sense of remorse in the act of apologizing (Vaish et al. 2011).

Psychodynamic theorists use a somewhat distinct definition of *guilt,* which is seen as connected to identifications with parental standards and to the formation of superego structure. Whereas the toddler dreads loss of the parent's approval and experiences shame when his or her behavior falls short of adult expectations, the oedipal child's internalized principles lead to fears about the potential loss of self-approval and self-esteem; failure to live up to internal standards leads to moral anxiety (guilt) rather than social anxiety (shame). As we discuss further in Chapter 5, these two emotions are often blended; narcissistic preoccupations about one's status and appearance in the eyes of others are inextricably linked to concerns about living up to inner values. Thus, shame often accompanies guilt. In addition, we discuss in Chapter 5 the way in which the oedipal child's possessive feelings toward the parents and fears about punishment, including specific concerns about bodily injury, relate to guilt and moral development.

As internal self-rewards and self-punishments, such as proud or guilty feelings, gradually take the place of external parental controls, the oedipal child's moral functioning becomes increasingly autonomous (Tyson and Tyson 1984). Once knowledge about right and wrong is consolidated, acts of misconduct, whether committed by the self or others, elicit inner discomfort and condemnation. Experimental conditions reveal that by age 3 years, children display preferential treatment of prosocially oriented peers (e.g., sharing toys more readily with playmates whom they perceive as generous); moreover, they manifest hesitation and uneasiness when confronted with potential "violations"—that is, behaviors that previously elicited adult disapproval (Kochanska 1994; Vaish et al. 2011). The 4-year-old child's more mature sense of empathy and understanding of others' needs further contribute to the process of socialization. In contrast to the toddler, who seeks concrete imitation of adult actions, the older oedipal child strives to follow the parents' more abstract standards and ideals; such notions as goodness, kindness, and helpfulness are increasingly understood and valued. Attachment to highly moralistic stories and fairy tales, whose characters vividly embody these qualities, reflects and reinforces children's interest in less tangible principles. During times of affective arousal, however, the ongoing support of parents remains highly influential. Active maternal involvement that emphasizes guidance rather than punitive reactions is correlated with good self-regulation; empathic parenting is a crucial underpinning for the child's development of prosocial feelings and behavior (Kochanska et al. 2000).

Emotional and Behavioral Self-Regulation

The slow, gradual process of autonomous self-regulation undergoes key changes during the oedipal phase. Psychodynamic thinkers (e.g., Winnicott 1958) suggest that the oedipal child's more organized mental representations and stable sense of self and others (object constancy) provide protection from affective upheavals; a soothing, integrated parental image is maintained, even when the adult is not physically present, leading to diminished emotional self-disruption during moments of distress. Moreover, as described in the preceding sections, the proliferation of symbolic resources—language, mentalization, and imaginary play—contributes hugely to the child's growing ability to maintain emotional stability. Within the empirical literature, self-regulation—defined as the ability to initiate and modulate personal behavior—is similarly viewed as crucial for the preschooler's earliest academic and social adjustment; the young child's capacities to engage in goal-directed action, adapt to the demands of the classroom, and participate in peer relations are all seen as predicated upon reliable self-control.

The defining shift from reliance on external controls of behavior (i.e., the presence of parents or other adults) toward internal self-regulation is a major focus of research (e.g.,Kochanska et al. 2001; Koenig et al. 2000). Many studies measure the child's self-management via demonstrated compliance with parental requests; adherence to adult injunctions, under experimental conditions where the parent has left the room, is seen as evidence for internalized rules of conduct and suggests that the child has attained a level of inner self-restraint. Underlying maturation in cognitive controls (e.g., deployment of attention, inhibition of automatic reactions) further contributes to improved self-management; for example, the capacity for deliberate engagement in self-distraction is hugely advantageous for tolerating frustration under circumstances wherein gratification must be deferred (Cole et al. 2011). The ongoing development of these mechanisms and the child's ever-increasing autonomous self-control help initiate *latency,* the next phase of development.

Early Superego Formation

- After age 3 years, moral feelings and reactions are increasingly integrated into the child's sense of self.
- The child begins to internalize more abstract parental values and interpersonal standards, such as goodness and kindness.
- Prohibited behaviors and urges elicit guilt feelings.
- As self-punishments and internal prohibitions substitute for external (parental) enforcement, the child's moral and self-regulatory capacities become more autonomous.

Key Concepts

The oedipal phase is a transformative period of development spanning ages 3–6 years. Enhanced awareness of and curiosity about those outside the mother-child dyad, and an increase in both sexual and aggressive urges toward the parents, lead to novel internal conflicts, anxieties, and resolutions. The young child's inner struggles are balanced by the emergence of myriad new cognitive, social-emotional, and self-regulatory capacities. Vastly improved symbolic abilities, reflected in such momentous achievements as narrative-making, mentalization, and imaginative play, open up creative ways to explore, organize, and integrate complicated feelings and fantasies. As the child begins to differentiate between his or her own and others' mental states and to make meaningful links between mind and behavior, internal representations of self and other become more nuanced, unified, and stable.

As the child gains new interest in *triadic* relationships, the parents' private bond, particularly their imagined sexual behaviors, becomes a source of avid curiosity, painful feelings of exclusion, and competitive fantasies. Increased genital excitement fuels a heightened interest in anatomical boy-girl differences and reproductive theories, along with a dawning sense of personal bodily limitations and inadequacies compared to the parents. Fears of punishment, often in the form of corporeal injury and loss of valued body parts, such as castration fears, accompany the oedipal child's romantic fantasies and jealous urges.

The child's sense of self is increasingly linked to morality; internalized behavioral standards and enduring identifications with the parents' qualities give rise to *superego formation*. As the oedipal phase draws to a close and the child approaches the years of intensive, school-based learning, he or she is progressively better able to relate to individuals outside of the family constellation, adhere to consistent standards of behavior, and manage internal feelings and conflicts.

- The oedipal child's verbal capacities soar, and language is increasingly separated from immediate actions and perceptual experience.

  - Preschoolers begin to comprehend ideas and engage in narrative building. Autobiographical stories help the child make meaning of complex events and enhance the sense of personal continuity.

  - Stories and fairy tales with relevant themes provide context for the child's own increased sexual and aggressive urges; romantic adventures, rewards for goodness, punishment for evil deeds, and the triumphs of naïve heroes and heroines are particularly satisfying as the oedipal child wrestles with intense wishes and fears.

- Pretend play, wherein children create elaborate story lines and assume imaginary roles, becomes a major mode of cognitive, emotional, and social development.

  - Play provides a safe, nonconsequential setting in which the oedipal child expresses and explores urgently felt wishes and impulses.

  - The attachment of affects, conflicts, and fears to imaginative narratives helps the child integrate and modulate their intensity.

  - Symbolic play offers opportunities to experiment with multiple roles and practice social perspective taking. Social-dramatic play with parents and peers increases relational skills, such as shared narrative creation, negotiation of roles, and joint planning.

- By age 4 years, most children have developed a theory of mind. They realize that each individual's experience is distinct and subjective, and they grasp the link between mental phenomena—thoughts, feelings, and wishes—and external behavior.

  - In developmental research, the child's ability to perform correctly on *false-belief tasks*—tests that require a child to accurately predict another's behavior—is considered a marker for this important achievement.

  - Children who understand mental states are better able to make meaning of complex behaviors and interpersonal events, and to self-regulate during moments of emotional upheaval; they tend to function better in social and academic settings.

  - Enhanced social understanding contributes to the oedipal child's dawning awareness of triadic relationships, and to the realization that he or she can be excluded from the connection between others. Feelings of jealousy and competition emerge.

- The mother-child bond remains essential to ongoing development. Mother-child dialogue, maternal empathy, and secure attachment facilitate the acquisition of narrative building, symbolic play, and theory of mind capacities and contribute to emotional self-regulation.

- As superego capacities are strengthened, the child is better able to regulate emotions and inhibit impulses in the absence of the parent. Guilty feelings and diminished self-esteem result from failure to adhere to behavioral ideals.

- Despite all of these advances, the thinking of the oedipal child is *preoperational*—that is, prelogical and concrete.

  - Young children tend to be overly influenced by a single, conspicuous element of complex problems or situations. Perceptual features, such as size, are given greater weight than are more subtle properties.

  - Such naïve cognition makes oedipal children vulnerable to simplistic theories about sexuality and reproduction, diminished self-esteem in relation to parental bodies and sexual apparatus, and concerns about talion forms of justice and bodily anxieties such as fears of castration.

REFERENCES

Abrams S: How child and adult analysis inform and misinform one another. Annual of Psychoanalysis 26:3–22, 1999

Alessandri SM: Play and social behavior in maltreated preschoolers. Dev Psychopathol 3:191–206, 1991

Auerbach JS, Blatt SJ: Self-representation in severe psychopathology: the role of reflexive self-awareness. Psychoanal Psychol 13:297–341, 1996

Bettelheim B: Oedipal conflicts and resolutions: the knight in shining armor and the damsel in distress, in The Uses of Enchantment: The Meaning and Importance of Fairy Tales. New York, Random House, 1975, pp 111–116

Birch M: In the land of counterpane: travels in the realm of play. Psychoanal Study Child 52:57–75, 1997

Blum HP: On the concept and consequence of the primal scene. Psychoanal Q 48:27–47, 1979

Bornstein MH, Haynes OM, O'Reilly AW, et al: Solitary and collaborative pretense play in early childhood: sources of individual variation in the development of representational competence. Child Dev 67:2910–2929, 1996

Cole PM, Tanz PZ, Hall SE, et al: Developmental changes in anger expression and attentional focus: learning to wait. Dev Psychol 47:1078–1089, 2011

Denham S, Blair K, De Mulder E, et al: Preschoolers' emotional competence: pathway to social competence? Child Dev 74:238–256, 2003

Donate-Bartfield E, Passman R: Relations between children's attachments to their mothers and to security blankets. J Fam Psychol 18:453–458, 2004

Fein GG: Pretend play in childhood: an integrated review. Child Dev 52:1095–1118, 1981

Fisher-Kern M, Buchheim A, Horz S, et al: The relationship between personal organization, reflective functioning and psychiatric classification in borderline personality disorder. Psychoanal Psychol 27:395–409, 2010

Fonagy P, Target M: Playing with reality, I: theory of mind and the normal development of psychic reality. Int J Psychoanal 77:217–233, 1996

Fonagy P, Target M: Attachment and reflective functioning: their role in self-organization. Dev Psychopathol 9:679–700, 1997

Fonagy P, Target M: Playing with reality, III: the persistence of dual psychic reality in borderline patients. Int J Psychoanal 81:853–874, 2000

Fraiberg SH: The Magic Years. New York, Fireside, 1996

Freud A: The concept of developmental lines. Psychoanal Study Child 18:245–265, 1963

Freud S: Three essays on the theory of sexuality (1905), in The Standard Edition of the Complete Psychological Works of Sigmund Freud, Vol 7. Translated and edited by Strachey J. London, Hogarth Press, 1962, pp 123–246

Freud S: Beyond the pleasure principle (1920), in The Standard Edition of the Complete Psychological Works of Sigmund Freud, Vol 18. Translated and edited by Strachey J. London, Hogarth Press, 1962, pp 1–64

Gergely G: Reapproaching Mahler: new perspectives on normal autism, symbiosis, splitting and libidinal object constancy from cognitive developmental theory. J Am Psychoanal Assoc 48:1197–1228, 2000

Gilmore K: Play in the psychoanalytic setting: ego capacity, ego state and vehicle for intersubjective exchange. Psychoanal Study Child 60:213–238, 2005

Gilmore K: Pretend play and development in early childhood (with implications for the oedipal phase). J Am Psychoanal Assoc 59:1157–1181, 2011

Ginot E: Self-narratives and dysregulated affective states: the neuropsychological links between self-narratives, attachment, affect and cognition. Psychoanal Psychol 29:59–80, 2012

Harris P, de Rosnay M, Pons F: Language and children's understanding of mental states. Curr Dir Psychol Sci 14:69–73, 2005

Hesse E, Main M: Disorganized infant, child and adult attachment: collapse of attentional system. J Am Psychoanal Assoc 48:1097–1127, 2000

Howe N, Petrakos H, Rinaldi C, et al: "This is a bad dog, you know...": constructing shared meanings during sibling pretend play. Child Dev 76:783–794, 2005

Knight R: Margo and me, II: the role of narrative building in child analytic technique. Psychoanal Study Child 58:133–164, 2003

Kochanska G: Beyond cognition: expanding the search for the early roots of internalization and conscience. Dev Psychol 30:20–22, 1994

Kochanska G, Murray KT, Harlan ET: Effortful control in early childhood: continuity and change, antecedents and implications for social development. Dev Psychol 36:220–232, 2000

Kochanska G, Coy K, Murray KT: The development of self-regulation in the first four years of life. Child Dev 72:1091–1111, 2001

Kochanska G, Koenig JL, Barry RA, et al: Children's conscience during toddler and preschool years, moral self, and a competent, adaptive developmental trajectory. Dev Psychol 46:1320–1332, 2010

Koenig A, Cicchetti D, Rogosch FA: Child compliance/non-compliance and maternal contributions to internalization in maltreated and non-maltreated dyads. Child Dev 71:1018–1032, 2000

Loewald HW: On the therapeutic action of psychoanalysis. Int J Psychoanal 41:16–33, 1960

Loewald HW: The waning of the oedipal complex. J Am Psychoanal Assoc 27:751–775, 1979

Loewald HW: Oedipal complex and development of self. Psychoanal Q 54:435–443, 1985

Lohmann H, Tomasello M: The role of language in the development of false belief understanding: a training study. Child Dev 74:1130–1144, 2003

Lyons-Ruth K: Play, precariousness and the negotiation of shared meaning: a developmental research perspective on child psychotherapy. J Infant Child Adolesc Psychother 5:142–149, 2006

Mahler M, Pine F, Bergman A: The Psychological Birth of the Human Infant: Symbiosis and Individuation. New York, Basic Books, 1975

Mahon E: The "dissolution" of the Oedipus complex: a neglected cognitive factor. Psychoanal Q 60:628–634, 1991

Marans S, Mayes L, Cicchetti D, et al: The child-psychoanalytic play interview: a technique for studying thematic content. J Am Psychoanal Assoc 39:1015–1036, 1991

Mayes LC, Cohen DJ: The development of a capacity for imagination in early childhood. Psychoanal Study Child 47:23–47, 1992

Mayes LC, Cohen DJ: Children's development of theory of mind. J Am Psychoanal Assoc 44:117–142, 1996

McCune LA: A normative study of representational play at the transition to language. Dev Psychol 31:198–206, 1995

Migden S: Dyslexia and self-control: an ego psychoanalytic perspective. Psychoanal Study Child 53:282–299, 1998

Nelson K: Emergence of the historical self, in Language in Cognitive Development: The Emergence of the Mediated Mind. New York, Cambridge University Press, 1996, pp 152–182

Passman RH: Attachment to inanimate objects: are children who have security blankets insecure? J Consulting Clin Psychol 55:825–830, 1987

Piaget J: The Language and Thought of the Child. New York, Harcourt Press, 1926

Piaget J: Play, Dreams and Imitation in Childhood. New York, Norton, 1962

Piaget J, Inhelder B: The Psychology of the Child. New York, Basic Books, 1969

Roby AC, Kidd E: The referential communication skills of children with imaginary companions. Dev Sci 11:531–540, 2008

Ruffman T, Slade L, Crowe E: The relationship between children's and mother's mental state language and theory of mind understanding. Child Dev 73:734–751, 2002

Senet NV: A study of preschool children's linking of genitals and gender. Psychoanal Q 73:291–334, 2004

Shatz M, Gelman R: The development of communication skills: modifications in the speech of young children as a function of the listener. Monogr Soc Res Child Dev 38:1–37, 1973

Slade A: A longitudinal study of maternal involvement and symbolic play during the toddler period. Child Dev 58:367–375, 1987

Solnit A: A psychoanalytic view of play. Psychoanal Study Child 42:205–219, 1987

Target M, Fonagy P: Playing with reality, II: the development of psychic reality from a theoretical perspective. Int J Psychoanal 77:459–479, 1996

Taylor M, Carlson SM, Maring BL, et al: The characteristics and correlates of fantasy in school-aged children: imaginary companions, impersonation and social understanding. Dev Psychol 40:1173–1187, 2004

Taylor M, Hulette AC, Dishion TJ: Longitudinal outcomes of young high-risk adolescents with imaginary companions. Dev Psychol 46:1632–1636, 2010

Trionfi G, Reese G: A good story: children with imaginary companions create richer narratives. Child Dev 80:1301–1313, 2009

Tyson P, Tyson RL: Narcissism and superego development. J Am Psychoanal Assoc 32:75–98, 1984

Vaish A, Carpenter M, Tomasello M: Young children's responses to guilt displays. Dev Psychol 47:1248–1262, 2011

Vygotsky LS: Thought and Language. Cambridge, MA, MIT Press, 1962

Vygotsky LS: Mind in Society: The Development of Higher Psychological Processes. Cambridge, MA, Harvard University Press, 1978

Wellman H, Cross D, Watson J: Meta-analysis of theory of mind development: the truth about false belief. Child Dev 72:655–684, 2001

Winnicott DW: Transitional objects and transitional phenomena: study of the first not-me possession. Int J Psychoanal 34:89–97, 1953

Winnicott DW: The capacity to be alone. Int J Psychoanal 39:411–420, 1958

Winsler A, De Leon JR, Wallace BA, et al: Private speech in preschool children: developmental stability and change, across-task consistency, and relations with classroom behavior. J Child Lang 30:583–608, 2003

Woolley J, Wellman H: Origin and truth: young children's understanding of imaginative mental representations. Child Dev 64:1–17, 1993

Yanof JA: Barbie and the tree of life: the multiple functions of gender in development. J Am Psychoanal Assoc 48:1439–1465, 2000

CHAPTER 5

The Oedipal Phase

Psychosexual Development,
Oedipal Complex and Constellation,
and Oedipal Phase Contributions to Mental Life

In this chapter, we focus in greater detail on the mental contents and conflicts of the oedipal phase. The advances in mental capacities outlined in Chapter 4, "The Oedipal Phase and Emerging Capacities," interface with, support, and augment the greatly increased complexity of mental life that characterizes the oedipal-age child. As noted earlier, the new developmental capacities allow the child to pursue researches and take in new information; to think and imagine, verbalize and pretend; to perceive and experience relationships; and to identify and name a hugely expanded repertoire of feelings. Children's naïve theories and interpretations in regard to the fundamental questions that now preoccupy them are incorporated into mental life and remain as central organizing fantasies throughout development (Erreich 2003).

Since the introduction of the concept, the oedipal complex has been viewed as foundational for human development; the triangular configuration represents the confluence of the child's growing capacity to experience nuanced, complicated emotions and to advance in object relations from dependency to love, desire, and rivalry. Moreover, it is accompanied by the last major addition to mental structure, the *superego*. The shift from dyadic to triadic relationships is profoundly significant for the development of object relations, as the child begins to recognize contenders for the mother's love, including the father and siblings. Intense possessiveness, jealousy, and painful feelings of exclusion, fluctuating fluidly from the focus on mother to

105

father and then to their relationship with each other, accompany the child's dawning realization that he or she is not entitled to be number one; this is associated with aggressive fantasies and urges aimed at doing away with the interloper. The fact that this third person is also loved or at least regarded as family creates conflict; introduces the emotions of ambivalence, guilt, and remorse; and presses toward utilization of the new defense of *repression* to push the entire reticulum of passionate feelings out of awareness. These events pave the way for the gradual shift toward *identification with the rival*. This entire process creates a template for intimate relationships, the *oedipal constellation* (Shapiro 1977).

Despite having detractors and undergoing many contemporary revisions, such as the relational perspective (Seligman 2003), the oedipal complex and the developmental phase in which it blossoms is considered a singular moment in development, with unique importance for future personality, for the content of (primarily unconscious) mental life, and for the outbreak of (nonpsychotic) mental illness (Elise 1998; Tucker 2008). After sketching the history of this idea, we explore current perspectives on central psychosexual-emotional-relational concerns of this age group and their role in subsequent personality development.

The Oedipal Complex in Freud's Theory

The oedipal complex was discovered by Sigmund Freud, in the year following his father's death, through self-reflection and his new technique of dream interpretation; these analytic tools allowed him to reconstruct his passionate childhood love for his mother and murderous competition with his father from derivatives of unconscious fantasy and dreams (Makari 2008). Freud recognized that the themes were embodied in Sophocles' retelling of the Oedipus myth, and he suggested that such intrafamilial tensions are universal in human development and form the basis for adult neurosis.

The oedipal complex is linked to some fundamental ideas that remained part of Freud's thinking throughout his intellectual evolution: 1) the notion of a *universal bisexual disposition,* based on the fantasy of being both male and female that permits love, desire for, and identification with both sexes (Heenen-Wolff 2011); 2) his binary dimensions of *masculine/feminine,* corresponding to *active/passive;* and 3) his first developmental theory of *psychosexual stages* (Freud 1905/1962). These notions informed his ideas concerning the oedipal experience and the differences in male and female development. Infantile bisexuality is gradually shaped and constrained into preference for one sex over the other, but the bisexual core ensures the dual nature of the oedipal complex. The coalescence of masculinity with activity and femininity with passivity is not absolute (Freud 1915/1962), because this bisexual core is more or less accessible throughout life; a combination of activity and passivity in both sexes is typical. Nonetheless, subsequent masculine and feminine elements in development tend to be identified in this way (Gediman 2005).

In regard to psychosexual development, the biological progression of bodily erotogenic zones, wherein pleasure and excitement are focused sequentially on the *oral, anal,* and *phallic* areas, organizes key aspects of mental development and human relatedness up to the oedipal phase. *Developmental anxieties* follow a roughly corresponding sequence: fear of loss of the object, fear of loss of love of the object, and fear of bodily injury with special focus on the genital, and finally fear of the superego, which is internalized at the resolution of the oedipal conflict. Because Freud saw the development of the boy and girl up to the phallic stage as identical and libido as active and therefore masculine, *castration anxiety* applied to both sexes. He felt that the vagina was unknown and thus the girl could only compare her clitoris to the boy's more impressive organ and feel that castration had already happened. Even in his lifetime, Freud's ideas about the developmental differentiation of boys and girls were challenged by some of his followers, especially Karen Horney (see section "Contemporary Views of the Oedipal Complex and Its Variations" later in this chapter), and today they are viewed as limited by the phallocentric cultural zeitgeist of his day.

Freud implicitly recognized the cognitive advances of the oedipal child by his observations of accelerated curiosity in this period, developing in concert with the interest in and excitement about genitals and genital differences. By the time the child is 3 years old, his or her questions and sexual researches begin to focus on fundamental mysteries with sustained reverberations on self-experience as gendered; these include the difference between the sexes, the difference between the generations in terms of size and bodily functions, the way babies are made and born, and the secrets of parental intimate relations. Children's dawning insights, inevitably colored by immature cognition, are all pivotal in the unfolding of oedipal fantasy. Naïve theories abound regarding the anatomical differences between boys and girls and the imagined possibility of loss of a highly valued organ; the nature of parental coitus and its links to excitement, pregnancy, and birth; and the narcissistically mortifying reality that adult prerogatives must be consigned to the future.

In the original formulation of male development, Freud asserted that the boy's primary love for his mother transforms from dependency into incestuous desire. The new focus on the genitals as a source of pleasure, phallic pride, and inevitable anxiety about loss accompanies his longings. Simultaneously, the boy recognizes a rival in his imposing father, whose size and authority are further evidence of the boy's own insignificance; he struggles with intense hostility and murderous feelings. Consistent with the greater emotional complexity that emerges during this time, rivalrous feelings coexist with love and admiration for his father; thus, the boy must grapple with his first deep experience of *ambivalence*. In Freud's original theory, the intense valuation of the penis and the fear of bodily injury (i.e., *castration*, which referred primarily to loss of the penis) play a key role in the resolution of this familial force field for the boy. Genital masturbation leads to castration threats (the boy "knows" that this is "possible" because he has just recently realized the penis-less state of the girl), and he renounces his designs on his mother in order to ward off his anxiety. He accepts the promise of future gratification with a woman of his own generation "when he grows up" and moves toward a closer identification with his father as his model of masculinity and the representation of the *reality principle* (in contrast to the *pleasure principle*). The prohibitions around oedipal desire form the kernel of the superego.

The oedipal complex for the girl was understood to be roughly comparable, with an important distinction as to etiological sequence. Freud maintained that the girl is unaware of her own genitals until the oedipal phase; he posited that the revelations accompanying her explorations and researches are devastating realizations of her comparatively inadequate genital equipment, creating the female castration complex, which in turn ushers in the oedipal complex and sets it in motion. According to this early theory, when the girl observes that the boy has something she does not have, namely a penis, she is bitterly disappointed. She experiences *penis envy* and resentment of the mother, who not only did not properly endow her daughter but also seems to prefer someone who possesses what the little girl lacks. In defeat, the girl turns to the father with hopes of obtaining a penis, but eventually renounces this ungratified wish in favor of a wish for a baby. She forgoes her masculine interest in activity and assumes a passive role. Because the girl already feels punished by virtue of not having a penis, she has no motivation to internalize parental prohibitions. She is therefore possessed of a weaker and less objective superego (Freud 1925/1962). However, some identification with the same-sex parent for girls, similar to that for boys, provides the basis for conscience.

The oedipal complex denotes the end to infantile omnipotence as both boys and girls experience intense narcissistic mortification by either observing or imagining the parental couple's intimacy (*the primal scene*) and feeling entirely excluded and insignificant. By virtue of its relative incomprehensibility to the mind of the child, the primal scene also gives rise to sadomasochistic theories of sexual intercourse. The intense feelings stirred up by the triangle, in which the formerly gratified baby finds himself or herself unimportant, unwelcome, and unwanted, is the impetus for revenge motives that can dominate the personality (Arlow 1980). Both boys and girls have castration complexes—the boy fears castration, and the girl feels it has already happened; for the boy, this leads to the demolition of the oedipal complex, whereas for the girl, this feeling marks the entry into the oedipal complex as she turns away in disappointment from her primary love object, the mother, to the father (Freud 1925/1962).

Consistent with the supposition of universal bisexuality, Freud observed that both boys and girls also have *negative oedipal complexes.* Freud suggested that boys can desire their fathers and view their mothers as rivals, and girls can do likewise with their mothers, eschewing interest in their fathers. These vectors of desire and rivalry and of activity and passivity add to the intensity of feelings stirred up in the hotbed of family life for the oedipal child. In the 2–3 years of the child's passage through the oedipal phase, the complex must be "resolved" by repression of forbidden desires and conflictual emotions and the establishment of the superego; many classical thinkers theorize that while the positive oedipal complex gives rise to the superego, the negative oedipal complex, with its overvaluation of the same-sex parent, is resolved into the *ego ideal.* This latter term, referring to a component of the superego, is inconsistently used in psychodynamic literature, including in Freud's writings. It sometimes refers to an impersonal moral barometer (Milrod 1982) but more often to a narcissistic ideal self-image (also known as the *wished-for self-image,* as discussed in Chapter 3, "The Toddler") based on a grandiose fantasy of same-sex parent (Blos 1974). We take the position that these two perspectives both apply; the internalized exalted representation of the self is most often the amalgam of both narcissistic and moral ideals. Thus, the intrapsychic events associated with repression of the oedipal complex introduce the last developmental structural changes in the mental life (the addition of the superego and ego ideal) and bring about the sexually quiescent stage of *latency.*

This early formulation underwent considerable modification and criticism in the evolution of psychodynamic development thinking over the last century. As we demonstrate in the remainder of this chapter, we continue to find the oedipal complex an illuminating insight about this crucial watershed in human development (Altman 1997; Gilmore 2011) but we subscribe to a modified version of its nature and appearance.

Freud's Original Formulation of the Oedipus Complex

- When a child is between 3 and 6 years of age, the genitals become the focus of interest and excitement following psychosexual progression through the oral, anal, and phallic stages.

- Sexual research leads to questions about the difference between the sexes and where babies come from; this results in genital anxieties (i.e., castration anxiety) as the child concretely observes that boys have something girls lack and girls fear the safety and integrity of their genitals.

- Triadic relationships emerge as the child becomes interested in and desirous of the opposite-sex parent and rivalrous with the same-sex parent (positive oedipal constellation). Primal-scene fantasies, narcissistic mortification, and revenge fantasies are woven into the child's imagination regarding intimate parental activity.

- Because of universal bisexuality, the negative oedipal complex emerges simultaneously. This is the inverse of the positive: the boy desires the father and the girl the mother.

- The oedipal complex "dissolves" under the threat of castration (or the conviction thereof in the girl) when the child renounces desire and accepts the promise of future gratification, yielding to generational and gender differences.

- The child identifies with the parent of the same sex and internalizes the prohibiting parental voice to form the superego.

Contemporary Views of the Oedipal Complex and Its Variations

Contemporary revisions of Freud's original formulation have been extensive. In this section, we elaborate a modern view of the developmental conflicts and anxieties of this important phase. Although we strongly endorse the idea that the maturation and interaction of multiple systems of development are responsible for the emergence of the oedipal complex and the characteristic features of the oedipal-age child, we continue to use the traditional terminology as a meaningful shorthand for this momentous developmental period. Moreover, although we reject the notion of a "normal" prescriptive passage through oedipal conflicts (Auchincloss and Vaughan 2001; Chodorow 1994), we do see this phase as a turning point in the nature and organization of mental life: the intensity of emotional and physical feelings, the new relevance of gender and the specifically sexed body, the shift in cognitive capacities, the establishment of complex, nuanced relationships in which others are ultimately recognized as separate subjectivities, and finally, an exploding capacity to represent all of these developments in symbolic forms—language and play (Gilmore 2011). These transformations bring the child into the "moral order" of humanity (Loewald 1985, p. 437) in a profound and significant developmental moment. From the vantage point of the child, these developmental issues—the body and its sensations, the intrafamilial rivalries and passionate desires, the powerful feelings of loss associated with the simultaneous end of babyhood and the recognition of smallness, and the requisite delay of gratification—all infuse daily experience, while not eclipsing the importance of ongoing concerns about attachment security and other fundamental needs.

The relationship of this drama to the experience of one's body (one's *biological sex*), the construction of personal meanings of masculine and feminine (*gender*), and the directions of sexual orientation (*sexuality*) are seen differently today than when the concept of the oedipal complex was introduced over a century ago. The general consensus among psychodynamic theorists is that there are a variety of determinants of sexual identity, gender, and orientation whose etiologies are not fully understood. The range of developmental outcomes and the unique individuality of sexuality underscore that any notions of "normalcy" are largely cultural. This is becoming increasingly apparent in contemporary Western society, where the traditional family paradigm in which the Oedipus is embedded is undergoing radical transformation. As conventional domestic arrangements decline, the intrafamilial force field in which the oedipal conflict is played out is splintering into a multiplicity of variants. How this affects mental development is only recently being considered from a psychodynamically informed developmental viewpoint (Seligman 2003). Circumstances such as single-sex parents, single parents, blended families, technological advances that delink conception and sexuality, surrogate mothers, donor eggs, and the like undoubtedly alter the unfolding oedipal drama. The repercussions on mental development are the challenge of thinkers in the twenty-first century (Seligman 2007). Therefore, even though there is little in-depth examination of these issues as yet (Heenen-Wolff 2011), it is possible to develop hypotheses or simply identify specific facets of the oedipal experience that may be affected, such as the link between the primal scene and fantasies about conception.

Clarification of Terms

Although the terms *oedipal complex, oedipal constellation,* and *oedipal configuration* are not used with complete consistency among psychodynamic thinkers, they are generally employed in the following ways: *Oedipal complex* usually refers to the network of feelings, fantasies, and relationships that emerge during the oedipal phase. The term is used popularly to refer to evidence of these in children and adults alike, as in Maureen Dowd's (2012) *New York Times* op-ed piece "Oedipus Rex Complex," referring to the generational struggles between fathers and sons in American politics. As noted, duality was very much part of the original theory, and the complex and its positive and negative manifestations are considered universal. The *oedipal constellation* is the residual "core fantasy" (Laufer 1978), "central fixation point" (Tolpin 1970), or "psychic organizer of mental life" (Auchincloss and Samberg 2012)) that remains as the child moves forward in development. *Oedipal configuration* refers to the idiosyncratic variations that inevitably occur in human development and therefore takes into account the specific nature of the child's circumstances and predominant mode of experience. Thus, *oedipal configuration* may signify the ascendance of the negative or positive oedipal complex in mental life for a given individual, but more frequently refers to the specific aspects of the situation such as birth order, divorce, parental death, adoption, blended families, and so on.

Some writers suggest that these terms refer not only to the child's feelings and fantasies but to the parents' as well. The implication is that this phase encompasses a broader dynamic in the family than the intrapsychic experience of the child alone (see Ross 1982 for a description of the reciprocal Laius complex). References to the individual's Oedipus complex would then include aspects of the parent's mental lives that are communicated to the child, such as preferences of one over others or over the spouse, the parent's own oedipal conflicts, or the parent's use of the child to substitute for the parent's own oedipal objects. This introduces an intergenerational component to oedipal conflicts.

Such variations illuminate the vast diversity in a complex that nonetheless seems recognizable from individual to individual. In nonlinear systems theory, it may thus be more accurate to consider the oedipal complex as a *strange attractor state,* characterized by two important features: 1) these states have predictable overall forms, even though made up of unpredictable details, and 2) the strange attractor appears to be a product of its own evolving system but simultaneously organizes that system (Scharff 2000).

Contemporary Views of Sex Differences, Gender Identity, and Genital Anxieties

Children between ages 2 and 3 years are usually very clear about their sex (by which we refer to biological sex) and can offer very simple notions of gender role (the idiosyncratic notions of masculine and feminine as they are defined culturally) as these have been communicated implicitly and explicitly in their families; if asked, very young children know their own and other people's sex most of the time. This knowledge is the bedrock of primary feelings about oneself as boy or girl (Elise 1997) and is inevitably composed of the experience of the body and its immediate interface with the environmental response to it. It forms the foundation for evolving notions of masculine and feminine, which are densely determined. Very young children have, from the moment of sex assignment, fledging notions of what it means to be a boy or a girl as defined by their cultural milieu and developing mental lives. In addition, they are well aware of their own genital sensations. However, they do not yet understand the fixed correspondence of genital and biological sex and have not yet linked genital sensations to the categorization of boy and girl. Their notions of what it means to be male or female—that is, their notions of masculinity and femininity—are largely created by the dynamic interplay of early maternal responses to sameness or difference, parental attitudes that further differentiate these gender concepts, the ways they are dressed and responded to, and their own observations of men and women. These influences well precede any demonstrable understanding of the crucial genital difference. For example, maternal attitudes toward aggression vary significantly with the gender of their child (Alink et al. 2006) and clearly contribute to boy-girl differences in expression of aggression. However, all of these messages, influences, and sensations do not create the link between sex, gender identity, and anatomy until children achieve a certain level of cognitive maturity.

Children's understanding of the connection between their sex and their genitals consolidates as they approach age 36 months. This observation has been demonstrated in a simple study in which children were asked to identify which anatomically correct doll was like themselves and then a little later asked to distinguish the boy and girl dolls and explain on what basis they did so (de Marneffe 1997). The coalescence of the idea that the genitals are decisive in determining one's sex is reliable only at age 36 months and beyond. This timing has great import for the oedipal phase because it confirms that the genitals takes on their importance as a marker of difference late in the ongoing childhood process of knowing one's sex. And in fact, *gender constancy*—that is, the comprehension that one's sex is unchangeable—is not achieved until the close of the oedipal phase (Egan and Perry 2001).

Both de Marneffe's (1997) research and a subsequent study by Senet (2004) show that although there is certainly interest in genital differences as children become aware of them, there is little evidence that the girl is irretrievably crestfallen because she has no penis, as in Freud's original phallocentric theory. Although both boys and girls are given the word *penis,* they are not typically provided the proper language for the complicated and partly internal female genitalia. Certainly, a girl may complain, upon visualizing a boy's naked body, that he has something she lacks; this is determined by the child's immature cognition wherein a penis seems more impressive than a multipart organ that is difficult to visualize, lacks a clear name, or is named only for its interior component (i.e., the vagina) (Lerner 1976). Similarly, upon observing the genital difference, boys may fear that a precious body part could be lost. Some thinkers believe that such an exposure is universally traumatic for the boy (Lewes 2009). Nonetheless, the growing awareness of difference does not lead to denial or avoidance of the appropriate identification of one's own sex. Senet's (2004) study, which examined the link in young children's minds between their sex and anatomy, shows that although 3- and 4-year-olds have no trouble recognizing anatomically correct dolls as boys or girls and even creating them when pressed to do so, if they are given the opportunity to construct their own dolls, they create figures with genitals of both sexes simultaneously, "revealing a free flow of play with ideas, wishes, fears" (p. 310). As noted, full gender constancy, the conviction of the permanence of anatomical sex, is not reliably present until age 6 or 7 years (Egan and Perry 2001). Boys and girls both "know" what sex they are because, from the moment it is ceremoniously announced at birth ("It's a girl!" or "It's a boy!"), it is relentlessly reinforced by culture. Girls and boys both have pleasurable genital sensations from early infancy that become incorporated into a specifically sexed and gendered self-representation. However, despite these demonstrable behaviors, they continue to imagine, when given the freedom to do so, that there need not be a committed choice for some time.

Developmental genital anxieties specific to girls have been extensively addressed in more recent literature, but even from early in the history of the field, Horney (1933) insisted that the girl has genital awareness, sensations, and desires for penetration; she suggested that an expressed preference to be a boy is more likely a defense against the anxiety engendered by *penetration fantasies*. Especially since the 1970s, discourse about both male and female genital anxieties and the impact of bodily anxieties on the mind and representations of gender have been a crucial part of psychodynamic theorizing. In 1976, Stoller made the important point, obvious to any child observer, that little girls, well before the oedipal phase, are possessed of a sense of "primary femininity" (Stoller 1976); this confident sense of being a girl is rooted in communications that begin at the moment the baby's sex is known, supported by the effect of circulating hormones and the innumerable identifications and imitations in which she engages, in the context of the culturally determined conditioning influences that accrue around her. Her feminine identity is clearly evident in her color and clothing choices, her physicality, and her play in the second year of life. Her recognition of difference from the boy emerges as her awareness of the gender-genital link consolidates. Following Stoller's idea, Mayer (1995) suggested that girls have two lines of affect-defense configurations that characterize their evolving gender identity:

primary femininity and *phallic castration anxiety.* Anxieties related to the former are dangers to the genitals the girl possesses, whereas phallic castration anxiety concerns her belief that her genitals are a damaged version of what boys have.

As little boys and girls recognize genital differences, they struggle to make sense of them, and their conclusions *can* result in feelings of inferiority and fear or anxiety. Although feelings of envy and loss may be present in girls, these are not their core gender representation. Boys worry about the safety of their valued penises; they identify with larger-than-life masculine figures (such as superheroes) and gradually distance themselves from girls over the course of childhood as counterphobic attempts to differentiate and regulate their anxieties (Harris 2008). Moreover, boys and girls alike are awed by and envious of adult roles and sexual characteristics (large penises, breasts, pregnant bellies, beards, etc.) and grapple with their interest in the genitals they have (Mayer 1995), their range of different worries about them (Bell 1961; Bernstein 1990; Lewes 2009), and their recognition of them as a source of excitement and pleasure.

The term *gender role identity* refers to the self-representation as a gendered person, consolidated during this phase; this is an amalgam of multiple sources of input, such as the body, parental views, sibling cohort, and cultural surround, and includes the specific anxieties related to genitals. As children grasp the real anatomical distinction between the sexes and consider the permanence of their categorization, already extant notions of themselves as gendered cohere and become solidly integrated with bodily sensation and identifications in the matrix of conscious and unconscious communications from and interactions with the important others in their environment. The little boy who, of course, knew he was a boy all along because he was so named and responded to since birth, draws together all of the impressions and meanings associated with "boyness," plus the attitudes and interactions of parents and siblings vis-à-vis his and their own sex, and constructs a gendered identity, a dynamic assembly that transforms over the course of development (Harris 2008). If there are discordant elements and he chafes, in terms of his self-experience and/or bodily sensations, against his own expectations and those he interprets as arising from others, he struggles to feel himself to be simultaneously a "proper boy" and his own unique self. Similarly, the little girl assembles a complex experience of her femininity, with its origins in the early influences of body and environment. Although every child's construction is a unique representation that evolves and transforms, it is also recognizable, at least superficially, as similar to that of other boys and girls in the same cultural milieu; children who visibly deviate from expectation may be diagnosed as having a *gender identity disor-*

der, called *gender dysphoria* in DSM-5 (American Psychiatric Association 2013), depending on onset and severity. As development unfolds, gender is a highly fluid aspect of self-representation that is revised and reissued with developmental change, at times more or less affected by parents, peer group, media, social norms, and so on.

The potential impact of technological innovations in regard to conception is as yet uncharted territory. With the loosening of the link between sexual intercourse and reproduction, the watershed moment where genital differences, biological sex, sexuality, and reproduction converge is unquestionably affected. From time immemorial, children have denied their parents' sexual relationship, because it excites, frightens, confuses, and excludes them. Coming to terms with its central role in their conception has been assumed to be part of the oedipal crisis. For children whose parents' sexuality has no direct link to their birth or the birth of their siblings, the mysteries of sexual intimacy and how babies are born are, from the vantage point of current social norms, bewilderingly separated. Moreover, the typical consolations understood to mollify the oedipal child's wounded narcissism (e.g., "You will grow up and make a baby with your husband/wife someday") have decidedly less relevance, at least at the bodily level, because there may be very different models available for adult love, sex, pairing, and reproduction. How this will change as increasing numbers of children are conceived differently remains to be seen.

Sex, Gender, Core Gender Identity, and Gender Role Identity

- *Sex* refers to biological sex, male and female; it is assigned at birth, based on perception of the genitalia, and sets in motion an array of environmental responses.

- *Core gender identity* is the conviction of belonging to the sex assigned at birth (or a different one), which becomes linked to anatomy by age 36 months and consolidates as a fixed feature of the self. Despite its establishment and the (usual) connection to a specific genital, some fluidity about the body persists in imagination into latency.

- *Gender* incorporates the constructed idiosyncratic meanings associated with each sex, masculinity and femininity. These are strongly determined by culture, but also psychologically influenced and unique in each individual despite shared features.

- *Gender role identity* incorporates core gender identity but is a dynamic evolving notion of how one measures up as a masculine or feminine person. It is shaped by the body, socialization, mental life, sexual fantasy, and so on; it is changeable over time. It reflects the subjective relationship to the concept of gender.

Contemporary View of Siblings and the Oedipal Complex

The prevalent downplaying of the role of the sibling in human development has received attention among researchers from a range of disciplines. Some have suggested that this remarkable oversight reflects a degree of denial in regard to the powerful emotions that are contained in that relationship and its derivatives in adult life, such as civil wars and tribal warfare. For example, an entry in the *Cambridge Dictionary of Sociology* notes that the "quality and nature of siblings' relationships with each other is not identified as having socially significant consequences" and that siblings are only noticeable in problematic circumstances (Turner 2006, p. 550). This neglect has been described within child developmental research (Kolak and Volling 2011) and in psychodynamic theory, despite the fact that siblings have always occupied considerable attention in the clinical situation (Jalongo and Dragich 2008; Mitchell 2011), in popular texts (Bank and Kahn 2003; Kluger 2011), in literature ranging from the Bible to J.D. Salinger's *The Catcher in the Rye*, and in other media. In recent decades, there have been efforts to redress this curious blind spot in regard to a highly influential yet underresearched and undertheorized arena of childhood experience.

Sibling relationships and their impact on individual psychology and adaptation are now studied more extensively, and a developmental progression in their evolution over childhood has been proposed (Sharpe and Rosenblatt 1994). Considerable data support both the positive impact of siblings—for example, on prosocial behaviors (Jalongo and Dragich 2008; Pike et al. 2005), the process of separation-individuation (Leichtman 1985), and development of theory of mind (Dunn et al. 1996; Fagan and Najman 2003; Hardy 2001; Ostrov et al. 2006). During the oedipal phase, the amount of time spent in interactions, expressions of emotion, and imaginary play with siblings far exceeds time spent with mothers (Dunn et al. 1996). Several psychodynamic contributors have suggested that the evolving complexity of the relationship to siblings, the uninhibited emotions it invokes, and the inevitable rivalry for the mother's love may be the earliest form of triangular relations, preceding the triad of mother, father, and child.

In fact, Juliet Mitchell (2003, 2011), a psychoanalytic scholar, proposes "sibling trauma" as a universal experience occurring in the second year of life. She uses the term *trauma* to capture the shock-like and ubiquitous recognition that one can be usurped by another much like the self (Mitchell 2003). The birth of a sibling within the family, the realization that siblings already exist and can fully occupy the mother to the exclusion of the self, or simply the awareness of pregnancies and babies born somewhere within the family orbit (e.g., the extended family, family friends, the preschool environment) are concrete and common examples. However, it is the universal "dawning awareness" of the existence of others much like the self that brings on the "crisis of nonuniqueness" (Vivona 2007, p. 1193). The realization that one is not "His majesty the baby" (Freud 1914/1962) (or in other words, the supreme and only baby) is a harsh one, radically altering the infantile grandiose self.

In past theorizing, this so-called *lateral dimension* was often understood as a deflection of attention from the parents, but there is plenty of evidence that siblings occupy much of the oedipal child's time and attention, carry considerable developmental weight, and foment intense emotions of love and hate because, in the mind of the child, they are "equals" (Sharpe and Rosenblatt 1994; Vivona 2007) and are not entitled to preferential treatment. Because this awareness predates the evolving capacity to experience nuanced emotions, the hostility can prove to be alarming, certainly to parents. Although the ongoing role of the sibling in the development of mentalization and reciprocity is well documented (Jalongo and Dragich 2008), the early experience of the sibling poses a challenge for the very young child who as yet lacks the mental capacity to comprehend and appreciate others' subjectivities. The observation of the mother in an intimate relation to a sibling—such as nursing (Kumar 2009), bathing, or cozily reading a book in bed—is a forecast of the primal scene and can only mean exclusion to the child who has not mastered patience and who does not fully grasp the idea of "sharing," "having a playmate," "being all loved the same but differently," and other routine consolations. The various family configurations and birth order all have impact on the unfolding family drama as the oedipal complex begins to take shape. Moreover, in regard to the elaborated sense of self that emerges from this matrix, the role of *differentiation* from similar others may play a part comparable to identifications with the parent (Vivona 2007). The need to distinguish oneself from the pack can result in the hypertrophy of aspects of personality that differentiate the child from siblings and the extended group of other children, all of whom can stand in for siblings. In addition, it can contribute to the need to polarize within sibling cohorts or in the larger family system, constraining development to conform to expectation (as in "Jamie is the smart one, and Sophie is the creative one") (Sharpe and Rosenblatt 1994).

The following vignette describes the reactions of an older child when faced with the birth of a sibling.

> Jimmy was 30 months old when his brother Chris was born. A previously exuberant boy who was an ardent student of trucks and loved his own little toy vehicles, Jimmy was also "in love" with his mother and delighted in pointing out and explaining all the trucks in the neighborhood and doing "tricks" on his scooter. He responded to Chris's arrival with a kind of disconsolate dis-

engagement and could find nothing that interested him. He circled his mother and the nursing baby and cried, especially when admonished to keep a certain distance. His attitude toward Chris was to ignore him as much as possible. But he demanded his mother's attention more and objected to his father's "rights" to her, uncharacteristically entering the parents' bedroom at night. On several occasions, he threw toys when he observed his parents practicing their ballroom dancing. He became much more controlling of the entire family, making everyone wait while he procrastinated. As he developed a passion for baseball at age 5 years, he and his father bonded and he became "Daddy's little boy." He adamantly excluded Chris from this interest, and indeed throughout early and middle childhood was not invested in their developing a playing relationship. He said Chris was babyish and "dumb."

The experience of siblings has infinite variations. Rather than the already multifaceted oedipal complex emerging as a "single planetary" organization in relation to the parents, it is a "miniature universe" of great complexity (Graham 1988, p. 91) as the multiplicity of triangulations unfolds in a given family. Especially today, when family structure is increasingly complicated, this universe can feel byzantine and baffling to young children. For example, multiple births, blended families, adopted and foster children, and surrogate mothers can confound children trying to understand how these "others" arrived, what determines when and why they come and go, and what they mean to the parents. Twins pose special problems for parents because their close and intense access to shared experience and special communication can exclude parents and make them seem superfluous (Bank and Kahn 2003). Twins and especially triplets and higher-order multiple births linked to assisted reproductive technology (Cook et al. 2011) complicate the struggle for individual identity and the tendency to substitute siblings as objects of desire. Siblings who are disabled, siblings who die in infancy or childhood, and siblings who are previously deceased are other complications of the lateral dimension, because these particular contexts heighten aggressive fantasies, guilty feelings, and the defenses against them, such as precocious maturity, massive inhibition of aggression, and parentification. All of these circumstances contribute to the pressure to differentiate or identify. Thus, siblings can be seen as universal contributors to an individual's oedipal configuration, by virtue of their presence, absence, and special features.

Variations in Oedipal Configuration Related to Divorce, Death, and Alternate Forms of Parenting

Divorce, a common reality in contemporary Western society, is often coincident with early childhood and can alter the unfolding of the oedipal phase and subsequent development (Wallerstein and Resnikoff 1997). While statistics concerning age of children at divorce are difficult to come by, a 2005 survey in the Netherlands reported that 19% of divorces affect children ages 0–4 (CBS Statistics Netherlands 2012). Children's adaptation to divorce depends on many factors, but the reality that, in the United States, 50% of marriages end in divorce and a high percentage of divorced parents remarry suggests that offspring must manage a more complex developmental trajectory than those in intact families (Ahrons 2007; Kleinsorge and Covitz 2012). Protracted custodial disputes, exposure to parental acrimony, subsequent remarriages, and blended families are ongoing sources of new and changing demands for adaptation. Not only does the familial landscape shift and change, but the meanings of each change are rewritten in the child's mind with each developmental epoch. As a consequence, such changes lend themselves to misinterpretation, confusion, and misattribution.

Divorce early in a child's life is correlated with future difficulties in adaptation, according to broad epidemiological surveys (Leon 2003). Many variables contribute to the impact of divorce on oedipal dynamics, including the child's age at the point of separation, the ongoing role of each parent in the child's life, the degree of hostility and aggression expressed in the household before, during, and after divorce, and the subsequent timing of remarriages.

Inevitably, the specific effect of divorce on the oedipal complex is highly individualized, but some overriding themes are generalizable. Parental dissension and separation are meaningful disruptions in the daily life of children ages 3–6 years, who rely on predictable routines for their sense of safety. Contact with both parents, however lopsided, is part of the rhythm of their experience. Significantly altered financial and living circumstances may not be fully grasped, but changes in these are noted and interpreted according to the child's cognitive capacity.

Parents' attitudes toward the children are complicated by marital failure; some parents struggle with wishes to obliterate the whole enterprise and the child with it. Parents can also come to depend on the child to manage their loneliness and depression (Wallerstein and Resnikoff 1997). Most importantly for the current discussion, the child's management of oedipal feelings is altered by the actual rupture in the parental unit, which can produce a heightened experience of oedipal triumph or failure, distorted views of parental power and privilege, and interference in the internalization of prohibitions. Self-regulation and the management of impulses in these circumstances are often not supported by parental example or support, thus leaving children to manage these developmental challenges at a very young age. Moreover, a parent who feels jilted, wounded, or overwhelmed can often turn to the child, even a very young one, for comfort, deforming the nature of the generational hierarchy by casting the child in a parental or spousal role. Equally problematic is the pressure to assume contradictory and polarizing positions in relation to each parent, as in the following example.

> Justine's parents, two high-powered, successful executives, separated acrimoniously when Justine was under age 2 years. Paternal visitation was often disrupted by her mother's accusations toward the father (of intoxication or irresponsibility) and physical scuffles over the child. Justine became anxious at her father's arrival, despite her apparent affection for him as a "playmate." Her father was increasingly inclined to gratify her wishes in order to stay in her good graces. While the custodial arrangements were revisited continuously in court, the child was torn in terms of her loyalty to her dad as her mother regularly questioned her about the father's state during visits. This was further compounded when, as Justine turned 4, the mother reconnected with an old boyfriend, Gary, who himself was divorced with three children: two older girls and one boy, Alan, close in age to Justine. Justine became engaged in a network of rivalries: with the boyfriend for her mother, with Alan for the affection of his sisters, even with all three of Gary's children for the interest and favor of his appealing ex-wife. Seen in consultation at age 4 years 10 months as part of the divorce proceedings, Justine was bossy and rather disdainful; she played out repetitive stories of families in which the children had to deal with foolish and misguided parents who completely underestimated the kids' capacities, dressed them in ridiculous outfits, and left them in the care of stupid and even dangerous nannies. However, the kids were possessed of magical powers and extraordinary intelligence and would typically escape to a country where parents did not exist.

Justine's oedipal conflict was distorted by the acrimonious divorce, leaving her confused about her role, unable to come to terms with the complications of triadic relationships, lacking confidence about the future, and unable to safely desire and be angry with her parents.

The oedipal complex can be similarly affected if a child is raised by a single parent. Of course, single-parent families are multiply determined, and some divorces can result in the disengagement of the noncustodial parent. In fact, a consistent finding in Wallerstein's research has been the relative loss of the father in divorce (Wallerstein and Kelly 1980). Abandonment, death, artificial insemination, and single-parent adoption are other ways that a single-parent family comes about, and each one has specific features and unfolds differently depending on multiple factors, including the psychology of the caregiving parent. Certainly, the hardships of raising a child or children alone, as well as the idiosyncratic meaning to the parent of parenting solo, contribute to the implicit or explicit communications to the child. To the degree that children continue to see their origins as the result of a parental union, they can become preoccupied with the missing parent. If biological origins and sexual congress are increasingly delinked due to technological advances, these connections may change. However, the desire to, at the very least, imagine a second parent and/or a differently gendered parent is still evident in many children of same-sex marriages, single parents, and adoptive parents (Corbett 2001). This longing can override any sense of oedipal triumph but simultaneously induce guilt around individuation and separation because such children often feel they are essential to the well-being of the single parent (Erreich 2011).

Adoption and the Oedipal Complex

Adoption is not a unitary phenomenon, and its many versions and details figure into its impact on the oedipal phase. Contemporary adoption occurs in heterogeneous circumstances with varying degrees of transparency. Today, open access to biological parents after age 18 is widely available and increasingly common, spearheaded by movements such as Bastard Nation, which calls for the "full human and civil rights of adult adoptees," including their access to information about their birth. Adoption remains relatively rare, affecting about 2.5% of children under age 18, as determined by the 2000 U.S. Census, which included "adopted son/daughter" as a kinship category (Kreider 2003). Accurate statistical accounts are not readily available, however, because no federal oversight exists. Public agencies are estimated to manage less than half of known adoptions, whereas most others are arranged by private agencies and "independent" placements. Documentation is most accurate in regard to foreign adoptions, because citizenship must be granted; in 2002, there were 20,009 foreign adoptions in the United States, more than triple the number reported a decade earlier. Kinship adoptions constitute roughly half of all adoptions and, depending on cultural expectations, are conceptualized differently by the participants than is adoption by strangers (Brodzinsky et al. 1998).

The humane service that adoption provides—that of offering a loving home to a child who needs one—is considerable. However, the impact of being adopted on the mind of the child is not insignificant, and it is important for parents to tolerate and help their child adjust, a process that is a work in progress throughout development. This process usually begins in toddlerhood, because information about adoption is frequently introduced early, long before a child can contemplate and understand the concepts involved. Adopted toddlers become familiar with terminology and specific details through stories explaining their own adoption or adoption in general, photographs, and/or the introduction of cultural artifacts of the child's origins, if different from those of the parents. Although there are undeniable advantages to addressing adoption early, especially if the fact of adoption is obvious to others (through appearance or parent circumstances), the young child's capacity to understand the complexity of the human drama involved is inevitably colored by cognitive organization, which even at age 4 years is not up to the task of comprehending the facts, however softened or elaborated by parents (Brinich 1995; Wieder 1977). The negative connotations of being "given away" are heightened by the young child's limited cognition; in the mind of a toddler, "given away" means gotten rid of, like garbage or dirty diapers (Wieder 1977). The child's capacity to grasp the distinction between birth mother and adoptive mother is immature at best; often the message is absorbed in a simplified form: "I am not your real mother or father." These naïve interpretations contribute to a background of insecurity and the preeminence of separation issues. Moreover, such ideas can be especially disorienting for children grappling with the mystery of how babies are born and the more personal question of how they themselves came to be. The notion that babies are acquired, bought and sold, or kidnapped often appears in the child's fantasy and play. Regulation of anger and ambivalence is complicated by the fear of being abandoned; negative feelings are sometimes directed solely at the birth parents, who are conceptualized as bad, dirty, naughty, and the like. Alternatively, adopted children can turn anger against their adoptive parents, testing their devotion and commitment to keep them "no matter what"; getting into trouble is the vehicle for ascertaining love.

The challenge permeates the parents' mental lives as well, because the adopted child who is disappointing can be easily distanced (e.g., "He's just like his [biological] parents"). Indeed, many fairy tales and myths pivot on the hostility of parents, both biological and adoptive, toward their children, including Hansel and Gretel as well as Oedipus himself (Brinich 1995). Some of the taboos that guard against abuse, physical and especially sexual (in terms of incest), are turned on their head in the adoption situation, because the adoptive parents are not kin and may feel under less compunction to protect their child. Similarly, adopted children are faced with the dilemma that their blood relations could be anywhere else but in the home where they were raised. A 5-year-old adopted girl, who enjoyed a warm relationship with her father but frequently engaged in angry exchanges with her mother about who her "real mother" was, situated her doll play in a magical land where girls married their fathers, claiming "That's allowed in Barbie land!"

These features complicate the oedipal experience in a number of ways. On a very fundamental level, attachment insecurity casts a shadow over the capacity to manage ambivalence and tolerate the intensity of the oedipal drama. In addition, because the incest prohibition is less secure, the adoptive parents may be defensively pictured as asexual and/or pure, whereas the birth parents are viewed as sex-crazed and depraved; ambivalence is not integrated into emotional attachments, but rather feelings are split between "good" and "bad" parents. Sibling rivalry is not tempered by a sense of blood bond and can become intensely hostile, coldly indifferent, or overtly sexual. The "consolation" of growing up and having one's own partner and one's own babies lacks a symmetry with the experience of the adoptive parents and can invoke guilt for envisioning greater success than the parents. The same 5-year-old whose dolls married their fathers in Barbie land decided that she would never have babies of her own, but she would be a clever nanny who took care of other people's babies. This represents a condensed fantasy that manages her guilt about the possibility that she would bear babies more successfully than her adoptive mother; to forgo this idea, she deliberately chose a child-rearing (as opposed to a childbearing) role (Novick 1988). She could not be the oedipal victor, a better baby maker than her mother. She was nonetheless still furious at her adoptive mother because she experienced the latter as critical and judgmental, but this only added to her burden of guilt.

Oedipal Configuration and Identity Development

These variations on the oedipal configuration have an impact on the conflicts and solutions of this phase, and they also affect the child's identity and sense of self. Elements of identity are achieved through the ego identifications that occur over the course of development and are reworked as an essential part of the adolescent identity crisis. Components related to certain external circumstances are relatively fixed, however, and these are not subject to revision of their factual existence. These elements, such as gender, race, and nationality, are built into the fiber of the self. Also included among these are adoption, sibling configurations, and divorce, when this occurs in early childhood. As one young boy said plaintively, upon hearing his parents were separating, "I don't want to be divorced!" He rightfully complained that this fact would be part of who he was forever. These enduring issues affect the oedipal conflict and continue to have a role as each developmental phase unfolds. In psychopathology, these features are exaggerated.

The following vignette illustrates the ongoing impact of oedipal distortion (in this case due to adoption and attachment insecurity) on the mental life of an adult.

> Will was in his late 20s when he sought treatment because he was blocked in his career and love life. He had reluctantly married his high school sweetheart a year earlier, but they were living apart while she finished graduate school. He was irritated by her and spoke about her with some disdain, seeing her as completely unsexy and kind of ditzy, despite her apparent brains,

beauty, and devotion. She was "dim." In regard to work, he had just quit a job he hated, a low-level position in a field of his father's choosing, and was at a loss as to what to do next. He was drinking too much and occasionally using cocaine.

Will had been adopted at birth by an affluent and prominent older couple. His father was a brilliant and successful politician and businessman, admired by Will's self-effacing mother and everyone else in their circle. Will was pressured "from infancy" to live up to his father's fantasies of what "his son" should be like. He was tutored in reading at age 3 and was expected to show an array of academic capacities precociously. Will's native athletic talents were encouraged by the father, but only in regard to sports that his father considered "classy," such as squash and tennis. Will's mother was much warmer and more forgiving, and she seemed to understand that Will's interests and predilections might take him in different directions. However, from as early as he could remember, Will had distanced himself from his mother. For example, as a separation-anxious young boy, he would fervently wish for his parents' safe return and offer up his mother as sacrifice in his fantasied negotiations with God for his father's safety. He felt guilty and puzzled by this pattern, especially because his mother died in his adolescence and he missed her terribly; in fact, his unresolved bereavement was a major focus of treatment. He gradually understood that his anxiety about "belonging" was due to his childhood understanding of his adoption as reflecting his birth mother's rejection, for which he punished his adoptive mother. This was compounded by his fears that his father was painfully disappointed not to have "his own son." In what was eventually understood as a desperate bid to please his father and identify with the aggressor, Will joined his father in mocking disdain for his mother, especially in regard to the traits that made her so appealing and consoling (i.e., her gentleness and absence of critical judgment). He came to understand that even as a very young child, he acted as if he had to eschew his love and yearning for his mother and ally himself with his feared and oppressive father in order to placate him and "be kept." Clearly, his own wife bore the legacy of this dynamic with his mother, as she was denigrated and desexualized. In addition, Will could not bear to exclude himself from his father's approval, and thus he repeatedly chose jobs that were completely unsuited to his talents and interests. His congealed rage at his father was deeply threatening to this young man who still reacted powerfully to separations because, without the regular contact and approval of his father, he was "entirely alone, floating in space with no gravitational pull anywhere."

This vignette shows the sequelae of an oedipal configuration distorted by attachment insecurity related to this young man's adoption and adoptive mother's death, and a disavowal of his positive oedipal feelings because they interfered with his anxious idolization of his father. His posture toward his mother was re-created in his marriage, as was his very specific need to keep sexuality out of his domestic relationship. This man's self-defeating behavior, which had been a persistent feature of his academic and work history, is part of a very complicated developmental course with multiple sources of trauma, including his mother's death while he was young, his father's verbal abuse, and his own rageful inner life. As is inevitable, the layering of influences affecting this man's mental experience was dense and intricate and took many years of treatment to sort out.

Superego

The Role of Gender in Superego Development

As the so-called "heir to the Oedipus complex" (Freud 1923/1962, p. 48), the superego has been traditionally described as a mental structure that emerges from resolution of oedipal conflict and brings with it the powerful affect of guilt. In the classical literature, the superego "forms" as a new structure by identification with the same-sex parent after anxiety-induced renunciation of oedipal desire and aggressive impulses. However, Freud himself recognized that the deepest roots of the superego are identifications with parents much earlier in life, establishing what he originally called the *ego ideal* (Freud 1914/1962). His subsequent explanation of same-sex identification as a consequence of castration anxiety or, in the case of a little girl, conviction of castration, does not make developmental sense to many contemporary thinkers (Chodorow 1994; Westen 1986).

We believe that superego development and the oedipal progression of boys and girls can be best understood by rethinking the superego as a structure with a long preoedipal history whose coalescence occurs in the course of oedipal conflict. As illustrated in Chapters 2, 3 and 4, the origins of self-regulatory capacities begin in mother-infant exchanges, as the mother attempts to manage infant states through affect displays and verbalizations. Myriad "dos" and "don'ts" are communicated from earliest infancy by caregivers who shape behavior, show empathy, and selectively reward (with evidence of approval and delight) desirable behaviors (Emde et al. 1991; Litowitz 2005). Undoubtedly, some of the communications about right and wrong, aggression, and the like are culturally sex specific, so that gender, as a complex, cultural, and idiosyncratic aspect of self-experience, is often laden with messages about rules of behavior. This kind of reinforcement of gender stereotypes begins with the announcement of a baby's sex and continues throughout development. Differential identifications with the parents as gendered, in addition to internalizations of nongendered parental injunctions, predate the oedipal conflict. The superego is thus the result of many different types of identifications with both parents (Westen 1986), even though gender role differences are simultaneously being communicated and processed.

The Role of Defenses in Superego Structuralization

The partial internalization of the parental voice and desire for parental approval facilitate the management of impulses in the toddler period, during which the willful child elicits the imposition of rules conveyed verbally and by physical restraints. In toddlerhood, the defenses of *reaction formation* and *identification with the aggressor* can be seen in a child's actions. Reaction formation helps the young child disavow forbidden impulses to mess and attack; identification with the aggressor involves the gradual process of taking in and adopting the stern parental prohibitions, epitomized by a child like Julia (described by Fraiberg [1996] and discussed in Chapter 4, "The Oedipal Phase and Emerging Capacities") who self-admonishes on the brink of committing a transgression. Moreover, imitation and identification serve to assuage the wounds to very young children's narcissism when they realize they do not partake of their parents' powers, skill, and privileges (Milrod 2002). All of these processes serving to self-regulate and bolster the sense of self of the child form a kind of "undergraduate superego" (Sandler 1960, p. 152) that still requires parental supervision to be effective. Ultimately, this fledging is incorporated into the formation of a newly organized agency in the mind: the superego. The internalization of "dos and don'ts," moral principles of right and wrong, and the guiding function that seeks to maintain parental approval thus have a long preoedipal history; the superego that coalesces in the oedipal period is presumably at a different level of structuralization, on the way to autonomy in maintaining its direction giving, limiting, and punitive/rewarding functions (Milrod 2002). There is an advance in mental organization that includes both a more gendered self-representation and an internalized sense of right and wrong.

Shame and Guilt

Ultimately, two emotions, shame and guilt, are closely associated with superego function. *Shame* begins in toddler conflicts and can be seen in the 18- to 24-month-old child, identified by a universal physical posture, averted gaze, and dropped head (Sheikh and Janoff-Bulman 2010). Shame typically contains an element of being seen in a humiliating and weak position and is associated with violation of prescriptive injunctions by parental authority. In psychodynamic thinking, moments of shame have narcissistic qualities, often connected to the sense of being rapidly deflated from an elevated state. Although early shame feelings are elicited in technically nonmoral situations, such as messing and temper tantrums, shame eventually is folded into "moral emotions," as in failing to live up to standards or disappointing others (Auchincloss and Samberg 2012; Sheikh and Janoff-Bulman 2010); these dynamics are therefore rightfully considered superego precursors (see Chapter 3, "The Toddler"). *Guilt* is inherently related to concern for others, such as early prosocial behaviors wherein young children demonstrate empathy and concern, identifying with the nurturing qualities of the caretaker. The parental messages in regard to these moral values, such as kindness and respect for others' boundaries, are fundamental to early, preoedipal moral strivings (Blum and Blum 1990). Guilt optimally inspires remorse and reparative efforts, whereas shame typically leads to retreat, often with attempts to externalize blame.

In the context of oedipal conflict and evolving ego capacities—defenses, cognition, theory of mind, and language—parental injunctions are incorporated into the relatively autonomous mental structure, the superego. This structure's independence of parental enforcement is facilitated by the introjection not simply of rules and regulations or "dos and don'ts," but of parental *authority*, which endows the superego with power to eventually regulate in the absence of the parent (Sandler 1960). While the superego is immature and subject to much reworking as development proceeds, it achieves its first level of internal coherence and independence from the parents and forever alters the nature of individual psychology. Although the superego is classically described as primarily focused on issues of morality (specifically concerning incest and parricide or matricide—sex and aggression), these are admixed with narcissistic aspirations throughout the lifespan. In practice, it is often difficult to tease apart moral concerns and guilt from narcissistic strivings and shame. As the child comes to terms with the fact that he or she does not share the power and glory of the idealized parents of infancy (or the idealized grandiose self), an inflated wishful self-representation is formed that is immature and oriented toward libidinal gratifications, such as wealth, beauty, power, and the like. This representation can be easily observed in fantasy play, as when a child plays at being Superman, "the man of steel," with X-ray vision and the power to fly, or Wonder Woman, with her magic lasso of truth, superhuman strength, and power to communicate with animals. The rapid deflation of such grandiose fantasies—for example, due to their sudden interruption by an admonition to "Take off your cape and come to dinner" or a scolding like "Look what a mess you made throwing around that rope!"—is experienced as shaming and humiliating. Strivings of this type are different from goals of moral goodness, where failure is associated with guilt and remorse. However, the clear differentiation of narcissistic and moral ideals is not always so easy, especially because living up to one's moral code is rewarded with some degree of self-satisfaction. The little boy who identifies with Superman may be as interested in his moral compass and determination to benefit mankind, as he is in his cape and strength (De-Souza and Radell 2011). In the most mature form of superego guidelines, the features of spiritual goodness are depersonified and abstracted, but not necessarily detached from human considerations.

A trajectory toward coherence in superego components has been observed in developmental studies that show that compliance with rules gradually becomes integrated with moral emotions—empathy and guilty feelings—by age 45 months (Aksan and Kochanska 2005). It is important to note that the superego's presence is a source of positive self-feeling, as well as restraint and punishment. To the extent that the child's ego strives to meet the standards imposed by the superego, self-esteem and self-love are maintained both in terms of narcissistic and moral feelings (Schafer 1960).

The Role of the Superego in the Management of Sex and Aggression

The superego, in its limiting function and ultimately its punitive function, is involved in the management of impulses; despite the emphasis on the sexual urges of this period in traditional formulations, "aggression looms larger than sex" (A. Freud 1972, p. 168) in the lives of most children. Aggression usually meets a variety of decisive interventions by parents, whereas sexual excitement, curiosity, and desire are more typically ignored or deflected (Fonagy 2008). Studies of trajectories of aggression and sexual activity in normal children show that the oedipal phase is indeed a turning point in the overt expression of both (Alink et al. 2006; Friedrich et al. 1998; Mayes and Cohen 1993). Hitting, kicking, biting, and other forms of overt violence, typically in response to frustration of desires and at least initially without intent to harm, usually appear by age 12 months and increase markedly between ages 24 and 36 months, after which these behaviors decline. This type of aggression is considered normative, as is its gradual successful containment. By age 4 years, overtly aggressive acts are rare. Sex differences are present as early as 12–24 months, with boys exceeding girls in physical aggression; explanations for this gender differentiation consider the impact of earlier language acquisition, cultural expectations, and greater sensitivity to approval in girls (Murray-Close and Ostrov 2009). Relational aggression (defined as damage to relationships or the threat to do so) requires a higher level of cognition, language skills, and intent to harm, and appears to increase as physical aggression declines, especially among girls (Crick et al. 2006). Mothers tend to tolerate relational aggression far more comfortably than physical aggression (Werner et al. 2006). Studies of aggression in young children concur on the shaping and inhibiting effect of internalization of rules, gender socialization, moral compunctions, improved language skills, self-regulation, and theory of mind.

Sexual activity, which is studied primarily in terms of mothers' reports of a broad range of behaviors indicating interest and/or excitement, shows a trajectory roughly similar to aggression, peaking between 2 and 5 years of age. Masturbation before adolescence is most commonly reported at age 4, when "the child learns that stimulation of the genitalia will consistently provide a pleasurable sensation" (Leung and Robson 1993, p. 238). Boys exceed girls in this and in other categories of observed sexual activity (touching others' genitals or breasts, trying to look at others when naked, overt manual masturbation). This differential may be due to genital anatomy that makes masturbation more obvious in boys (Friedrich et al. 1998; Kellogg 2010), but it may also reflect parental attitudes toward gender. Thereafter, as norms of behavior are better internalized and controls stabilize, sexual behavior appears to decline or certainly becomes less visible. When children violate social expectations by behavior no longer tolerated in their age group, such as excessive masturbation or frankly coercive sexual actions, they are viewed as reflecting behavioral disturbance and inadequate socialization. The vast majority of children bring their sexual impulses under control by the end of the oedipal phase.

These observations support the idea that the oedipal phase is a time of arousal and excitement in the lives of children. Urges and impulses are heightened, while internalization of controls is only just developing. Feelings are expressed in the context of the family; passionate love, rivalrous hate, and bodily anxiety are powerful challenges for children who are just becoming aware of their relative smallness, insignificance, lack of adult privileges, and limited knowledge and experience. The emotional drama of the oedipal complex is made possible by the multiple developmental advances that converge during this period.

As with many aspects of classical Freudian theory, the original developmental observations are remarkable for their insights, but the etiology in psychosexual conflict is too narrow; the oedipal period marks the emergence of a new organization of the mind, but not primarily due to the specifically sexual tensions and anxieties of this age, despite their prominence and intensity. These emotions are indeed stormy and pose a huge challenge for children—but their management and resolution are not achieved primarily through castration anxiety or disappointment about not having a penis. Such feelings may be present, but they are not what propel development toward a new mental organization. The superego appears because the child's cognition, object relations, theory of mind, affect tolerance, self-observation, language development, reality orientation, narcissistic vulnerability, and ongoing identifications are evolving and all contribute to the maturation of the mind (Gilmore 2008; Westen 1986). And just in the nick of time! The child who is grappling with a new repertoire of intense emotions also has an evolving mental capacity to help manage it. There is no doubt that sexual and aggressive impulses are both important foci for superego activity, but they do not produce it.

THE OEDIPAL COMPLEX IN CONTEMPORARY PSYCHODYNAMIC THINKING: IS IT STILL IMPORTANT?

Contemporary American psychodynamic schools can be differentiated according to their developmental theories and what they consider the fount of psychological health and illness. Some theorists continue to argue for the role of conflict and drive; others advance the preeminence of dyadic relationships, most specifically the mother-infant relationship; and still others proffer mixed models such as the relational-conflict model (Greenberg and Mitchell 1983). Among these theorists are those who think that the overvaluation of the Oedipus creates a mistaken emphasis on "irrational drives" and a predetermined "transformational moment" (Seligman 2003, p. 498). We continue to think that the oedipal narrative recurs as an organizing factor in mental life, but it can only emerge from a prior mother-infant relationship providing "relatedness [that] is the psychic matrix out of which intrapsychic instincts and ego and extrapsychic objects differentiate" (Loewald 1978, p. 503; see also Chodorow 2004).

Given the current status of the oedipal concept in contemporary theorizing, one might argue that it has outlived its usefulness in psychodynamic developmental thinking. The reality is that references to the oedipal complex, oedipal conflict, oedipal phase, and preoedipal-oedipal psychopathology, in addition to a multitude of ancillary terms, such as penis envy, positive and negative oedipal constellations, castration anxiety, and so on, are still ubiquitous in theoretical and clinical papers from almost all schools of psychodynamic thinking. These references vary in terms of their degree of acceptance of traditional implications or their attempts at modernization. It is the reader's challenge to approach this terminology with an eye to contemporary modifications. We argue here for retaining oedipal terminology not only for the sake of communication in the field (Phillips 2003) but also because it serves as an evocative designation of a momentous period in development, characterized by an unprecedented level of emotion in the context of cherished familial relationships, a new capacity to symbolize and create meaningful narratives, and an enlarged facet of identity in regard to gender. While promoting the continued usage of this terminology, we hasten to emphasize that 1) the oedipal complex is embedded in an intricate network of interacting developmental systems and familial relationships, without which it could not be evoked, and 2) many aspects of the original conceptualization are no longer tenable. We no longer see the oedipal complex as marking the first subjective experience of differentiation in gender; nor do we think it "produces" the superego and thereby ushers in latency. Also, despite the pervasive tendency for psychopathology to be differentiated according to the preoedipal-oedipal continuum, we believe that these designations do not faithfully reflect actual developmental experience.

Contemporary Views of the Oedipal Complex

- Emerging capacities introduce a new range of affects, sexual desire, and curiosity about the mysteries of life: the difference between the sexes and the facts of birth.

- The new focus on the genitals and genital pleasure inevitably brings anxieties about their loss or damage.

- The force field of family life creates the setting for intense longings and rivalries in triadic forms that can include any configuration of family members and important others influenced by the idiosyncratic circumstances of each child's family.

- Superego precursors coalesce to form the superego proper, which facilitates the repression of the oedipal drama and progression toward latency.

- The new affects of guilt, shame, and ambivalence are closely associated with oedipal resolution.

THE OEDIPAL COMPLEX AND "UNIVERSAL FANTASY"

Fantasies derived from the oedipal complex are ubiquitous in Western culture and are present, in derivative form, in dreams, pretend play, and literature. A handful of leitmotifs derived from the oedipal situation are recurrent themes in the fantasy and dreams of children and adults alike. Because such elements are subject to vast individual variation and figure differently in terms of their importance in a given person, they are generalizable only in schematic form. Many of these recurrent motifs are reflections of children's naïve cognition and do not conform to rational thinking or mature mentation; however, they are woven into culture in all their infinite variations and are recognizable to the receptive ear and eye.

One central theme concerns the nature of intimate sexual relationships: fantasies of violent, sadomasochistic parental intercourse, dominance and submission, and various forms of bodily, specifically genital, injury are typical in oedipal children and can be discovered in the dreams and fantasies of adults. The experience of the child as the excluded onlooker to an event of awesome mystery and excitement is captured in recurrent *primal scene* fantasies that take countless forms and frequently have the aura of voyeuristic intrigue and secrecy. Despite the pleasure associated with such fantasies, narcissistic mortification is often the accompanying experience and can be observed in many people who seem to experience exclusion at every turn and who show exquisite sensitivity to belittlement. These predilections can produce a powerful revenge motive that organizes the personality and in some cases obscures the underlying humiliation. Another set of derivative fantasies, observed both in oedipal-age children and in adult dreams and fantasy, concerns childish misconceptions regarding the way babies are born. For example, notions of anal birth or fears of dreadful bodily injury are unconscious fantasies that are observable in people at all ages. In fact, despite enlightened sex education offered at a very young age, many children harbor fantastical notions of conception and birth until adolescence. Similarly, castration fears persist in mental life, associated with fantasies of punishment for assertiveness and ambition. Female genital anxieties likewise can be observed in subsequent development. These fears are typically represented symbolically; a classic metaphor for this kind of bodily damage is the Little Mermaid's lost voice or Oedipus's clubfoot. Finally, while the incest taboo may arise from evolutionary or other mechanisms, it is hypothesized to achieve the level of moral imperative in the context of oedipal conflict; it certainly set the stage for Oedipus' own tragedy.

As noted in Chapter 4, many beloved children's stories are grounded in oedipal themes; the parental persona is often split into all-bad or all-good figures, dismantling the hard-won tolerance of ambivalence required to come to terms with one's own oedipal drama. For example, Cinderella has a benevolent fairy godmother and wicked stepmother and stepsisters, and Little Red Riding Hood has the evil, sexual Big Bad Wolf and the heroic woodsman who saves her in the end. Oedipal themes are also woven into adult movies, plays, and books. Although it has been argued that these themes are unique to Western literature, some thinkers have suggested that variants of (profoundly repressed) oedipal themes are evident in Eastern cultures as well (Gu 2006). Shakespeare's *Hamlet* is frequently cited as a masterpiece of oedipal drama. Another timeless tale of oedipal exclusion and revenge in adult literature is Alexandre Dumas's (1844) *The Count of Monte Cristo*, in which a young and handsome merchant sailor, arrested on his wedding day and unfairly imprisoned by cruel, envious rivals (bad fathers), is educated and given access to untold riches by a loving old man, the Abbé, a fellow prisoner and victim of injustice (the good father). After a breathtaking escape from prison, the hero spends the remainder of his life pursuing artful revenge. The *Star Wars* series is a modern example of this kind of narrative, replete with castration imagery when the evil father, Darth Vader, cuts off the arm of his son Luke Skywalker. These narratives are, of course, present in myths, such as that of Oedipus Rex itself. On a more mundane level, such themes are readily observed in children's persistent wish to penetrate the parental bedroom, their feelings of injury when excluded, and the associated fear that, for example, robbers will break in and defeat (steal, kill) the rival parent.

• **See the video "4-Year-Old Girl," also cited in Chapter 4. In addition to illustrating emerging capacities, the girl's imaginary play shown in this video has oedipal themes (Cinderella with her evil stepmother and fairy godmother; concerns about bodily injury).**

Key Concepts

We continue to see the oedipal complex as an important organizer of mental life, provided it is conceptualized in the updated form we have elaborated in this text. The oedipal complex creates the template for adult triadic relationships, by which we refer not only to romantic and rivalrous feelings but also to the capacity for complexity and nuance in adult object relations. Although not the linchpin of adult personality organization as was once believed, the complex does leave its imprint on many components of mental life: the management of sex and aggression; sexual orientation and gender role identity; the modulation of love and hate; the tolerance of ambition, competition, and success; and defeat and humiliation. The complex can have reverberations in lifetime self-actualization or self-denial. The superego, the mental agency that emerges contemporaneously with this phase and facilitates development beyond it, represents the internalization of regulatory capacities and the emotions of shame, guilt, and remorse that introduce children into the adult moral world.

- Freud's original description of the Oedipus complex has undergone significant revision, but his insight into the human drama of this phase of life is remarkable and his psychosexual developmental schema is still useful clinically (Michels 1999).

- In modern thinking, the oedipal phase is not the product of a unitary developmental progression; it originates from the multiple developing systems of the 3- to 6-year-old child, as does its so-called heir, the superego.

- These interacting systems include the following:
  - Increasing genital sensations and excitement about the body
  - New complexity in emotions, object relations, and cognition
  - An explosion in semiotic capacity including language and symbolic play
  - A deeper awareness of individuation or the separate self

- Through the passionate experience of the oedipal phase, the child achieves a sense of being individual and self-contained, and is recognized as such by adults who henceforth assume the presence of motivation and responsibility for actions (Loewald 1985).

- The experience of the oedipal phase, with its focus on the genital, sex, and gender differences, has reverberations specifically on how children see themselves as sexed and gendered individuals.

- The oedipal constellation wanes in importance as a new mental organization is achieved in latency. However, it remains a core unconscious template or structure that affects the following (Tolpin 1970):
  - Future object relationships
  - Sexuality
  - Sense of self
  - Management of aggression
  - Moral convictions

- By the close of this phase, theory of mind is established, contributing to empathy and the sense of morality.

- The superego, which consolidates into a mental agency during the oedipal period, is by no means a fully formed or mature structure by the close of this phase. However, it is internalized and based upon moral principles, albeit simplistic ones. It is never absolutely reliable and consistent, and it rarely operates on purely moral grounds; narcissistic strivings are often commingled. The superego begins to contribute to the shape of character and brings with it the associated affect of guilt.

REFERENCES

Ahrons C: Family ties after divorce: long-term implications for children. Fam Process 46:53–65, 2007

Aksan N, Kochanska G: Conscience in childhood: old questions, new answers. Dev Psychol 41:506–516, 2005

Alink LRA, Mesman J, Van Zeiji J, et al: The early childhood aggression curve: development of physical aggression in 10- to 50-month-old children. Child Dev 77:954–966, 2006

Altman N: The case of Ronald: oedipal issues in the treatment of a seven-year-old boy. Psychoanal Dialogues 7:725–739, 1997

American Psychiatric Association: Diagnostic and Statistical Manual of Mental Disorders, 5th Edition. Washington, DC, American Psychiatric Association, 2013

Arlow JA: The revenge motive in the primal scene. J Am Psychoanal Assoc 28:519–541, 1980

Auchincloss E, Samberg E: Psychoanalytic Terms and Concepts. New Haven, CT, Yale University Press, 2012

Auchincloss E, Vaughan S: Psychoanalysis and homosexuality: do we need a new theory? J Am Psychoanal Assoc 49:1157–1186, 2001

Bank SP, Kahn MD: The Sibling Bond. New York, Basic Books, 2003

Bell A: Some observations on the role of the scrotal sac and testicles. J Am Psychoanal Assoc 9:262–286, 1961

Bernstein D: Female genital anxieties and typical mastery modes. Int J Psychoanal 71:151–165, 1990

Blos P: On the genealogy of the ego ideal. Psychoanal Study Child 29:43–88, 1974

Blum EJ, Blum HP: The development of autonomy and superego precursors. Int J Psychoanal 71:585–595, 1990

Brinich PM: Psychoanalytic perspectives on adoption and ambivalence. Psychoanal Psychol 12:181–199, 1995

Brodzinsky D, Smith DW, Brodzinsky A: Children's Adjustment to Adoption: Development and Clinical Issues. Thousand Oaks, CA, Sage, 1998

CBS Statistics Netherlands: Six out of ten divorces involve children. Available at: http://www.cbs.nl/en-GB/menu/themas/bevolking/publicaties/artikelen/archief/2006/2006-1976-wm.htm. Accessed April 22, 2013.

Chodorow N: Femininities, Masculinities, Sexualities: Freud and Beyond. Lexington, University Press of Kentucky, 1994

Chodorow N: The American independent tradition: Loewald, Erikson, and the (possible) rise of intersubjective ego psychology. Psychoanal Dialogues 14:207–232, 2004

Cook JL, Geran L, Rotermann M: Multiple births associated with assisted human reproduction in Canada. J Obstet Gynaecol Can 33:609–616, 2011

Corbett K: Nontraditional family romance. Psychoanal Q 70:599–624, 2001

Crick N, Ostrov JM, Burr JE, et al: A longitudinal study of relational and physical aggression in preschool. J Appl Dev Psychol 27:254–268, 2006

de Marneffe D: Bodies and words: a study of young children's genital and gender knowledge. Gender and Psychoanalysis 2:3–33, 1997

De-Souza D, Radell J: Superheroes: an opportunity for prosocial play. Young Child 66:26–32, 2011

Dowd M: Oedipus Rex complex. New York Times, January 3, 2012, p A23

Dunn J, Creps C, Brown J: Children's family relationships between two and five: developmental changes and individual differences. Social Dev 5:230–250, 1996

Egan SK, Perry DG: Gender identity: a multidimensional analysis with implications for psychosocial adjustment. Dev Psychol 37:451–463, 2001

Elise D: Primary femininity, bisexuality, and the female ego idea: a re-examination of female developmental theory. Psychoanal Q 66:489–517, 1997

Elise D: The absence of the paternal penis. J Am Psychoanal Assoc 46:413–442, 1998

Emde RN, Biringen Z, Clyman RB, et al: The moral self of infancy: affective core and procedural knowledge. Dev Rev 11:251–270, 1991

Erreich A: A modest proposal: (re)defining unconscious fantasy. Psychoanal Q 72:541–574, 2003

Erreich A: More than enough guilt to go around: oedipal guilt, survival guilt, separation guilt. J Am Psychoanal Assoc 59:131–150, 2011

Fagan AA, Najman JM: Association between early childhood aggression and internalizing behavior for sibling pairs. J Am Acad Child Adolesc Psychiatry 42:1093–1200, 2003

Fraiberg SH: The Magic Years. New York, Fireside, 1996

Fonagy P: A genuinely developmental theory of sexual enjoyment and its implications for psychoanalytic technique. J Am Psychoanal Assoc 56:11–36, 2008

Freud A: Comments on aggression. Int J Psychoanal 53:163–171, 1972

Freud S: Three essays on the theory of sexuality (1905), in The Standard Edition of the Complete Psychological Works of Sigmund Freud, Vol 7. Translated and edited by Strachey J. London, Hogarth Press, 1962, pp 123–246

Freud S: On narcissism: an introduction (1914), in The Standard Edition of the Complete Psychological Works of Sigmund Freud, Vol 14. Translated and edited by Strachey J. London, Hogarth Press, 1962, pp 67–102

Freud S: Instincts and their vicissitudes (1915), in The Standard Edition of the Complete Psychological Works of Sigmund Freud, Vol 14. Translated by Strachey J. London, Hogarth Press, 1962, pp 110–140

Freud S: The ego and the id (1923), in The Standard Edition of the Complete Psychological Works of Sigmund Freud, Vol 19. Translated and edited by Strachey J. London, Hogarth Press, 1962, pp 1–66

Freud S: Some psychical consequences of the anatomical distinction between the sexes (1925), in The Standard Edition of the Complete Psychological Works of Sigmund Freud, Vol 19. Translated and edited by Strachey J. London, Hogarth Press 1962, pp 241–258

Friedrich WN, Fisher J, Broughton D, et al: Normative sexual behavior in children: a contemporary sample. Pediatrics 101:e9–e18, 1998

Gediman HK: Premodern, modern, and postmodern perspectives of sex and gender mixes. J Am Psychoanal Assoc 53:1059–1078, 2005

Gilmore K: Psychoanalytic developmental theory: a contemporary reconsideration. J Am Psychoanal Assoc 56:885–907, 2008

Gilmore K: Pretend play and development in early childhood (with implications for the oedipal phase). J Am Psychoanal Assoc 59:1157–1182, 2011

Graham I: The sibling object and its transferences: alternative organizer of the middle field. Psychoanalytic Inquiry 8:88–107, 1988

Greenberg J, Mitchell S: Object Relations in Psychoanalytic Theory. Cambridge, MA, Harvard University Press, 1983

Gu MD: The filial piety complex: variations of the Oedipus theme in Chinese literature and culture. Psychoanal Q 75:163–195, 2006

Hardy M: Physical aggression and sexual behavior among siblings: a retrospective study. J Fam Violence 16:255–268, 2001

Harris A: Gender as Soft Assembly. London, Routledge Press, 2008

Heenen-Wolff S: Infantile sexuality and the "complete oedipal complex": Freudian views on heterosexuality and homosexuality. Int J Psychoanal 92:1209–1220, 2011

Horney K: The denial of the vagina—a contribution to the problem of genital anxieties. Int J Psychoanal 14:57–70, 1933

Jalongo MR, Dragich D: Brothers and sisters: the influence of sibling relationships on young children's development, in Enduring Bonds. Edited by Jalongo MR. New York, Springer, 2008, pp 35–96

Kellogg ND: Sexual behaviors in children: evaluation and management. Am Fam Physician 82:1233–1238, 2010

Kleinsorge C, Covitz LM: Impact of divorce on children: developmental considerations. Pediatr Rev 33:147–155, 2012

Kluger J: The Sibling Effect: What Brothers and Sisters Reveal About Us. New York, Riverhead Books, 2011

Kolak AM, Volling BL: Sibling jealousy in early childhood: longitudinal links to sibling relationship quality. Infant Child Dev 20:213–226, 2011

Krieder R: Adopted children and step-children: census 2000 special reports. Available at: http://www.census.gov/prod/2003pubs/censr-6rv.pdf. Accessed April 22, 2013.

Kumar M: Recasting the primal scene of seduction: envisioning a potential encounter with otherness in Laplanche and Sudhir Kakar. Psychoanal Rev 96:485–513, 2009

Laufer M: The nature of adolescent pathology and the psychoanalytic process. Psychoanal Study Child 33:307–322, 1978

Leichtman M: The influence of an older sibling on the separation-individuation process. Psychoanal Study Child 40:111–161, 1985

Leon K: Risk and protective factors in young children's adjustment to parental divorce: a review of the research. Fam Relat 52:258–270, 2003

Lerner HD: Parental mislabeling of female genitals as a determinant of penis envy and learning inhibitions in women. J Am Psychoanal Assoc 24(suppl):269–283, 1976

Leung AK, Robson WL: Childhood masturbation. Clin Pediatr (Phila) 32:238–241, 1993

Lewes K: Psychoanalysis and Male Homosexuality: Twentieth Anniversary Edition. New York, Jason Aronson, 2009

Litowitz BE: The origins of ethics: deontic modality. International Journal of Applied Psychoanalytic Studies 2:249–259, 2005

Loewald HW: Instinct theory, object relations, and psychic-structure formation. J Am Psychoanal Assoc 26:493–506, 1978

Loewald HW: Oedipal complex and development of self. Psychoanal Q 54:435–443, 1985

Makari G: Revolution in Mind: The Creation of Psychoanalysis. New York, Harper-Collins, 2008

Mayer EL: The phallic castration complex and primary femininity: paired developmental lines toward female gender identity. J Am Psychoanal Assoc 43:17–38, 1995

Mayes LC, Cohen DJ: The social matrix of aggression—enactments of loving and hating in the first years of life. Psychoanal Study Child 48:145–169, 1993

Michels R: Psychoanalysts' theories, in Psychoanalysis on the Move: The Work of Joseph Sandler (New Library of Psychoanalysis, Vol 35). Edited by Fonagy P, Cooper A, Wallerstein R. London, Hogarth Press, 1999, pp 187–200

Milrod D: The wished-for self image. Psychoanal Study Child 37:95–120, 1982

Milrod D: The superego: its formation, structure, and functioning. Psychoanal Study Child 57:131–148, 2002

Mitchell J: Siblings: Sex and Violence. Cambridge, UK, Polity Press, 2003

Mitchell J: Unpublished discussion for the Sibling Symposium, presented at the Western New England Psychoanalytic Institute and Society, March 2011

Murray-Close D, Ostrov JM: A longitudinal study of forms and functions of aggressive behavior in early childhood. Child Dev 80:828–842, 2009

Novick KK: Childbearing and child rearing. Psychoanalytic Inquiry 8:252–260, 1988

Ostrov JM, Crick NR, Stauffacher K: Relational aggression in sibling and peer relationships during early childhood. J Appl Dev Psychol 27:241–253, 2006

Phillips S: Homosexuality: coming out of the confusion. Int J Psychoanal 84:1431–1450, 2003

Pike A, Coldwell J, Dunn JF: Sibling relationships in early/middle childhood: links with individual adjustment. J Fam Psychol 19:523–532, 2005

Ross J: Oedipus revisited: Laius and the "Laius complex." Psychoanal Study Child 37:169–200, 1982

Sandler J: On the concept of the super-ego. Psychoanal Study Child 15:128–162, 1960

Schafer R: The loving and beloved superego in Freud's structural theory. Psychoanal Study Child 15:163–188, 1960

Scharff DE: Fairbairn and the self as an organized system: chaos theory as a new paradigm. Canadian Journal of Psychoanalysis 8:181–195, 2000

Seligman S: The developmental perspective in relational psychoanalysis. Contemp Psychoanal 39:477–508, 2003

Seligman S: Social psychoanalytic research and the twenty-first century family: comment on Wallerstein and Lewis. Psychoanal Psychol 24:459–463, 2007

Senet NV: A study of preschool children's linking of genitals and gender. Psychoanal Q 73:291–334, 2004

Shapiro T: Oedipal distortions in severe character pathologies: developmental and theoretical considerations. Psychoanal Q 46:559–579, 1977

Sharpe SS, Rosenblatt AD: Oedipal sibling triangles. J Am Psychoanal Assoc 42:491–523, 1994

Sheikh S, Janoff-Bulman R: Tracing the self-regulatory bases of moral emotions. Emot Rev 2:386–396, 2010

Stoller R: Primary femininity. J Am Psychoanal Assoc 24S: 59–78, 1976

Tolpin M: The infantile neurosis: a metapsychological concept and a paradigmatic case history. Psychoanal Study Child 25:273–305, 1970

Tucker S: Current views of the oedipal complex. J Am Psychoanal Assoc 56:263–271, 2008

Turner BS: The Cambridge Dictionary of Sociology. Cambridge, UK, Cambridge University Press, 2006

Vivona J: Sibling differentiation, identity development, and the lateral dimension of psychic life. J Am Psychoanal Assoc 55:1191–1225, 2007

Wallerstein J, Kelly J: Surviving the Break-Up. New York, Basic Books, 1980

Wallerstein J, Resnikoff D: Parental divorce and developmental progression: an inquiry into their relationship. Int J Psychoanal 78:135–154, 1997

Werner NE, Senich S, Przepyszny KA: Mothers' responses to preschoolers' relational and physical aggression. J Applied Dev Psychol 27:193–208, 2006

Westen D: The superego: a revised developmental model. J Am Acad Psychoanal Dyn Psychiatry 14:181–202, 1986

Wieder H: On being told of adoption. Psychoanal Q 46:1–21, 1977

CHAPTER 6

The Latency Phase

Cognitive Maturation, Autonomy, Social Development, and Learning

INTRODUCTION TO THE LATENCY CHILD

Entry into middle childhood, which roughly spans ages 6–10 years, marks a quantum shift in the child's mental organization, relationships, and behavior. Sigmund Freud (1905/1962) applied the term *latency* to this developmental phase to capture an overall quieting of sexual and aggressive urges; in his view, the latency years represent a relatively calm era between the manifest turbulence of the oedipal period and the inevitable arrival of pubertal pressures. The typical latency child evokes the image of a "good citizen"; cooperation, industry, and avid interest in achievement are highly visible social-emotional and behavioral trends (Erikson 1950).

Despite the child's outwardly dutiful and compliant attitude, modern psychodynamic theorists recognize latency as a vibrant period of cognitive growth, inner conflict, and elaborate fantasizing. Transformations of the child's *ego structure*—comprising such mental functions as symbolization, psychological defenses, and fantasy formation—and increasingly autonomous superego capacities bring about greater independence, more reliable self-regulation, and strengthened identifications with adult values (Sarnoff 1971). These developments allow the latency child to turn attention toward the reality-based tasks of education, rule-bound activities, and group socialization. The confluence of brain maturation, sweeping changes in cognition and emotional self-regulation, diminishment of oedipal phase pressures, and increasing societal demands generates this critical period of childhood.

The latency youngster's special propensity for learning is universally noted. At around age 7 years, children are assigned new roles and responsibilities within society (Shapiro 1976). Newly acquired skills and expanded opportunities—sports and games, reading and writing—serve as *sublimations*—that is, structured, socialized channels or intellectual outlets for the child's aggressive feelings and sexual inquisitiveness. Increasingly reliable self-management, intense motivation for mastery, a growing sense of morality, and greater awareness of others' needs make the latency child amenable to classroom values and goals. Uneventful separation from parents, sustained attention and compliance throughout the school day, control over bodily functions, participation in group activities, and absorption of a huge body of academic knowledge are among the formidable achievements of the grade school years.

Dramatic shifts in the latency child's cognitive, social, and self-regulatory capacities lead to novel challenges and vulnerabilities. An increasingly internalized "voice" of moral authority disposes the child to guilty feelings and feelings of disappointment in the self. Superego-based attitudes and self-reproaches are energetically rejected in the early years of latency, often leading to *externalization* of moral conflicts; common manifestations include eager scrutiny of others' mistakes and transgressions, and attempts to elicit outside sources of punishment. Moreover, as the older child's social world expands—toward teachers, friends, and other members of the community—nonfamilial relationships and peer group status are inextricably linked to the quality of self-regard. Learning dominates the latency child's experience; regardless of personal strengths and weaknesses, the grade-school student is required to engage in and master multiple subjects and activities. For the anxious child, or the one who is hampered by reading delays and attentional weakness, the relentless performance required in school environments can interfere with a sense of pride and efficacy. New sources of shame and embarrassment proliferate in the classroom and on the playground, where teachers inspect the child's progress and young peers measure each other's competence. Highly visible skills, such as handwriting and athletics, confer status within the group; the shy, watchful child may not achieve popularity as easily as the outgoing baseball player or the successful student. Parental love and approval remain critical as a source of emotional security and contentment but are no longer sufficient for the latency child's happiness and positive self-esteem.

Cognitive Maturation and the Mind of the Latency Child

The Concrete Operational Phase

Between ages 5 and 7 years, with entry into the period of *concrete operations*, an internal "cognitive revolution" begins to transform the latency child's intellectual and social-emotional life (Mahon 1991; Piaget and Inhelder 1969). The hallmark of this phase is an increasing capacity for mental rather than action-based problem-solving. In simple cognitive tasks, such as counting, the child's growing freedom from touching and manipulating objects is easily observed. More broadly, the momentous shift from overt action toward inner assessment vastly expands the child's emotional resourcefulness and self-regulation. The latency child begins to substitute thought for action, think through the consequences of behavior, and avoid impulsive reactions when emotionally aroused.

Strengthened capacities for logic and premeditation, as well as the maturation of *effortful control* (the ability to direct attention and inhibit behavior), contribute to the school-age child's highly visible new powers of intellectual and emotional self-management. Latency children are increasingly able to direct their attention to relevant material, maintain information in working memory, inhibit automatic reactions, and practice repetitive tasks. These myriad recently acquired skills are initially shaky but support the child's growing capacity to plan and organize personal behavior with diminished parental input; the child begins to defer desire for a special treat, arrange a play date, pay attention to a lesson, and raise a hand rather than blurt out the answer to a question. Quintessential latency pastimes and hobbies (e.g., collecting, sorting and trading cards or trinkets, playing board games with extensive rules, building models from complex diagrams), very familiar to parents and educators alike, reflect a newfound fondness for order and categorization. Such activities provide important cognitive and social opportunities to practice basic skills such as memory and classification; to learn strategies; and to strengthen tolerance for frustration.

During the latency phase, a child's approach to cognitive and social situations is increasingly *decentered*—that is, the child is less influenced by conspicuous, tangible factors and can more easily grasp others' perspectives (Piaget 1932). The widely known *tests of conservation* (Piaget and Inhelder 1969) vividly illustrate such cognitive advances. In this series of experiments, children make judgments about quantity, weight, or number after observing shifts in the appearance of liquids or solids. For example, a researcher pours water from one beaker into another of dissimilar shape and then poses questions about the volume of liquid. The younger, *preoperational*, child is most influenced by prominent aspects of the beakers' physical form; he or she concludes that the second beaker contains more water if it is taller or wider than the first. By contrast, the concrete operational child is not fooled by appearances, grasps that the researcher's actions are reversible, and correctly assesses that the volume of liquid is unchanged.

As children's logical and problem-solving capacities mature, they begin to apprehend multiple aspects of reality. The latency child's dawning realization of life's practical limitations—such as time and money—contrasts sharply with the naïve, impressionistic, and fantasy-laden thinking of the previous oedipal phase. Concepts of past and future are increasingly accessible and woven into conversation and thinking; a deepening understanding of personal continuity and awareness of the course of the life cycle add meaning to the latency child's sense of self. By around age 8 years, children grasp the concept of time and make use of such tangible measures as calendars and clocks (Colarusso 1987). They learn the relative values of coins and bills and gradually absorb the practical role of money in society. These myriad pragmatic issues create new worries for the latency child ("Will I be late for dance class?" or "How long will it take me to save up for a new sled?") but also help establish common ground for engaging with peers and participating in group projects, because the child can follow a set of steps, anticipate deadlines, and work toward common goals.

Cognitive Maturation and New Defensive Strategies

Unlike the oedipal-phase youngster, whose conscious experience is suffused with fantasy, intense feelings, and bodily preoccupations, the school-age child is intently focused on pragmatic engagements, such as learning and rule-bound activities, and is less susceptible to internal disruptions. Relative freedom from immediate inner pressures, as well as the child's maturing cognitive apparatus, allows for the proliferation of sublimated outlets that expand and enhance defensive strategies; sustained concentration for the reading or writing of engrossing stories, prolonged focus on classroom projects, or patient participation in mastering a musical instrument or sport brings a sense of mastery and gratification and provides a new, socially acceptable outlet for feelings and impulses. Bodily anxieties and intense interest in adult sexuality are transformed; whereas the oedipal child attempts to gain entry to the parents' bedroom, seeking direct gratification of sexual curiosity, the latency child experiences a "thirst" for knowledge and conducts academic researches or diverts competitive and aggressive feelings into structured group competitions (e.g., spelling bees) and athletics. Creative outlets such as writing poems and short stories serve as highly effective vehicles for self-expression. One sensitive fifth-grade teacher, noting a highly verbal 9-year-old girl's writing talents as well as her continued trouble managing her temper in the classroom, suggested diary keeping and presented her with a small notebook; this was taken up with a passion by the child, who named the diary Scheherazade, composed nightly letters to "her" in which she faithfully recorded daily events and feelings, and thereby began to gain better control over her daytime reactions.

Obsessional Tendencies

Despite the sweeping cognitive advances of this phase, fundamental aspects of the latency child's thinking are rigid and concrete. People and behaviors are judged categorically: the self and peers are good or bad, teachers are kind or mean, situations are fair or not (Westen 1986, 1990). Normative obsessive and compulsive defenses and behaviors are highly characteristic of the school-age child (Jemerin 2004). One 7-year-old girl began to insist on sharpening her pencils and then lining up her clothing, shoes, and backpack every night before school, in a specified order on her rug, and became quite upset if her younger sister interfered with the layout; such careful but inflexible planning helped assuage her anxieties about being prepared for school and her fears that she would arrive without the necessary equipment.

Obsessional phenomena, which reflect unyielding, age-typical intellectual trends as well as the child's reduced tolerance for oedipal-phase impulses, nonetheless contribute to cognitive practice and growth (Chused 1999). These universal tendencies are easily discernible in latency youngsters' ritualistic, repetitive rhymes and games such as hopscotch and jumprope, or in their adherence to irrational prohibitions such as avoiding cracks in the sidewalk. However, when such proclivities encroach upon the child's activities or relationships, impede mastery of new skills, or result in a proliferation of ritualized behaviors (e.g., hand washing or repetitive checking), they exceed normative levels and veer toward clinical psychopathology. Often, the novel stress of school, with its demands for performance and separation, uncovers such difficulties. For example, an 8-year-old boy with an emerging obsessive-compulsive disorder, whose parents ultimately sought professional consultation, refused to use school toilets and adhered to an absorbing sequence of repetitive hand washings after any contact with communal materials such as toys or sports equipment; not surprisingly, such behavior posed a serious interference to his life in the classroom and on the playground, often leading to paralyzing anxiety when he could not immediately clean his hands.

Categorical Thinking and Attitudes Toward Gender

During the years immediately following the oedipal phase, when the young latency child remains vulnerable to impulses and affective eruptions, the combined presence of concrete cognition and a shaky sense of self-control create an affinity for clear-cut, easily grasped rules and uncompromising attitudes (Tyson and Tyson 1990). Overly simplistic, judgmental reactions are quickly revealed when the child ponders complex constructs such as gender or analyzes social and moral dilemmas. "Black-and-white" thinking, rather than an appreciation for subtle distinctions and nuanced interpretations, leads to discomfort with perceived nonconformities and fuels an intense desire to engage in conventional behavior. Actions, appearances, or attitudes that seem outside of the established norms stir up anxiety and are often self-righteously criticized and rejected. As a result, the child whose dress, demeanor, or interests are slightly unfamiliar or whose academic struggles fall outside the mainstream may encounter little sympathy from peers. Rather, the young latency child often seeks to belong to an easily labeled, well-defined group of overtly like-minded associates, such as gender-segregated classmates.

Indeed, a highly observable gender divide, wherein boys and girls self-select into same-sex groups, begins to materialize in preschool and peaks during the latency years (Maccoby 2002). Attitudes toward perceived gender characteristics and views of the opposite sex reflect the grade school child's categorical thinking; often, the habits and preferences of the other gender are devalued. For example, it is common for grade school girls to label boys as "yucky" or boys to insist that girls have "cooties." Organized patterns of beliefs about girls' and boys' tendencies—such as the conviction that boys are more likely to exhibit physical aggression—deeply influence the child's social thinking and are resistant to change, even when the child is confronted with situations that challenge existing notions (Giles and Heyman 2005; Theimer et al. 2001).

Deep feelings and beliefs about gender identity are affected both by the child's cognition and by the increasing exposure to the world of peers, non-familial adults, and culture. Even though children make the link between their biological sex and their anatomy at around age 3 years, some fluidity in their thinking continues. Certainly, by the close of the oedipal phase the vast majority of children attain full gender constancy—that is, they grasp the stable, enduring nature of gender and realize that superficial alterations, such as hair or clothing styles, do not fundamentally change one's status as a boy or girl (Egan and Perry 2001). Nonetheless, they are influenced by an overriding eagerness to conform to perceived rules and conventions and by anxiety about maintaining the strict gender differentiations that pervade latency culture. One tearful second grader, whose ongoing battles with head lice caused her mother to assert that her long hair would have to be cut, burst into tears and sobbed, "I can't cut my hair. When Lucy cut hers, everyone whispered that she looked just like a boy." When her mother expressed dismay over this piece of unkindness and asserted that "girls can have short hair just like boys," the daughter responded, "I know they *can* have short hair, but they're not *supposed* to!"

Moral Reasoning and the Child's Gradual Acquisition of Insight

The latency child's efforts at moral reasoning reveal similar limitations in comprehending complex and nuanced situations, tendencies toward judgmental reactions, and occasional lapses into egocentric perspectives. A substantial literature on moral development has identified a maturational sequence, from hedonistic, self-focused moral judgments in early childhood toward higher-level, more abstract and nuanced conceptualizations in adolescence. During the latency phase, the child's absolutist thinking and preference for easily recognizable, stereotypically "good" behaviors are prominent, leading to highly conventional thinking about ethical principles and transgressions; in addition, the school-age child manifests keen awareness of authority figures and overt concern about potential punishments (see, e.g., Eisenberg et al. 1987; Kohlberg 1984; Piaget 1932). Strong condemnatory responses toward others' perceived transgressions, frequent cries of "that's not fair," and reactions of disgust are common; often, such attitudes coexist with the child's failure to reflect on his or her own personal flaws.

In fact, both psychodynamic and empirical writers note the young child's targeted interest and manifest pleasure in the misbehavior of others; the child eagerly reports on even the most minor infractions committed by peers (Loke et al. 2011; Tyson and Tyson 1990). As classroom teachers know well, tattling behavior peaks in preschool and the early years of grade school, reflecting children's social inexperience, dependency on adults, and strenuous efforts to consolidate moral identification with parents and other important adults. Although very young children demonstrate the capacity to distinguish between moral violations (such as mean behavior) and minor social transgressions (such as failure to say "thank you"), and they judge the former as more egregious, the contents of tattling tend to be nondiscriminatory (Loke et al. 2011). The younger child's poor tolerance for his or her own guilt-laden internal conflicts, lack of autonomy, limited peer experience, and immature cognitive controls all contribute to avid reporting on others' behavior.

Piaget's many brief, lively descriptions of children's verbal reasoning provide a window into the latency mind and reveal an ongoing struggle to grasp abstract features of complex moral dilemmas. For example, he presents the following pair of moral scenarios: 1) an intentionally mischievous boy makes a small ink puddle on his father's desk and 2) another boy accidentally creates a large ink spill (Piaget 1932, p. 122). Then, children are engaged in a conversation about which boy is more "naughty." The judgments of younger latency children are dominated by conspicuous perceptual features (i.e., size of the ink blots); these youngsters conclude that the second boy is more culpable despite a realization that his actions were accidental. In these children's judgments, the dimensions of the ink spills and the imagined ensuing reaction of the father are more influential than the boys' motivations.

Although we continue to find Piaget's examples very useful for highlighting latency tendencies, it is important to note that more recent research reveals that young children are capable of greater moral complexity and suggests that Piaget's theorizing about moral development requires revision. For example, children as young as age 4 years exhibit the ability to differentiate between different types of lies and to consider others' underlying motivations when they make moral judgments; in one study (Bussey 1999), preschoolers rated "antisocial" lies (such as falsehoods deliberately intended to hide a person's misbehavior) as more egregious than either "white" (largely small, social, and inconsequential) or "trick" (playfully deceiving) lies.

Potential discrepancies between girls' and boys' ethical thinking and behavior have been the subject of some controversy. Gilligan's (1977) seminal notions about the role of gender in moral development aimed to revise widely accepted notions about mature moral thinking, such as Kohlberg's (1984) emphasis on the acquisition of abstract, justice-oriented concepts. Gilligan suggests that girls, when confronted with complex social and moral dilemmas, reveal a unique moral voice; they are less concerned with abstract principles, placing higher value on maintaining relationships, caring for others' needs, and avoiding hurtful actions. Although a number of studies (e.g., Eisenberg et al. 1987) support the presence of a gender moral gap with different hierarchies of concern for boys and girls, some writers (e.g., Jaffee and Hyde 2000) raise doubts about these distinctions, suggesting that all children employ both care-oriented and justice-oriented reasoning.

During the latter grade-school years, due to a confluence of cognitive maturation, social experience, and more reliable self-regulation, the latency child's rigid attitudes begin to soften. An expanding capacity for reflection develops; children achieve a deeper awareness of others' perspectives and an increasing tolerance for their own uncomfortable feelings and conflicts, leading to greater empathy and more flexible social understanding. The tendency to focus on others' perceived rule violations diminishes, and more complex notions of reciprocity and mutual respect are integrated into children's sense of values and ideals. Moreover, as superego capacities gain in autonomy, self-responsibility is on the rise and the looming presence of adult authority is less of a presence in children's moral judgments.

The latency child's gradual acquisition of *insight* is an ongoing cognitive and affective process that continues well into adolescence; insightful capacities require that the child tolerate sustained self-observation and self-critique, endure inner discomforts, and avoid seeking external sources of blame and responsibility. Although older school-age children, like their younger counterparts, often embrace external, practical solutions for emotional problems, they begin to engage in introspection, reflecting on their own mental states and imagining more creative resolutions to complex social dilemmas (Jemerin 2004; Kennedy 1979; Schmukler 1999).

The following vignette depicts the typical thinking and behavior of the latency child when confronted with a challenging situation. In this case, a young girl's vivid imagination, developing sense of the wider world, and deepening empathy for the plight of others creates conflicts with more self-serving urges. Emma's yearnings to be good and to be acknowledged for moral actions makes her an eager participant in her school's social action projects. Nonetheless, she is affected by competitive feelings, a sense of gender superiority, and a rather concrete understanding of ethics. On this occasion, she happily assumes responsibility for her third-grade classroom's food drive, designed to provide relief for children who were victims of a foreign country's recent natural disaster.

Emma, age 8½ years, was an excellent student, a dedicated creative writer, and a popular playmate whose teacher described her as a "natural leader" within the classroom. Often, she could be found rallying her friends to perform a short skit she had written or volunteering to carry the attendance papers from her classroom to the office. She always remembered to bring a cupcake to the school secretary when a student celebrated his or her birthday at school. It was no surprise when the plight of one group of vulnerable children, brought to her attention by older, admired fifth-grade girls, captured Emma's imagination. Almost overnight, she assumed an organizing role for her classroom's food drive and began assigning tasks to her female friends. Emma spoke warmly about the afflicted youngsters who were suffering from hunger and disease. Of her own accord, she begged her parents to withhold a month's allowance and contribute it to a foundation that would direct her funds toward providing food and shelter. During the school day and before bed, she fantasized about a future meeting with a young girl she would sponsor. In this highly gratifying daydream, the girl and her family would journey to America and Emma would be awarded a special prize for saving her life; they would become permanent friends.

At first, Emma's teacher was pleased to allow Emma a familiar, prominent role in the collection of food and clothing. Soon, however, complaints began to pour in. A number of boys asserted that Emma would not let them do anything other than stack food cans. When the teacher questioned her, Emma defended these actions, claiming that the boys were "messy" and that "girls thought of the food drive first." Soon, however, a number of female third graders also criticized the arrangements as "unfair," protesting that Emma was reserving the most interesting jobs (i.e., writing letters to the children and accompanying the food to a local organizational center) for herself and her best friends. Once again, the teacher delicately approached Emma, who responded that the letters should be written by girls with the best handwriting, who happened to be her chums. The teacher gently explained that other children were feeling left out and reminded Emma that concern for the young population abroad was the main principle of the project. Emma grew teary but complied with the teacher's suggestion that everyone be allowed to participate in all aspects of the food drive. She even accepted the teacher's appointment of a male co-leader. Although Emma's outward behavior was compliant and conciliatory, she complained bitterly to her mother that night about the teacher's "meanness" and hotly protested Matthew's appointment as her partner in the project.

In this instance, a latency child's dawning social conscience and kindly inclinations are limited by a lack of emotional self-awareness and age-typical desires to be recognized and praised. Emma's sympathy for the distressed children is keenly felt, but her urge to convert those feelings into praiseworthy actions is more powerful than her capacity to recognize less than empathic behavior toward those closer to home. She does not question her own entitlement to a leadership role, her desire to elevate a close circle of best friends, her dismissive attitude toward boys, and her exclusionary behavior toward less favored girls. Her teacher tactfully rescues the situation and allows the child to retain a sense of self-respect and an important role in the project. Despite Emma's apparent resentment after the fact, she benefits from her private consultation with the teacher and from the proffered insight into her classmates' experience.

Cognitive Maturation During Latency

- Entry into the *concrete operational* period of cognitive development transforms mental life, increasing capacity for mental, rather than action-based, thinking.

- Children begin to plan, organize, and control personal behavior as well as regulate emotional reactions.

- New opportunities for *sublimations* proliferate, such as academic and creative channels.

- Attitudes toward gender roles and characteristics tend to be categorical and conventional.

- Moral and social reasoning is concrete and not yet autonomous. Children favor black-and-white rules, eagerly condemn others for perceived transgressions (while avoiding their own feelings of guilt and self-judgment), and heavily weigh anticipation of adults' reactions in their moral judgments.

- *Insight* and *self-reflection* are gradually achieved, leading to more flexible attitudes and acceptance of personal responsibility.

THE PHASES OF LATENCY

The period of latency has been usefully divided into two rough segments, elaborated in the following subsections. This division underscores the marked differences in maturity in the early and late grade-school years. The awkward and inconsistent relationship to self-regulation, the struggle to consolidate the internalized voice of conscience, the reliance on concrete thinking, and the confidence in managing peer interactions of the early latency years mature dramatically in the later period. The child's focus decisively turns away from family toward school and peer group. These internal shifts are accompanied by considerable changes in external expectations.

Early Latency and the Child's Struggle for Self-Control

The early phase of latency, between ages 6 and 8 years, is dominated by the child's recently acquired partial mastery over feelings and impulses. The turbulence of the oedipal phase is not yet safely in the distant past; the child's capacities for self-control and emotional regulation are easily taxed and frequently overwhelmed. Identification with parental values and repression of sexual and aggressive feelings are under way but not fully consolidated, and the child's self-management often breaks down. This brittle state of self-regulation disposes the child toward a rigid sense of rules and punishments; he or she feels most secure with very clear-cut guidelines and procedures (Mahon 1991; Tyson and Tyson 1990). One 6-year-old girl, whose inconsistent self-control led to deep satisfaction with the simplistic, easily accessible rules of pedestrian traffic, admonished her mother for crossing the street on a yellow light; when her parent casually responded that she was an adult and therefore able to judge what was safe, the child stamped her foot and retorted, "You can't cross until it's green. The crossing guard says so!" As the child's social world extends beyond the parents, new authority figures must be accommodated and integrated into the existing internal moral "voice."

Teachers, coaches, and community figures begin to assume increasing importance as admired sources of identification.

The young latency child's self-esteem and sense of competence is fragile. Struggles to acquire new skills, such as reading, often cause frustration; tears and protests over homework are common for the first and second grader. Moreover, the entry into grade school and the requirements of the lengthy academic day—prolonged separation from family, sustained periods of attention, academic tasks, and evaluations—are daunting after the relatively loose structure of the pre-elementary years. New methods for social engagement must be learned; expectations and responses from teachers and peers differ dramatically from those at home. Many children experience an internal sense of disconnection and aloneness and a feeling of having been "pushed out into the world outside their home" (Knight 2005, p. 186). The considerable demands of the nonfamilial world and the child's own fledgling inner resources contribute to an overall shaky sense of self (Freedman 1996).

Initially, the child experiences his or her increasing internal awareness of morality and personal wrongdoing as a burden. A child psychoanalyst, Berta Bornstein (1951), famously likened the nascent superego to the presence of a mental "foreign body." The intense novel discomfort of guilt feelings causes the youngster to engage in a number of defensive maneuvers, as he or she attempts to rid the self of unfamiliar and disturbing reactions. The externalization of superego struggles and attitudes, a process wherein children create environmental battles to avoid more painful inner feelings and conflicts, is a major mode of coping. For example, the young latency child may repeatedly provoke or resist adult authority, eliciting punishment from without rather than dealing with painful self-recrimination. Such actions cause considerable consternation in adults who are unprepared for the youngster's noncompliance; however, retribution from outside figures is less unbearable for children than their own harsh and inflexible self-reproaches.

The child derives intense satisfaction from scrutinizing and exposing the misdeeds of others; such revelations are a welcome relief from internal self-monitoring and guilt. Complaints of the world's unfairness are common. The inner superego "voice" is often attributed to persons outside of the self; for example, teachers are frequently experienced as mean or strict, even when there is little supporting evidence for such claims (Furman 1980). At the same time, the child's own behavior may be substantially out of sync with the standards he or she demands from others. As Tyson and Tyson (1990), two noteworthy child clinicians, observe, "the child may appear at one moment to be a budding delinquent with no internalized moral standards; at the next moment he may be excessively moral and, like a police officer, supervise and report on the transgressions of others..." (p. 221).

• **See the first two videos on latency, "7-Year-Old Girl" and "7-Year-Old Boy," for illustrations of children's discomfort with negative feelings, their concerns about fairness, and their tendency toward concrete or external sources of blame for conflicts.**

The following vignette illustrates typical, normative early latency behaviors and attitudes that parents often find puzzling. This 6-year-old child's complaints about unfair conditions, her rigid sense of rules, and her unfailing enthusiasm for tattling are highly inconsistent with her own minor but frequent transgressions. Her brittle self-esteem, ready tears, and angry refusals to acknowledge personal wrongdoing are frustrating to her parents, who maintain that she should assume greater personal responsibility for her own actions. The entire family often feels that they must tread carefully lest they set off a bout of Talia's crying and recriminations.

> Talia, age 6 years, had recently started first grade. She was happy and excited about school and loved playdates with her friends. She had adjusted extremely well to preschool and kindergarten, and her parents expected a similar adaptation to elementary school. However, late afternoons and early evenings were stressful; she was often fussy and fatigued after the school day. Moreover, although there was only a single, 10-minute homework assignment per night, this short period frequently ended in tears and protests; she would demand help from her mother or babysitter but then reproach herself by repeating, "My teacher wants me to do it all by myself." In a phone call with Talia's worried parents, the teacher recalled that she had once casually mentioned that students should attempt assignments on their own, but she had never intended to discourage them from seeking adult help if they felt stuck; she suggested that Talia might have interpreted her remarks too concretely but she would work to resolve the misunderstanding the next day. She further reassured the parents that Talia's academic progress was on target and that the behaviors they were describing, such as falling apart over homework, were typical of adjustment in early first grade.
>
> Although Talia and her 9-year-old sister had always been close, their play was now frequently interrupted by the younger child's recently increased crying and complaining. Often, she would run to her mother to announce that her sister was "mean" and to report on minor bickering and comments. Her sister was becoming impatient and sometimes called Talia a "tattletale," resulting in further crying. Talia's own unabashed name calling and rampant cheating at games contrasted sharply with her eagle eye for her older sibling's small errors and misbehaviors. Her mother found herself becoming annoyed at Talia; it was hard to reconcile the child's newfound independence, such as her insistence on setting out her own clothes and drawing her own bath, with these almost daily lapses into babyishness. To her chagrin, her mother realized she was losing her temper and scolding Talia much more frequently than in the past.
>
> Talia enjoyed pretend play, but she had recently developed a fondness for board games, particularly those that featured nonnegotiable rules governing

the gradual acquisition of material possessions. The entire family tensed when she insisted on playing such games, however. Talia's comprehension of the more complex procedures was limited, and she would regularly dissolve into tears if she lost or failed to procure the desired items. Often, she would beg her parents and sister to play with her and promise that she would neither cheat nor cry. However, such resolve would quickly fall apart once the game was under way. She would angrily accuse others of cheating and meanness and declare "that's not fair" whenever another player enjoyed an advantage. At the same time, she would insist on redoing her own turns and would furtively attempt to acquire small tokens and play money that she had not actually earned. Her parents attempted to reason with her and remind her of her promises. Her lack of personal responsibility and truthfulness bothered them, although they had witnessed similar trends with their older daughter and these were gradually outgrown. Most confusing was Talia's calm, cooperative attitude most hours of the day, her insistence that others follow rules and regulations, and her heartfelt desire to be good. Another brief conversation with the classroom teacher helped restore the parents' confidence that Talia's overall social and academic adjustment was typical and that she would soon develop better tolerance for frustration.

Despite their impatience and discomfort with her various behaviors, these parents draw on their memories of their older child and their positive relationship with Talia's teacher to gain empathy and reassurance. They realize that Talia is trying hard to accommodate the many challenges and novel demands of the school day and that it is a strain for her to maintain composure beyond the three o'clock bell; moreover, they can see that her rigid interpretations of parameters and her harsh, self-imposed standards are contributing to inner discomfort and external tensions. Such understanding helps them avoid criticizing and punishing her, reactions that would only gratify her desire to embroil the family in conflicts so as to avoid her own internal stress and guilt feelings.

By contrast, the next example depicts a child who required therapeutic intervention to resolve mounting social and behavioral problems. Eight-year-old Tom struggles to achieve the self-regulation that is necessary to meet early latency expectations, such as getting along with classmates and managing brief periods of unstructured time. His use of adults as external sources of punishment is intensifying, and he frequently engages in both verbal and physical aggression. On the playground, his reputation as a bully and a bother grows; almost daily, he interrupts the boys' kickball or dodgeball games by pushing or yelling about the rules. Both teachers and parents respond with a host of punishments and consequences, none of which seem terribly effective.

At the recommendation of his school, 8-year-old Tom's parents sought consultation with a child psychologist. Tom's verbal skills had been precocious, while his fine-motor development was somewhat slow. His parents noted difficulties with self-regulation in excess of what they observed in other children, but they assumed that maturity would bring improved self-control. His preschool and kindergarten experiences were mostly positive, although he had struggled with basic handwriting skills and had sometimes erupted in anger when his poor eye-hand coordination interfered with his activities. Increasingly, these bouts of anger involved blaming another student or the teacher for his failures. In first grade, he excelled at reading but continued to have trouble with writing, and his difficulty managing anger was more pronounced. His parents noticed that he began to refuse playdates, but he seemed content to play with his cousins on the weekends, so his parents were not unduly concerned.

However, almost from the first week of the second-grade year, his parents had been repeatedly summoned to his class for teacher conferences. In addition, a meeting with the school principal was arranged wherein she disclosed that Tom's behavior was becoming increasingly problematic. Tom's teacher described him as very bright but oppositional; often, he would defy her instructions or openly challenge her authority. On a couple of occasions, he walked out of the classroom. Despite his own lack of self-control, Tom would insist that other children adhere to the exact rules of board and sports games and would immediately complain if there were infractions. During recess, he interrupted games by relentlessly arguing and calling the other children "stupid"; on a couple of occasions, he pushed boys who had refused to listen to him. Inevitably, an adult would intervene, caution Tom about the need to calm down, and ultimately threaten him with expulsion from playtime. Tom would protest and occasionally retort with rudeness, ending in the now-routine consequence of no recess.

When a psychologist met with Tom, the child soon re-created a conflictual situation. He resisted the few rules of the psychologist's playroom, such as no hitting or breaking toys. Moreover, he was often rude and insulting, demeaning her knowledge and skill at board games and exclaiming over her ignorance of sports statistics. Her calm responses and failure to engage in punishment elicited anxiety in Tom. However, as they played together, she gently pointed out that he himself felt ignorant, feared the exposure of his own weaknesses, and suffered shame from his bouts of poor self-management. She found opportunities to elaborate his inner struggles to be good and linked these to his guilty desires for external punishment. Tom's parents and teachers were advised to provide him with structure and supervision and to initiate extra help for handwriting, but to avoid overreacting and harsh punishments so that Tom could gradually assume responsibility for his own behavior. In addition, he was referred for psychological testing to determine whether an underlying biologically based attentional problem might be contributing to his poor self-control. Continued play therapy helped him expand his tolerance for uncomfortable conflicts and feelings. Over the course of the second-grade year, Tom's provocative behaviors diminished gradually and he began to derive pride from his very considerable intellectual achievements in reading and classroom discussions.

In this case, Tom's underlying problems with attention and self-regulation, in combination with real weaknesses in fine-motor coordination, lead to deep self-esteem injuries, a greater than average intolerance for uncomfortable feelings and conflicts, and an intensified version of typical early latency behavioral difficulties. His externalizing tendencies, such as accusing others of weakness and ignorance, involving other children and adults in conflicts, and eliciting punishment from authority figures, are highly disruptive and interfere with his ability to engage in key developmental tasks of middle childhood, such as group socialization. Although he had been able to cope with the limited expectations of the preschool and kindergarten environments, the first- and second-grade classrooms require more structured writing skills and increased self-discipline, areas in which Tom suffers real deficits and a growing sense of inadequacy.

The Later Phase of Latency, the Shift Toward Self-Regulation, and the Role of Fantasy

Between ages 8 and 10 or 11, the years often referred to as *middle childhood,* the latency child is increasingly immersed in reality-based events and challenges. Academic achievement, extracurricular involvements, and peer relationships become major determinants of positive self-esteem. Augmented parental and societal expectations parallel the maturation of the child's ego capacities, such as self-regulation and impulse control. Outwardly, the older latency child appears far more competent, independent, and solid than the fragile, inconsistently self-contained 6- or 7-year-old. Internally, emotional investment gradually shifts away from the nuclear family and toward the widening world of classmates and other adults. A growing sense of confidence, autonomy, and desire for friendships creates a powerful push toward peers (Knight 2005). Inevitably, children's engagement in the surrounding culture and deepening experiences with people beyond the family lead to more realistic views of the parents; more realistic, less idealized parental images reinforce a sense of the self as separate and self-reliant, but also lonely and bereft.

• See the third video example of latency development, "10-Year-Old Male Friends" for an illustration of older children's more flexible, reflective capacity to contemplate relationships.

The shaky self-management and rigid, rule-bound outlook of the early latency period gradually yield to greater composure and more nuanced interpretations of interpersonal and moral situations. Less threatened by internal eruptions and better able to grasp multiple perspectives, the 8- to 10-year-old child is far better equipped to handle unpredictable or frustrating aspects of group situations with resourcefulness and flexibility. Exceptions to the rules, last-minute changes, or modifications to the known procedures are increasingly tolerated. As a result, social relationships and organized group activities are more rewarding and begin to assume enormous importance as sources of connection and pride.

In contrast to the 6- or 7-year-old, who may routinely engage in pretend play, the older latency child is increasingly drawn to more structured and challenging activities, such as board games and sports; unlike the freewheeling nature of fantasy-based play, rule-governed pastimes are precise and demand far greater self-control (Piaget 1962). Many children continue to enjoy pretend activities, but these are often diminished, restricted to solitary time or manifested only within certain peer relationships. Although less creative, the organized play of older children provides essential outlets for intense feelings as well as opportunities for socialization, identification, and self-regulation. Varied experiences and roles, such as loser and winner or leader and follower, help the older latency child practice self-discipline, develop empathy for others' situations, tolerate disappointing outcomes, and handle winning with graciousness. Moreover, as participants in well-defined teams or clubs, children achieve deepening identities with the common interests and goals of a nonfamilial community. These identifications provide a sense of belonging and shared values as the child's idealization of and dependency on the parents begins to decline.

Fantasizing and daydreaming are central to the latency child's private experience, providing emotional compensation for the inevitable frustrations and disappointments of the reality-based world (Knight 2005; Sarnoff 1971). Loss of the previously held idealized image of the parents and dawning realizations about personal strengths and weaknesses can be assuaged by the child's wishful adventures and identifications. A universal example is the *family romance*, a latency adoption fantasy wherein the biological connection to the real-life parents is denied; in its place, the child envisions a special heritage that has been lost but may at some point be regained (e.g., he or she was born of royal lineage, but somehow separated from the original mother and father; the current, very ordinary parents serve as temporary adoptive substitutes until the child can reclaim the special destiny of birth). Such fantasies allow latency youngsters to revert to an earlier developmental time when the parental figures were venerated; current ambivalent and disappointed feelings toward the real parents are avoided (A. Freud 1963). However, for the latency child with a true history of adoption, the family romance accrues additional meanings and functions and may not provide the same playful benefits (Bonovitz 2004; Brinich 1995). The entry into middle childhood brings increased awareness of the adoption situation; children are now able to contemplate the thoughts and feelings of both biological and adoptive parents, often leading to increased speculation about birth conditions and a more intensified realization of having been "given away." For some adopted children, the family romance fantasy reflects idealization of the birth parents and devaluation of the adoptive couple.

The latency child's enhanced awareness of and exposure to the world beyond the family broadens the potential contents of daydreams and imaginative scenarios. Independent reading brings exposure to an array of literary adventures with heroes and heroines; latency favorites tend to include stories about clever youngsters and teens who win the admiration of their peers by employing special powers, magical abilities, and their own wits to tackle adult-size dilemmas and solve mysteries that elude the older generation. In addition, children begin to esteem real-life characters, such as athletes or entertainers, whose achievements and widespread acclaim resonate with their own intense desires for mastery and recognition. Grandiose themes are common, and the child derives great satisfaction from daydreams in which fame and glory are attained; these imagined accomplishments help motivate grade-school students toward industry and perseverance as they cope with the frustrating and often rote repetitive tasks and practicing that pervade their daily lives (Novick and Novick 1996).

The Phases of Latency

- The early phase of latency (ages 6–8 years) is dominated by recently acquired, shaky superego capacities, leading to unreliable self-regulation and rigid attitudes.

- Intense discomfort with inner guilt feelings and self-blame leads to avid interest in others' rule transgressions and to externalization of superego attitudes.

- The later phase of latency (ages 8–10 or 11 years) is characterized by better self-regulation, greater flexibility, and more extensive involvement in peer socialization.

- Adventurous and grandiose fantasies, including the *family romance,* serve to compensate for the loss of idealized images of the parents and for fears of inadequacy as the child faces the myriad, often daunting tasks of latency.

THE EXPANDING SOCIAL WORLD OF THE LATENCY CHILD

The Importance of Peer Relationships and the Role of Emotional Self-Regulation

The capacity to form peer relationships is a critical social-emotional achievement for the latency child. One-on-one friendships and perceived status within the cohort are increasingly integrated into the child's self-feelings and sense of competence; indeed, the development of positive peer bonds during the grade school years is foundational for later social connections (Bemporad 1984). A desire for peer group acceptance begins to sharpen during middle childhood, fueled by decreased intimacy with the parents, desire for a sense of belonging, and heightened insight into others' feelings and opinions. Importantly, low friendship status and peer rejection during latency are antecedents for a wide range of psychological and behavioral difficulties; lack of "friendedness" creates vulnerabilities to loneliness and feelings of isolation in early adolescence (Pedersen et al. 2007). Moreover, chronic peer group rejection and maltreatment (e.g., forms of bullying) predict future disengagement from school (Buhs et al. 2006).

Social adjustment, emotional self-regulation, and positive self-regard are increasingly interrelated during the latency phase. The school-age child's enhanced superego functioning—that is, the capacity to cope with uncomfortable feelings, avoid impulsive reactions, and engage in increasingly independent self-management—forms the foundation for a "relatively autonomous and reasonable source of self-regulation and self-esteem" (Novick and Novick 1994, p. 158). A substantial body of empirical work suggests that poor behavioral and emotional control is linked to peer rejection in middle childhood, whereas high levels of self-regulation are correlated with competent social functioning (e.g., Contreras et al. 2000; Eisenberg et al. 1996, 1997; Pedersen et al. 2007). Those who are often in the company of school-age children can attest to their keen awareness of peers' relative success or failure at autonomous self-control; the latency child who cries inconsolably after losing a game or erupts into anger and verbal attacks when frustrated is vulnerable to both self-criticism and disapproving attitudes from others.

Gender-Divided Groups in Latency

Consolidation of gender identity and the acquisition of peer norms are major, interrelated tasks of childhood; whereas the former is deeply influenced by adult role models, the latter is primarily child generated (Sroufe et al. 1993; Tyson 1982). The social world of latency is visibly gender divided; a glance into elementary school yards quickly reveals the dominant social pattern, namely same-sex groups of children. Firm gender boundaries, often sustained via elaborate child-created rules and consequences, are prominent during the latency years (for example, one group of third-grade boys was heard loudly threatening to exclude a male friend from their daily game of tag if he invited girls to his birthday party). Large portions of free-play time are devoted to same-sex company, whether in groups or in one-on-one friendships. As the latency period draws to an end and prepubertal development commences, the social gender divide persists, but considerable interest in and conversation about the opposite sex begins to emerge (Sroufe et al. 1993).

Gender-based boundaries and behaviors provide developmental benefits, but the rigidity and conformity of latency society pose serious challenges for children whose feelings and behaviors defy neat gender categorization (Egan and Perry 2001). Contentment with one's biological sex, feelings of gender compatibility, and felt freedom to explore gender flexibility, if so desired, are correlated with positive social adjustment, whereas the experience of pressure to conform to gender stereotypes is a hindrance to social development (Egan and Perry 2001). However, consolidation of feminine and masculine identity, a sense of social pride, and feelings of gender compatibility are among the positive consequences of same-sex groups and their typical activities, such as girls' secret-telling and rope-jumping, boys' rough-and-tumble games, and the team sports of both groups (Friedman and Downey 2008; Kulish 2002). The tendency toward gender chauvinism in childhood may even contribute to greater feelings of belonging, self-definition, and self-esteem, while gender divisions also help the latency child shore up defenses against oedipal desires. As discussed in the section "Cognitive Maturation and the Mind of the Latency Child" earlier in this chapter, concrete and categorical views of gender are compatible with the school-age child's intellectual style; indeed, by the time they enter the latency phase, children already possess entrenched, inflexible views about gender qualities (Giles and Heyman 2005).

The protracted time spent in the company of same-sex peers provides constant reinforcement of gendered conventions and behaviors (Friedman and Downey 2000; Maccoby 2002). Boys' play is action oriented, often reflecting themes of danger and overt conflict; female games are often less physical and tend toward domestic and romantic contents. The quality of male and female relationships during latency is distinct as well: girls' friendships are more likely to involve intimate sharing about each other's lives, whereas boys' bonds are often rooted in mutual actions and activities, with minimal knowledge of each other's personal experiences and attitudes (Maccoby 2002). In groups, boys are observed to be competitive and exclusionary; hierarchical organization is common, topped by certain dominant males (Friedman and Downey 2000). Girls' groups are comparatively less aggressive and more tolerant, but female hostility is manifest via "relational aggression" (i.e., tight-knit cliques and mean-spirited attitudes toward nonmembers) (Crick and Grotpeter 1995; Friedman and Downey 2008).

As the latency child's dependency on the parent declines, membership in same-sex friendships and groups provides a powerful compensatory sense of community and connection (Knight 2005). Friedman and Downey

(2008) note that all-male peer groups appear to play an especially critical role in fostering "gender-valued self-esteem" for boys in middle childhood; failure to achieve such group affiliations can result in lowered self-worth and deep feelings of isolation. These authors suggest that for all children, "the painful effects of being ostracized or carrying a label of low status by same-gendered peer groups during middle and late childhood are often felt for life" (Friedman and Downey 2008, p. 153).

The following examples demonstrate gender-segregated play and attitudes that are commonly observed during middle childhood.

Three 6-year-old girls, who had each brought their small toy ponies and accoutrements from home, carried these carefully out to the schoolyard during recess. They began to brush the ponies' long hair and soon agreed on a pretend play scenario wherein the blue-haired pony would be a prince and the two pink-haired ponies would be princesses.

Two 9-year-old girls, known to the entire grade as best friends who often had playdates together, huddled in a corner of the school yard while making an origami fortune teller (a complexly folded paper construction with written "predictions"). Once it was assembled, they eagerly lured numerous other girls to engage in fortune-telling play. At one point, a few boys ran over to see what was going on, but the girls shrieked and insisted that they leave; after delivering some taunting remarks, the boys returned to playing kickball. The two best friends began to tell the fortunes of the other girls; with certain peers, they gleefully giggled when the predictions (most of which involved forecasts about marriage and family) were negative. At one point, a girl who received bad "news" began to cry; this caught the attention of the adult monitor, who scolded the two instigators, provided brief comfort to the distressed child, and confiscated the fortune teller.

Half a dozen 10-year-old boys spontaneously erupted into a game of tag, but disagreements soon arose over the location and rules of home base. Much shouting and gesticulating was involved; one boy, taller than the rest and known as a competent athlete, naturally assumed a leadership role, but even his pronouncements did not entirely put an end to the conflicts. The game was stopped and started numerous times as fresh quarrels broke out. Twenty minutes later, when recess was called to an end, the game had never really gotten under way. The boys were all annoyed, blaming each other for the loss of playing time.

Jenny, age 11 years, was the best female athlete in fifth grade, known throughout the school for her speed and skill. Although some of the girls referred to her as a tomboy, they nonetheless admired her ability to outrun the boys and took pleasure in the ensuing male frustration. During field day in late June, when girls and boys competed in a running event, Jenny's entire female cohort cheered her on as she raced past the finish line ahead of the boys.

A number of typical gender-segregated latency games and pastimes reveal children's use of ritual and symbolization to manage "freshly repressed desires" (Clowes 1996, p. 438). For girls, games with repetitive components—such as hand-clapping or jump-roping to accompanying rhymes—serve to assuage gender-related anxieties and provide expression for sexual and aggressive feelings; both the actions and verbalizations of these activities offer a structured, playful, and highly socialized channel for sensual movement and themes of sexuality, aggression, and rivalry (Goldings 1974). Similarly, the typically off-color, private joking of older latency boys often reveals oedipal themes and fears, such as sexual conquests, bodily injury, and feared loss of masculinity. Joking with peers and sharing overtly sexual material allows school-age boys to defuse deep-rooted apprehensions and redirect impulses in a safe setting; a sense of group support and affiliation further reduces the intensity of bodily based anxieties.

The Parent-Child Relationship

The latency child's increasing autonomy and engagement in nonfamilial life fuel a deepening sense of separateness from the parents. School-based achievements and new friendships bring feelings of pride and a sense of belonging, but the many hours spent away from home and the loss of parent-child closeness induce loneliness and a sense of being adrift. The child must adjust to the demands, expectations, and reactions of the peer group, all of which are dramatically different from those of parents and siblings (Friedman and Downey 2008). Often, parents push children toward self-reliance, encouraging activities beyond the home and enrolling them in various after-school pursuits (Knight 2005). As the child acquires more independent self-control and becomes less dependent on the parent's physical presence, the unique intimacies of the earlier parent-child bond are relinquished and mourned. This painful process engenders both guilt and satisfaction; the latency child comes to terms with a diminished view of the parents while discovering his or her own newfound competencies (Loewald 1979).

Despite the inevitable transition toward greater freedom and independence, however, a positive ongoing relationship with the parents and a history of strong parent-child bonding are instrumental for the latency child's autonomous functioning and broadening social horizons. Secure attachment, as measured in infancy, is highly correlated with age-appropriate self-regulatory capacities, relative freedom from behavioral difficulties, and social competence during middle childhood (Cohn 1990; Contreras et al. 2000). Moreover, parental support for the child's separateness and autonomy in early childhood has been shown to predict self-reliance and good academic adjustment during the school years (National Institute of Child Health and Human Development 2008). The specific role of fathers in the development of latency children is less well researched, but several studies suggest that the male parent increasingly provides a source of support and mentorship for boys in middle childhood (e.g., Diamond 1998; Knight 2005).

Empirical observation of mother-child attachment during latency suggests that secure and anxious patterns of relating are highly stable from infancy to middle childhood and continue to profoundly affect key social and emotional developments. Two major studies (Main and Cassidy 1988; Main et al. 1985) assessed latency children's attachment by measuring separation behavior and evaluating responses to a series of photos that depict impending parental departures. (In this latter condition, subjects were asked to describe how the children in the pictures might be feeling and to discuss hypothetical resolutions to separation.) Children who were previously classified as "securely attached" manifested open, emotionally rich verbal and nonverbal exchanges with their mothers; when reunited after a short separation, they demonstrated pleasure in the parent's return and engaged in fluent verbal discourse, often reporting on their activities during her absence. When confronted with separation photos, these well-attached youngsters talked freely about feeling states and engaged in problem-solving discussions. As noted by Main et al. (1985), "the secure six-year-olds seemed to have free ranging access to affect, memory and plans, whether in forming speech in conversation with the parent or in discussing imagined situations relevant to attachment" (p. 95). In contrast, insecurely attached children displayed controlling and critical attitudes toward the mother and manifested an overt lack of interest or ambivalent, approach-avoidance behavior upon her return. They responded to the pictures with muted or overly aroused emotional states, and their suggestions for behavioral solutions lacked coherence and relevance.

LEARNING AND THE IMPORTANCE OF ACADEMIC LIFE

Learning, Self-Esteem, and the Impact of Learning Disabilities

The latency child's cognitive maturation, enhanced self-control, and intense desire for mastery contribute to unprecedented availability for learning. Between ages 6 and 11, the primary school student is expected to absorb vast quantities of knowledge and master a diverse set of skills. In combination with familial and peer relationships, educational environments powerfully influence the child's evolving sense of competency and social connection; they provide an ongoing source of intellectual and interpersonal experience, and they are frequently the setting for creative and athletic pursuits as well. Major developmental achievements of the latency period include a capacity for industry, productivity, and perseverance in the face of frustration; sustained motivation and goal-oriented attitudes toward learning and work form an essential foundation for successful negotiation of the elementary years and beyond (Erikson 1950). In addition, the child's receptivity to learning hinges on calm inner states; his or her ability to cope with separation and performance anxieties and to manage personal feelings and impulses are major determinants of school adjustment. Not surprisingly, a number of learning, anxiety, and developmental disorders—such as school phobias and the range of academic and attentional problems—are uncovered (and may ultimately rise to the level of clinical concern) under the pressures and expectations of the school setting. Here, we briefly discuss some of the specific learning and developmental impediments that directly affect academic skills and more broadly impede ego capacities during the latency phase.

As one 9-year-old girl described, following a day when her ongoing struggles with reading were a subject of her peers' lively lunchroom discussion, the classroom can feel like "a fishbowl where I'm swimming around and everyone is looking, waiting to catch my mistakes." Individual strengths and weaknesses are vividly displayed and relentlessly evaluated in the school environment. As numerous writers have described (e.g., Gilmore 2002; Novick and Novick 2004; Rothstein 1998), the child's sense of self is increasingly intertwined with learning successes and failures. Learning delays, which typically manifest in the first or second grade, pose serious threats to the child's feelings of mastery and social acceptance, particularly as the latency peer group gains heightened awareness of individuals' skill levels. Even minor delays in achievement can profoundly affect the child's experience; slow oral readers or children with immature handwriting encounter daily and highly public reminders of their obstacles, making them vulnerable to social embarrassment, performance anxiety, and diminished pleasure in learning. Reading and writing delays are particularly painful for the latency child given the enormous emphasis that standard curricula place on assessing literacy and the typical classroom divisions of "high" and "low" reading groups. Grade-school children tend to be acutely conscious of such distinctions and are well aware of strong versus weaker reading students. On a less overt level, unconscious fantasies about personal defects, which deeply influence self-views long after the school experience is finished, may begin to coalesce around perceived limits and disabilities (Coen 1986).

Although definitions vary, *learning disabilities* currently are conceived as reflecting specific neurological impairments that hamper the child's acquisition of basic academic skills. Recent studies (e.g., Tanaka et al. 2011) employing functional magnetic resonance imaging support the presence of neural deficits. Such disabilities, which encompass a sweeping range of disorders in the areas of listening, spelling, reading, writing, and arithmetic, are estimated to affect at least 4%–6% of schoolchildren, although a number of studies suggest substantially higher percentages (Chalfant 1989; Kavale and Forness 2000; Shaywitz et al. 1992). Rates of comorbidity for depression, attentional problems, anxiety, social difficulties, and somatic complaints are elevated within the learning disabled population (San Miguel et al. 1996; Sideridis et al. 2006; Willcutt and Pennington 2000). In the following two subsections, we describe two common disorders and their far-reaching implications for the latency child's learning experience, social-emotional development, and maturing ego structure.

Reading Delays

Dyslexia is a common learning disability estimated to affect 5%–10% (some studies suggest considerably higher rates) of children in the elementary grades and to account for up to 80% of the general learning disabled population. The major feature of this disorder is weak phonological processing, often severely hampering the child's acquisition of reading fluency and spelling skills (Gabrieli 2009; Hudson et al. 2007; Lyon et al. 2003; Shaywitz 1998). Children with dyslexia frequently have comorbid conditions, such as problems with attention, further complicating their intellectual and psychological development. Reading delays, not all of which are related to dyslexia, are particularly challenging in the school environment, affecting a wide range of subjects. Whereas children with dyslexia often encounter immediate difficulty due to their weakness in language decoding, "late-emerging poor readers" initially demonstrate reading competence but then gradually fall behind in the later grades as comprehension demands increase (Catts et al. 2012). These slightly older children possess an even sharper sense of self-other comparison and must manage a peer group experience wherein concerns about personal status and social acceptance are on the rise.

Life beyond the classroom is fundamentally altered as well. The child in early or late latency who struggles with literacy and who associates reading with anxiety and frustration lacks easy access to developmentally appropriate tools for sublimation and self-regulation. Pleasurable reading and goal-oriented research, as well as the fantasizing that is evoked by fictional stories, are important ways in which the school-age child channels intense feelings and desires. When reading mastery is especially arduous, such activities are often avoided and may become mired in conflict; oppositional behavior at school or refusals to complete homework are common behavioral manifestations. Some children with reading delays seek to hide their struggles. For example, one 8-year-old boy, whose low reading level caused him considerable shame, determinedly sat with chapter books during his classroom's independent reading period, hoping to prevent his teacher and classmates from realizing that he could not comprehend the material. Furthermore, children with underlying language weakness have restricted capacity to recruit verbal self-expression for both communication and emotional regulation; the use of words to symbolize and modulate immediate experience is compromised, making children vulnerable to overstimulation (Arkowitz 2000; Weinstein and Saul 2005).

Attentional Problems

The prevalence of *attention-deficit/hyperactivity disorder* (ADHD) in school-age children is estimated at between 5% and 10%, with rates for boys as much as four times higher than those for girls (Biederman et al. 2002; Centers for Disease Control and Prevention 2010). This disorder, with primary symptoms of poor attentional and behavioral self-control, is highly variable in its presentation. Children with attentional weakness may appear markedly different depending on the setting; moreover, manifestations of the condition shift as children mature. ADHD is correlated with a wide range of functional impairments, including social and emotional delays and well-documented academic problems (Barkley 2006). Although distractibility and impulsivity are often first noted when children enter first or second grade, some studies (e.g., Loe et al. 2008) suggest that behavioral manifestations are evident in the preschool years. In addition to the outward signs of attentional deficits—restlessness, impaired concentration, and failure to complete demanding tasks—the presence of attentional problems impacts children's capacity to integrate and organize both intellectual and affective information, and can interfere substantially with the development of ego capacities and social relationships during the latency phase (Gilmore 2002).

Beginning in the first and second grades, the years when distractibility and impulsivity are often first noted, children are increasingly required to direct and sustain their focus, screen out distractions and extraneous information, and prioritize multiple tasks. Patience and persistence, planning, and management of internal frustrations are necessary to achieve success with typical classroom pursuits. A complex set of cognitive control processes (*executive functions*), which undergo substantial maturation during latency, typically guide the child's ability to adjust to diverse tasks and monitor self-performance, select certain strategies, and inhibit others. When attentional control is weak, children may impulsively respond before a task is fully understood, attend to irrelevant stimuli, or fail to correct obvious errors. Parents and educators often note organizational difficulties, poor time management, and lack of planning. Moreover, although decoding weakness is not a feature of attentional disorders, distractible children often manifest reading delays; they have trouble with such complex tasks as holding information in mind while looking back on the text, and often have gaps in their absorption of relevant material.

Just as importantly, in and out of academic settings, poor attentional and impulse control limits the child's capacity to discern subtle social cues, tolerate interpersonal disappointments, and flexibly adjust to complex, fast-paced peer situations. One very distractible, impulsive 10-year-old boy repeatedly employed a "strategy" for gaining the attention of other children whom he perceived as rejecting; this involved following boys around the classroom and poking them until they grew angry, acknowledged him (negatively), and then sought even further distance. He seemed unable to stop himself, to recognize the adverse consequences of such behavior, or to implement a different approach. This same youngster similarly struggled to absorb nuanced academic information, to refrain from blurting out answers in class, and to avoid distracting his peers through chatter and joking. Such children, highly familiar to classroom educators, often engender strong negative responses in teachers and peers alike as they increasingly experience academic failure and turn to maladaptive behaviors for a sense of acknowledgment and validation.

The Impact of Learning Delays on Social-Emotional Development and Autonomy

Challenges to language, perceptual-motor, memory, or attentional capacities inevitably influence children's developing personality, the quality of their relationships, and their inner sense of confidence and self-reliance. The impact of learning delays during early childhood, before formal learning is initiated, may begin to affect the experience of separation, autonomy, and self-regulation. For example, deficits in either communication or motor coordination can impede the very young child's emerging awareness of self-other differentiation; moreover, memory or perceptual processing delays may interfere with the toddler's and preschooler's growing realization that qualities of the self and others are stable and enduring (Rothstein 1998).

Learning problems manifest in multiple settings. A child's tendency toward social isolation, preference for much younger playmates, fearful or avoidant reactions to new academic activities, lying and cheating behaviors (beyond age expectations), and low tolerance for frustration are familiar social-emotional correlates of weakness in language systems or problems with executive functioning (Rothstein et al. 1988). Furthermore, the academically challenged youngster is often thrown back on adult assistance, requiring extra help to meet educational expectations. Such prolonged dependency interferes with the child's sense of autonomy and independence and with confident immersion in the world beyond the family. Beginning in the early grades, children's social status and acceptance within the peer group are positively linked to good school performance; indeed, successful students begin to select each other as playmates in the latter elementary years (Veronneau et al. 2010).

The following vignette illustrates the expansive social and emotional effects of a mild math delay in a normally developing 8-year-old girl whose overall intellectual capacities are within or beyond average levels. Even though Sharon's difficulty absorbing arithmetic does not formally meet criteria for a learning disability, the fallout from her placement in "special math" class is far-reaching.

> In preschool and kindergarten, Sharon enjoyed success in early readiness skills and social adjustment; however, in the beginning of first grade, she began to encounter difficulty with math. At the beginning of second grade, her teacher suggested that Sharon participate in extra math support, which involved being pulled out of her classroom once a day to attend a small group. For the first month of school, Sharon dissolved into tears nearly every day before and after school, protesting that she did not like being removed from class, that none of her friends were in the small group, and that the other children in her class whispered about her when she left. She insisted that she did not have problems with math and that the teacher made her go to "special math" because she was "mean." Her parents' gentle efforts to reason with Sharon were largely unsuccessful. Although the teacher has tried to assure them that their daughter seems happy enough during the school day, the parents are concerned because Sharon has begun to complain of stomachaches and headaches in the morning, sometimes claiming that she is too sick to go to school. Sharon's pediatrician could find no medical cause for her increasing, psychosomatic symptoms.
>
> Sharon, whose mild learning issues primarily affect arithmetic, nonetheless has begun to develop avoidant behavior toward school. Her headaches and stomachaches are a source of real concern to her parents, particularly because she has always been a child who loved school and looked forward to the social and academic activities of the classroom. She experiences the extra help she is required to accept as an unfair punishment, and feels exposed and embarrassed when she has to leave the mainstream class. Ultimately, support from her parents, reassurance and feedback from her special math and classroom teachers, and the numerous ongoing areas of academic and social satisfaction are sufficient for Sharon to gradually adjust to her situation. A year of extra math support, plus additional tutoring at home, helps her catch up, and she is ready to return to the mainstream group for third grade.

By contrast, the following description illustrates a third-grade child with a more serious and far-reaching learning challenge. Eric has poor attentional capacities that not only make it difficult for him to absorb large amounts of information and achieve good work routines, but also interfere with his overall behavioral, social, and emotional functioning.

> Eric's parents had always seen him as an active, very verbal, and somewhat hard to soothe child. He excelled at sports but sometimes went too far when roughhousing with friends, and had frequent "meltdowns" when frustrated. However, his excellent verbal skills, physical agility, and general good humor had been assets in preschool and kindergarten; there were only occasional complaints that he had trouble settling down or following the group activity. In first and second grades, however, there were more frequent and urgent comments that Eric had trouble following classroom routines and often blurted out answers, forgetting to raise his hand. Nevertheless, his verbal talents contributed to satisfactory academic results, and his parents assumed that he would "grow out of" his overstimulated states.
>
> From the beginning of third grade, the teacher had more serious concerns: Eric habitually distracted his neighbors, talked over the instructor during lessons, and rushed through assignments. His notebooks were a mess, and he was often missing homework. Moreover, he seemed to be developing a "class clown" persona, deriving excitement and satisfaction from disrupting his classmates and insisting on their attention during quiet times. His peers sometimes found him amusing, but many were beginning to express annoyance at his antics. He responded to his classmates' irritation by increasing his activity level, often to the point that the teacher would have to intervene. At home, homework time was becoming more and more unpleasant and conflictual; Eric could not focus on his assignments long enough to complete them and rushed through his work. Academic results were beginning to decline, despite his fine capacity for verbal ideas and conversation.
>
> Eric is unable to achieve the quiet, neutral inner states that are necessary for sustained, typical third-grade work. Unable to focus and increasingly aware of his restlessness and failure to follow the classroom rules, he begins to seek gratification in negative ways. His quick verbal thinking and reactions facilitate clever joking, and his classmates' occasional laughter spurs him on to further heights of overstimulation and jocular behavior. His internal response to his teacher's frequent scolding is immediate shame and regret; discomfort with these feelings leads to further defensive use of humor and action to avoid a sense of poor self-control. Ultimately, at the teacher's recommendation, Eric's parents seek a professional evaluation, leading to diagnosis and treatment for an attentional disorder.

Socialization and Learning During Latency

- Peer relationships, perceived social status, and learning mastery all acquire enormous significance in middle childhood.

- Peer acceptance during primary school is correlated with academic and social adjustments in adolescence.
- Connection to the peer group helps compensate for the latency child's loss of parent-child intimacy and the ensuing feelings of loneliness.
- Well-developed ego capacities, such as behavioral self-control and emotional self-regulation, provide a foundation for latency friendships and contribute to positive regard by self and others.
- Gender-divided group socialization serves to reinforce a sense of identity and belonging but also contributes to conventional and exclusionary attitudes.
- Boys' groups tend toward hierarchical organization, physical actions, overt competitiveness, and chauvinistic attitudes.
- Girls' groups tend toward greater personal intimacy but may employ relational aggression.
- Learning problems and learning disabilities, such as attentional deficits and dyslexia, not only affect the acquisition of academic skills but interfere with the child's sense of mastery and autonomy, socialization, behavioral self-control, and emotional self-regulation.

BRAIN MATURATION AND PHYSICAL DEVELOPMENT DURING LATENCY

The transforming mental developments of latency correspond with a notable frontal lobe growth spurt, reported to occur between ages 5 and 8 or ages 7 and 9 (Anderson 2002; Davies 2010). Although increased myelination, refinement, and efficiency of prefrontal connections are ongoing processes throughout childhood and adolescence, this distinct period of brain maturation is intimately connected to the school-age child's entry into the concrete operational period, unprecedented availability for learning, and increased orientation toward reality. Memory systems, cognitive controls, integration of intellectual processes, absorption of new information and skills, and processing speed are all significantly enhanced (Anderson 2002; Eaton and Ritchot 1995).

The physical growth of the latency child is far less dramatic than during infancy or puberty, but steady gains in stature lead to substantial size changes between ages 7 and 11 years; moreover, growth spurts in middle childhood have been noted at ages 7, 9, and 10 years, with boys beginning to lag behind once girls' earlier pubertal onset gets under way (Butler et al. 1990; Davies 2010; Eaton and Ritchot 1995). Locomotive skills are vastly improved (running, skipping, bicycling), as are fine-motor and visual-motor capacities (e.g., ball handling, handwriting). With increased public health concern over rising rates of childhood obesity, which is estimated to affect nearly one-fifth of U.S. children (Davies 2010), a number of studies have begun to track the lasting effects of sedentary versus active habits during middle childhood (e.g., Janz et al. 2005).

Key Concepts

The child's entry into the period of latency, which roughly spans the ages between 6 and 10 years, signals a momentous shift in mental organization, behavior, and relationships. In contrast to the turbulent oedipal phase, when the child's passionate yearnings and outspoken sexual interests are dominant, the hallmarks of the latency period include cooperation, industrious attitudes, and intense interest in rules and behavioral standards. Children begin to absorb and master a dazzling array of skills and knowledge; their myriad newfound abilities, such as literacy and sports, provide a range of *sublimations* for underlying feelings and conflicts. Moreover, the child's emotional investment and self-esteem are increasingly tied to the world of school, social activities, and peer friendships. The cognitive advances of the *concrete operational* period and concomitant brain maturation, the gradual repression of sexual and aggressive impulses, newfound self-regulatory capacities, and the expectations of the surrounding culture all contribute to the emergence of the latency period.

Within psychodynamic theory, two phases of latency are identified. In the early phase, between ages 6 and 8 years, the child's experience is dominated by recently acquired superego capacities. Self-management is tenuous and fragile and frequently breaks down. However, between ages 8 and 10 years, the child's *ego structure,* composed of coping mechanisms, fantasies, and self-regulatory functions, acquires greater stability. Self-control is far more reliable, and children are better able to engage fully in the world beyond the family. As children traverse latency, feelings about the parents shift toward greater ambivalence and diminished idealization; the *family romance* is a universal latency fantasy wherein the child imagines a more extraordinary family of origin.

Maturation of cognition and self-control, increased independence from the parents, expanded awareness of others' perspectives, and intense desire for mastery create unprecedented availability for learning and group socialization. The formation of same-sex groups, often based on rigidly defined parameters, is a highly visible trend of latency socialization. Success in school, friendships, and status within the peer group are major sources of pride and positive self-regard during middle childhood, with consequence for later academic and social adjustment. The presence of learning challenges or learning disabilities can impede underlying ego capacities and peer relationships as well as acquisition of academic skills.

- A hallmark of the child's entry into the cognitive period of concrete operations is increasingly mental rather than action-oriented problem solving.

  · Myriad cognitive advances and improvements in self-control make the child highly amenable to classroom learning and structured group activities.

  · However, the concrete, "black-and-white" thinking of latency children limits their reasoning about complex notions, such as morality and gender. They tend toward rigid rules and categorical distinctions.

- The early phase of latency (ages 6–8 years) is heavily influenced by the recent acquisition of superego structure and by fragile, incomplete mastery over oedipal desires and impulses.

  · The child erects powerful, rigid defenses against the threat of regressive wishes, leading to insistence on inflexible rules.

  · Externalization of superego attitudes is a major defense.

- The late phase of latency (ages 8–10 years) is characterized by greater internal stability and more reliable inner controls.

  · The child begins to grasp more subtle aspects of morality, understands reciprocity, and adopts a softer stance toward rules.

  · Autonomous functioning and immersion in group socialization are more apparent.

- Peer relationships gain enormous importance during the latency years, helping to compensate for the loss of parent-child intimacy.

  · School-age children who fail to establish close peer connections are vulnerable to diminished self-esteem and feelings of loneliness, both during the latency years and beyond.

- Peer rejection during the primary school years is correlated with an eventual decline in school engagement.

- Emotional and behavioral self-control are important capacities for friendships and peer acceptance.

- A highly visible, child-imposed gender divide leads to
same-sex groups and friendships.

- The child's sense of self and self-esteem are increasingly tied
to competence and success in the learning environment.

  - Learning problems are often first revealed during early years
  of grade school and may have far-reaching consequences
  for the child's academic, social, and self-regulatory development.

  - Dyslexia is a common language-based learning disorder that
  impedes the child's phonological processing and causes
  delays in reading; in addition, underlying linguistic delays
  may lead to problems with self-regulation.

  - Attentional deficits interfere with learning, self-regulation,
  and socialization.

REFERENCES

Anderson P: Assessment and development of executive function (EF) during childhood. Child Neuropsychol 8:71–82, 2002

Arkowitz SW: The overstimulated state of dyslexia: perception, knowledge, and
learning, J Am Psychoanal Assoc 48:1491–1520, 2000

Barkley RA: Attention-Deficit/Hyperactivity Disorder: A Handbook for Diagnosis
and Treatment, 3rd Edition. New York, Guilford, 2006

Bemporad JR: From attachment to affiliation. Am J Psychoanal 44:79–97, 1984

Biederman J, Mick E, Faraone SV, et al: Influence of gender on attention deficit hyperactivity disorder in children referred to a psychiatric clinic. Am J Psychiatry
159:36–42, 2002

Bonovitz C: Unconscious communication and the transition of loss. J Infant Child
Adolesc Psychother 3:1–27, 2004

Bornstein B: On latency. Psychoanal Study Child 6:279–285, 1951

Brinich PM: Psychoanalytic perspectives on adoption and ambivalence. Psychoanal
Psychol 12:181–199, 1995

Buhs ES, Ladd GW, Herald SL: Peer exclusion and victimization: processes that mediate the relation between peer group rejection and children's classroom engagement and achievement? J Educ Psychol 98:1–13, 2006

Bussey K: Children's categorization and evaluation of different types of lies and
truths. Child Dev 70:1338–1347, 1999

Butler GE, McKie M, Ratcliffe SG: The cyclical nature of prepubescent growth. Ann
Hum Biol 17:177–198, 1990

Catts HW, Compton D, Tomblin JB, et al: Prevention and nature of late-emerging poor readers. J Educ Psychol 104:166–181, 2012

Centers for Disease Control and Prevention: Increasing prevalence of parent-reported attention-deficit/hyperactivity disorder among children—United States, 2003 and 2007. MMWR Morb Mortal Wkly Rep 59:1439–1443, 2010

Chalfant JC: Learning disabilities: policy issues and promising approaches. Am Psychol 44:392–398, 1989

Chused JF: Obsessional manifestations in childhood. Psychoanal Study Child 54:219–232, 1999

Clowes EK: Oedipal themes in latency analysis of the "farmer's daughter" joke. Psychoanal Study Child 51:436–454, 1996

Coen SJ: The sense of defect. J Am Psychoanal Assoc 34:47–67, 1986

Cohn DA: Child-mother attachment of six-year-olds and social competence at school. Child Dev 61:152–162, 1990

Colarusso C: The development of time sense: from object constancy to adolescence. J Am Psychoanal Assoc 35:119–144, 1987

Contreras JM, Kerns KA, Weimer BL, et al: Emotion regulation as a mediator of association between mother-child attachment and peer relations in middle childhood. J Fam Psychol 14:111–124, 2000

Crick NR, Grotpeter JK: Relational aggression, gender, and social-psychological adjustment. Child Dev 66:710–722, 1995

Davies D: Child Development: A Practitioner's Guide. New York, Guilford, 2010

Diamond M: Fathers with sons: psychoanalytic perspectives on "good enough" fathering throughout the life cycle. Gender and Psychoanalysis 3:243–299, 1998

Eaton WO, Ritchot KF: Physical maturation and information-processing speed in middle childhood. Dev Psychol 31:967–972, 1995

Egan SK, Perry DG: Gender identification: a multidimensional analysis with implications for psychosocial adjustment. Dev Psychol 37:451–463, 2001

Eisenberg N, Shell R, Pasternack J, et al: Prosocial development in middle childhood: a longitudinal study. Dev Psychol 23:712–718, 1987

Eisenberg N, Fabes RA, Guthrie IK, et al: The relations of regulation and emotionality to problem behavior in elementary school children. Dev Psychopathol 8:141–162, 1996

Eisenberg N, Fabes RA, Shepard SA, et al: Contemporaneous and longitudinal prediction of children's social functioning from regulation and emotionality. Child Dev 68:642–664, 1997

Erikson EH: Childhood and Society. New York, Norton, 1950

Freedman S: Role of selfobject experiences in affective development during latency. Psychoanal Psychol 13:101–127, 1996

Freud A: The concept of developmental lines. Psychoanal Study Child 18:245–265, 1963

Freud S: Three essays on the theory of sexuality (1905), in The Standard Edition of the Complete Psychological Works of Sigmund Freud, Vol 7. Edited by Strachey J. London, Hogarth Press, 1962, pp 123–246

Friedman RC, Downey JI: The psychobiology of late childhood: significance for psychoanalytic developmental theory and clinical practice. J Am Acad Psychoanal 28:431–448, 2000

Friedman RC, Downey JI: Sexual differentiation of behavior. J Am Psychoanal Assoc 56:147–175, 2008

Furman E: Transference and externalization in latency. Psychoanal Study Child 35:267–284, 1980

Gabrieli JDE: Dyslexia: a new synergy between education and cognitive neuroscience. Science 325:280–283, 2009

Giles JW, Heyman GD: Young children's beliefs about the relationship between gender and aggressive behavior. Child Dev 76:107–121, 2005

Gilligan C: In a different voice: women's conceptions of self and of morality. Harv Educ Rev 47:481–517, 1977

Gilmore K: Diagnosis, dynamics, and development: considerations in the psychoanalytic assessment of children with AD/HD. Psychoanalytic Inquiry 22:372–390, 2002

Goldings HJ: Jump-rope rhymes and the rhythm of latency development in girls. Psychoanal Study Child 29:431–450, 1974

Hudson RF, High L, Otaiba SA, et al: Dyslexia and the brain: what does current research tell us? Read Teach 60:506–515, 2007

Jaffee S, Hyde JS: Gender differences in moral orientation: a meta-analysis. Psychol Bull 126:703–726, 2000

Janz KF, Burns TL, Levy ST: Tracking of activity and sedentary behaviors in childhood: the Iowa bone development study. Am J Prev Med 29:171–178, 2005

Jemerin JM: Latency and the capacity to reflect on mental states. Psychoanal Study Child 59:211–239, 2004

Kavale KA, Forness SR: What definitions of learning disabilities say and don't say: a critical analysis. J Learn Disabil 33:239–256, 2000

Kennedy H: The role of insight in child analysis: a developmental viewpoint. J Am Psychoanal Assoc 27(suppl): 9–28, 1979

Knight R: The process of attachment and autonomy in latency: a longitudinal study of ten children. Psychoanal Study Child 60:178–210, 2005

Kohlberg L: Essays on Moral Development, Vol 2: The Psychology of Moral Development. San Francisco, Harper & Row, 1984

Kulish N: Female sexuality: the pleasure of secrets and the secret of pleasure. Psychoanal Study Child 57:151–176, 2002

Loe IM, Balestrino MD, Phelps RA, et al: Early history of school-aged children with attention-deficit/hyperactivity disorder. Child Dev 79:1853–1868, 2008

Loewald HW: The waning of the oedipal complex. J Am Psychoanal Assoc 27:751–775, 1979

Loke IC, Heyman GP, Forgie J, et al: Children's moral evaluations of reporting the transgressions of peers: age differences in evaluation of tattling. Dev Psychol 47:1757–1762, 2011

Lyon GR, Shaywitz SE, Shaywitz BA: A definition of dyslexia. Ann Dyslexia 53:1–14, 2003

Maccoby E: Gender and group process: a developmental perspective. Curr Dir Psychol Sci 11:54–58, 2002

Mahon E: The dissolution of the Oedipus: a neglected cognitive factor. Psychoanal Q 60:628–634, 1991

Main M, Cassidy J: Categories of response to reunion with the parent at age 6: predictable from infant attachment classifications and stable over a 1-month period. Dev Psychol 24:415–426, 1988

Main M, Kaplan N, Cassidy J: Security in infancy, childhood and adulthood: a move to the level of representation. Monogr Soc Res Child Dev 50:66–104, 1985

National Institute of Child Health and Human Development, Early Child Care Research Network: Mothers' and fathers' support for child autonomy and early school achievement. Dev Psychol 44:895–907, 2008

Novick J, Novick KK: A developmental perspective on omnipotence. J Clin Psychoanal 5:129–173, 1996

Novick J, Novick KK: The superego and the 2-system model. Psychoanalytic Inquiry 24:232–256, 2004

Novick KK, Novick J: Postoedipal transformations: latency, adolescence, and pathogenesis. J Am Psychoanal Assoc 42:143–169, 1994

Pedersen FV, Barber ED, Borge AIH: The timing of middle childhood peer rejection and friendship: linking early behavior to early adolescent adjustment. Child Dev 78:1037–1051, 2007

Piaget J: The Moral Development of the Child. New York, Harcourt, 1932

Piaget J: Play, Dreams and Imitation in Childhood. New York, Norton, 1962

Piaget J, Inhelder B: The Psychology of the Child. New York, Basic Books, 1969

Rothstein A: Neuropsychological dysfunction and psychological conflict. Psychoanal Q 67:218–239, 1998

Rothstein A, Benjamin L, Crosby M, et al: Learning Disorders: An Integration of Neuropsychological and Psychoanalytic Considerations. Madison, CT, International Universities Press, 1988

San Miguel SK, Forness SR, Kavale KA: Social skills deficits and learning disabilities: the psychiatric comorbidity hypothesis. Learn Disabil Q 19:252–261, 1996

Sarnoff C: The ego structure of latency. Psychoanal Q 40:387–414, 1971

Schmukler A: Use of insight in child analysis. Psychoanal Study Child 54:339–355, 1999

Shapiro T: Latency revisited: the age 7 plus or minus 1. Psychoanal Study Child 31:79–105, 1976

Shaywitz BA, Fletcher JM, Holahan JM, et al: Discrepancy compared to low achievement definitions of reading disabilities. J Learn Disabil 25:639–648, 1992

Shaywitz S: Current concepts: dyslexia. New Engl J Med 338:307–312, 1998

Sideridis GD, Mouzaki A, Simos P, et al: Classification of students with reading comprehension difficulties: the roles of motivation, affect, and psychopathology. Learn Disabil Q 29:159–180, 2006

Sroufe AL, Bennett C, Englund M, et al: The significance of gender boundaries in preadolescence: contemporary correlates and antecedents of boundary violation and maintenance. Child Dev 64:455–466, 1993

Tanaka H, Black JM, Hulme C, et al: The brain basis of the phonological deficit in dyslexia is independent of IQ. Psychol Sci 22:1442–1451, 2011

Theimer CE, Killen M, Stangor C: Young children's evaluations of exclusion in gender stereotypic peer contexts. Dev Psychol 37:18–27, 2001

Tyson P: A developmental line of gender identification, gender role and choice of love object. J Am Psychoanal Assoc 30:61–86, 1982

Tyson P, Tyson RL: Psychoanalytic Theories of Development: An Integration. New Haven, CT, Yale University Press, 1990

Veronneau MH, Vitaro F, Brendgen M, et al: Transactional analysis of the reciprocal links between peer experiences and academic achievement from middle childhood to early adolescence. Dev Psychol 46:773–790, 2010

Weinstein L, Saul L: Psychoanalysis as cognitive remediation: dynamic and Vygotskian perspectives in the analysis of an early adolescent dyslexic. Psychoanal Study Child 60:239–262, 2005

Westen D: The superego: a revisited developmental model. J Am Acad Psychoanal 14:181–202, 1986

Westen D: The relations among narcissism, egocentricity, self-concept and self-esteem: experimental, clinical and theoretical considerations. Psychoanalysis and Contemporary Thought 13:183–239, 1990

Willcutt EG, Pennington BF: Psychiatric comorbidity in child and adolescent reading disabilities. J Child Psychol Psychiatry 41:1039–1048, 2000

CHAPTER 7

Preadolescence

Bodily Challenges, Changing Relationships, and the Transition to the Teen Years

INTRODUCTION TO PREADOLESCENCE

Between ages 10 and 12 years, as the latency phase draws to a close and adolescence looms, children enter the brief but turbulent period of prepubertal development. Preadolescence begins during late childhood and ends with the events of puberty, spanning the months of increasing hormonal levels and the first signs of sexual maturity. Both subjective and tangible physical changes, such as accelerations of weight and height, the appearance of secondary sexual characteristics, and novel internal pressures, create confusion and perceived loss of control; these upheavals disturb the calm, compliant demeanor of the latency phase. Infantile longings and fears from the oedipal and preoedipal phases are revived (Blos 1958; Dahl 1995). At the same time, preadolescents' enhanced cognition, greater capacities for autonomy, and shift to middle school culture draw them into a complex social and academic environment. Newly buffeted by these progressive and regressive forces, the child's internal equilibrium is disrupted; a "normative crisis" (Erikson 1956) ensues, wherein conflictual feelings, outward restlessness, and mood instability are dominant trends.

The preadolescent's mind is increasingly capable of complex, abstract problem solving and self-reflection. Often referred to as the transition to *formal operational thinking* (Inhelder and Piaget 1958), these gains in cognitive and social understanding allow the child greater control over his or her own mental processes, more ready engagement in systematic and scientific reasoning, and a heightened awareness of what is possible (Kuhn 2006; Westen 1990). Intangible social and psychological dimensions of the self and others assume greater importance than more concrete qualities (Auerbach and Blatt 1996; Westen 1990). Whereas the latency child seeks playmates based on shared activities, the preadolescent begins to value self-expression and conversation in relationships that provide a sense of mutuality and validation. Enhanced capacity for *mentalization,* the ability to reflect on one's own and others' mental states (Fonagy et al. 2002), enriches the older child's relational world but sharpens self-awareness and self-consciousness, leading to vastly increased concern about the opinions of others. The preadolescent must adjust to greater cognizance of the world beyond family and community, more realistic appraisals of the self and others, and knowledge about the consequences of actions.

The entry into preadolescence signals a fundamental shift in the child's relationship to the family and peer group. Separation from the intimate ties of childhood and reworking of the parent-child bond are major tasks of the teen years; as noted, Peter Blos (1967) refers to this process as the "second individuation." Unlike the gradual process of increasing autonomy and diminished idealization of parents that characterizes latency-phase development, the preadolescent's separation is more urgent and dramatic. Increased conflicts with the parents, especially with mothers, are commonly reported (Blos 1958; Paikoff and Brooks-Gunn 1991). As children remove themselves from the potentially regressive pull of parental ties, they turn powerfully toward the peer group for companionship, excitement, and a sense of belonging.

THE CENTRALITY OF THE BODY IN MENTAL LIFE

Deep concerns about the unknowable, irrepressible, and potentially disappointing outcomes of puberty are central to the preadolescent experience. Fears of conspicuously early or late maturation are prominent. Heightened self-consciousness and self-awareness, along with intense desires for peer acceptance, create a tension-filled environment for children who fear that their particular bodily characteristics will be noticed by everyone. Indeed, research on preadolescent groups suggests that children are readily able to pinpoint their own and their peers' progression in the line of pubertal development (Brooks-Gunn and Warren 1988).

Along with premonitory sexual feelings, these changes often engender an internal sense of fear, confusion, and overstimulation in the child. The poignancy of this developmental phase and the often lonely position of the preteen, caught between childhood and adolescence, are movingly captured in *The Member of the Wedding,* Carson McCullers's timeless fictional portrayal of 12-year-old Frankie; bodily changes cause this young protagonist to feel like one of the "freaks" she encounters at the local fair and to dread the inevitable arrival of further pubertal transformations. In the midst of a growth spurt, Frankie calculates her eventual height and concludes that she will ultimately exceed 9 feet (McCullers 1946).

Although fears about menstrual "accidents" and unwanted erectile reactions are more common during the next stage of development, when puberty has been achieved, the preadolescent suffers a number of bodily concerns and potential humiliations, such as heightened sexual arousal, overt changes in weight and height, novel odors, and body hair. For the girl, menarche arrives late in a highly visible sequence of maturational events; well before puberty, she must adjust to a rapid growth spurt, increase in body fat, and other significant changes in bodily contour (Brooks-Gunn and Warren 1988). One particularly tall 10-year-old girl, who had been weighed and measured by the school nurse along with her classmates, was mortified to learn that her "statistics" were the subject of rumor throughout the day, eventually becoming a chorus among the boys who themselves were embarrassed to be significantly shorter than their female counterparts. Similarly, an 11-year-old boy related that while changing his clothes in the gym locker room after playing basketball, he became aware of a highly unpleasant, unfamiliar odor; to his horror, it slowly dawned on him that this was emanating from his own body. As he slunk back to math class, he was terrified that others would identify him as the source of the offensive smell.

Defensive Trends and Behaviors of Preadolescence

The child's intense fears about loss of bodily control, shameful reactions to masturbatory urges, and desires to avoid the reality of physical changes lead to a number of normative defensive trends. Many children exhibit signs of *asceticism* and *intellectuality*, two ego attitudes that reflect attempts to escape the body and repudiate sexual feelings (Sandler and Freud 1984). Abstinent behaviors, such as vegetarianism or others forms of restricted eating, provide a sense of self-control and mastery over instinctual urges, while redirecting the child's anxious focus from sexual to oral preoccupations. One 12-year-old girl and her best friend, after studying an indigenous culture in which beds were unknown, insisted on forsaking their own comfortable sleeping arrangements in favor of mats on their bedroom floors. Such self-denial was deeply satisfying to these girls, conferring a sense of shared pride and self-sacrifice, particularly at night when masturbatory urges were intensified. Similarly, the preadolescent often recruits increased conceptual capacities in the service of intellectual escape; a flight from the body to the mind, via newly grasped abstract ideas and philosophies, brings relief from biological pressures. The potential for such trends to veer toward psychopathology is significant as those children who are already vulnerable due to genetic loading, neurodevelopmental disorders, deleterious environmental events, and innumerable other contributions now grapple with a disruptive and disorienting transformation.

Preadolescent culture embraces a number of normative styles, behaviors, and activities that represent attempts to mask, avoid, or master the body's changes and pressures. Baggy clothing or gender-neutral fashions are sometimes employed to hide weight gain or deny gender-defining contours. The preteen's typical adoration of technology, particularly of social media, serves as a "retreat into cyberspace" (Lemma 2010), creating distance and relief from bodily sensations and pressures. Often, preadolescents seek increasing involvement in structured physical and athletic activities; girls' well-known affinity for horseback riding and boys' and girls' engagement in sports can serve needs to sublimate aggression, master powerful urges, and discipline the body while enjoying physically stimulating outlets.

Boy-Girl Similarities and Differences

Physically and psychologically, boys enter the period of preadolescence 1–2 years later than their female counterparts (Knight 2005; Paikoff and Brooks-Gunn 1991). Although both genders share in the emotional, environmental, and bodily pressures that define this developmental phase, differences in their respective biological timetables are only one of several meaningful distinctions. Restlessness, increased moodiness, a drive toward action, and a powerful turn to peer groups are familiar hallmarks for boys and girls alike, but their particular fears and fantasies, their modes of behavioral expression, and the qualitative nature of their relationships are distinguishable.

As the older latency child begins to be buffeted by sexual urges, he or she experiences an inevitable regression to earlier phases of development; the resurgence of oral, anal, and oedipal trends, all of which were largely repressed during the relatively peaceful years of middle childhood, is a defining aspect of preadolescence (Blos 1958, 1967). The child's struggle against such regressive forces is partly determined by gender; for example, boys' increased affinity for scatological and sexual humor and girls' growing preoccupation with foods and diets are typical modes of expression (Blos 1958; Fischer 1991). Boys are pressured by more intense sexual drives and an earlier immersion in sexual fantasies (Friedman and Downey 2008); these factors may contribute to the more obviously regressive and action-oriented behaviors that characterize preadolescent male groups (Blos 1958). Many previously tidy, compliant children of both genders begin to resist bathing, causing friction with parents who bemoan their children's loss of hygienic habits.

As preadolescent children immerse themselves in groups and friendships, further gender distinctions are visible. Often, boys prefer large, hierarchically organized same-sex "packs"; a sweeping avoidance of females, both young and old, is a central tenet of these groups and their activities (Blos 1958; Friedman and Downey 2008; Sroufe et al. 1993). Unlike preteen girls, who may seek out brief, pseudosexual relations with the opposite gender, preadolescent males rarely align themselves with females. Boys' heightened sexual drive reawakens earlier fears of bodily injury, along with a dread of passivity and submission, particularly vis-à-vis strong female figures; preadolescent males often describe girls and women as mean, possessive, and even dangerous. The realities of boy-girl physical differences, such as girls' much earlier growth spurt and tendency to tower over boys during the prepubescent years, only serve to reinforce a boy's sense of peril and powerlessness and drive him forcefully toward the felt safety of unisex groups. Once surrounded by same-sex age-mates, boys typically engage in loud and rowdy activities, sexual innuendos, and more grossly offensive language. Blos's (1965) somewhat outdated but lively, highly recognizable description of preteen boys captures key aspects of this attitude: "You will probably recognize this kind of boy if I remind you of the many therapy hours you have spent with him while he was playing with, drawing, or impersonating battleships and bomber planes, accompanying their attacks with a gunfire of onomatopoetic noises in endless repetition. He loves gadgets and mechanical devices, he is motorically restless and jumpy, usually eager to complain about the unfairness of his teacher, assuring us that the lady is out to kill him..." (p. 148). In the context of the mother-son relationship, the boy's aversion to females is often expressed as avoidance and withdrawal; resistance to physical contact, which may have previously been tolerated or even sought, is enacted with vigor. One 11-year-old boy's mother wistfully described his sudden refusal to share the sofa with her after many years of mutual enjoyment and close physical proximity as they watched his favorite nighttime television programs.

The preadolescent girl's struggles and confusion as she heads toward bodily maturation are experienced and expressed in ways that differ from her male counterparts: Resistant attitudes toward the inevitable feminization of the body, resentment about the need to renounce tomboyish activities, and a reluctance to accept the limits imposed by pubertal changes are common. In contrast to boys, however, girls tend to evince a greater sense of gender exploration and flexibility. One child clinician, anticipating the arrival of a young girl who would alternately present herself as an unkempt tomboy and a glamorous starlet, wrote, "I never knew who would enter the office" (Fischer 1991, p. 462).

Like boys, preadolescent girls turn sharply away from mother-daughter intimacy and toward same-sex peers, driven by a fear of dependency and the dread of reengulfment in infantile satisfactions. Girls' struggles often take the form of overt fighting and argumentative attitudes; mothers of preteen girls are highly familiar with the conflicts and high emotionality that often result from well-meant, seemingly casual maternal overtures and attempts to reestablish formerly close, mutually pleasurable bonding. Critical, rejecting reactions toward the mother and an ensuing sense of loneliness go hand in hand with the preadolescent girl's craving for peer companionship. In contrast to males, however, girls often seek smaller same-sex groups. Often, very intimate but fleeting "best friend" relationships are eagerly pursued; these intense female bonds, which tend to be transient and interchangeable rather than enduring, help compensate for the preadolescent's loss of mother-daughter closeness (Fischer 1991). Certain girls prematurely seek out pseudosexual contact with boys in an attempt to solidify a sense of femininity, disavow "tomboyish" behaviors and feelings, gain status within the peer group, and renounce the intimate bond with the mother; the need for intimacy and affirmation of feminine qualities, rather than sexual desire, are typically the driving forces in such relationships (Blos 1958).

COGNITIVE AND SOCIAL DEVELOPMENT DURING PREADOLESCENCE

In their seminal work on cognitive development, Piaget and Inhelder (1969) define preadolescence as a specific period of intellectual growth that marks the end of childhood and ushers in the adolescent's increasing orientation toward reality and the future. Although the notion of discrete, successive unfolding cognitive stages has been revised by recent research, many psychodynamic and developmental writers draw from Piaget's notion of formal operational thinking to describe the preadolescent's mental achievements. The following characteristics are widely noted: increasingly flexible and abstract thinking, the advent of hypothetical reasoning, enhanced self-reflection and awareness of others' needs and perspectives, an orientation toward future possibilities, and a grasp of the multiple outcomes and consequences that may follow events (Barkai and Hauser 2008; Granic et al. 2003; Spear 2000; Westen 1990). Moreover, the older child demonstrates greater control over his or her own intellectual processes and reactions (Kuhn 2006).

The preteen's enhanced mentalization capacities facilitate a growing ability to interpret and reflect on complicated social and emotional behavior (Fonagy et al. 2002). In contrast to the younger child's more simplistic grasp of emotional states, the preadolescent comprehends such concepts as conflict and ambivalence; for example, he or she recognizes that an upcoming summer trip arouses both anxiety and excitement in the same individual. Although the acquisition of such insight about the self and others is not always evident in the day-to-day behavior of the preadolescent child, deeper cognitive and emotional understanding of mental states ultimately facilitates more thoughtful and less action-oriented responses to unexpected or confusing social situations. Despite the parent-child distance characterizing this phase of development, parent-led discussions about emotionally laden events are positively linked to the preadolescent's capacity for social-emotional insightfulness (Marin et al. 2008).

The child's greater awareness of others' perspectives and increasing capacity to incorporate these into the self-concept lead to more realistic and sometimes harsher self-appraisals (Molloy et al. 2011). Feedback from important others, such as teachers and especially peers, is more keenly attended and felt than in the latency phase, and both objective and idiosyncratic criteria for self-measurement—such as grades, popularity, and results of athletic competitions—have greater emotional consequence; a newly informed sense of personal strengths and weaknesses inevitably follows. In the context of the preteen's intense desire for social validation and group acceptance, enhanced awareness of personal limits and others' opinions leads to considerable preoccupation and comparison of the self with others. Slight physical flaws and concern about how these are perceived by peers assume enormous importance; similarly, mild social mishaps are replayed in the child's mind and are enthusiastically discussed and relentlessly analyzed by the group. Even the previously confident, self-assured latency child may experience a sharp increase in self-consciousness and self-doubt.

At the same time, an increased focus on others' mental lives expands the preadolescent's capacity for empathy, social conscience, and more mature, reciprocal social relationships. The latency child's tendency toward rigid, rule-bound judgments and behaviors has significantly softened, and a greater appreciation of individualistic and nonconventional attitudes emerges. Awareness of the world beyond the self and concern for unknown others increase, leading to intensified interest in community service and social causes. In their immediate peer relationships, preadolescents evince a greater focus on friends' abstract qualities; a desire for shared feelings and mutual validation gains importance. The preteen's interest in conversation and common attitudes begins to take precedence over the notion of peers as playmates (Buhrmester 1990).

Changes in the preadolescent's thinking and social understanding affect the family and transform previously well-accepted rules and parent-child hierarchies. The rigidity of existing structures and routines, once diligently followed by the latency child, may now be resisted. Roles, responsibilities, and parental authority are no longer upheld without question. The young adolescent will seek greater involvement in decision making and a more equal balance of power.

Bodily and Cognitive Changes in Preadolescence

- Emergence of secondary sexual characteristics, premonitory sexual and aggressive urges, and subjective sense of bodily change disrupts the calm latency demeanor and revives long-repressed infantile wishes.

- Bodily changes predispose the preadolescent to restlessness, moodiness, fears of out-of-control growth, and a sense of shameful exposure.

- Children avoid or deny the body through normative defensive trends (*asceticism* and *intellectualization*), or involvement with technology.

- Boys manifest negative views toward females, seek the company of same-sex groups, and engage in sexual or scatological talk.

- Girls may focus on food restrictions and prematurely seek heterosexual connections.

- Preadolescents seek distance from the regressive pull of mother-child closeness.

- Increased mentalization capacities enhance empathy but lead to preoccupation with others' opinions.

THE SOCIAL AND FAMILY LIFE OF THE PREADOLESCENT

Changing Family Relationships

Both psychodynamic and empirical writers describe preadolescence as a uniquely challenging, vulnerable period of development. Internal pressures, physical changes, and the inevitable loss of parent-child intimacy engender a profound sense of restlessness and instability; such feelings powerfully propel the child toward peers and external outlets (Barrett 2008; Knight 2005). In *The Member of the Wedding*, 12-year-old Frankie declares that she has become an "unjoined person" and soothes herself with fantasies about sharing a life with her older brother and his fiancée; she is devastated when this fails to materialize (Dalsimer 1979; McCullers 1946). The preadolescent's fear of revived childish needs and his or her concomitant dread of passive surrender to adults set the stage for frequent child-initiated conflict (Dahl 1993, 1995). Moreover, parents' uneasiness about their child's maturing body and dawning sexuality, discomfort with his or her more confrontational and less compliant stance, or unresolved issues from their own adolescent years further encumber the parent-child relationship.

The process of autonomy and the gradual de-idealization of the parents beginning in the latency years accelerate sharply as the child enters the preadolescent phase. Intensifying sexual urges reawaken long-dormant oedipal feelings; the child experiences an urgent need to escape incestuous, hostile, and dependent wishes, all of which are repressed for the duration of middle childhood (Blos 1958, 1962, 1967). Physical closeness to the parents feels inexplicably threatening. Moreover, the preadolescent's enhanced awareness of the world beyond the family, immersion in the reality-based environment of school, and growing connection to peers all serve to challenge previous unrealistically held notions about the parents. Anna Freud (1949) observes that the "family romance," a universal latency fantasy wherein real-life parents are replaced with elevated, royal, or magical figures (discussed more fully in Chapter 6), is merely "the forerunner of the more complete, more ruthless disillusionment concerning the parents which characterizes preadolescence" (p. 102).

The preteen's physical changes and bodily anxieties are therefore endured mostly alone, against the background of shifting parent-child relationships. Younger children tend to seek adult reassurance during stressful circumstances, but preadolescents' need and desire for adult counsel and sympathy are a source of mounting conflict, challenged by their intense vulnerability to shame, drive toward autonomy, and concomitant fears of revived dependency. Moreover, deep shame about masturbatory urges and sexual excitement increase preadolescents' resistance to seeking out parental involvement. Indeed, the mother's empathic responsiveness and mirroring—formerly the child's major source of bodily and emotional self-regulation—are completely unavailable in the arena of emerging sexual feelings (Fonagy 2008). Rather, the child must manage novel stimulation, accompanying fantasies, and bodily worries in the absence of familiar maternal ego support.

These same internal pressures predispose the child to create conflict with the parents, further reducing the likelihood of eliciting maternal reassurance. For example, a somewhat late-developing 11-year-old girl, who had been teased by a female classmate about her immature body, insisted that her mother take her shopping for bras, declaring that she was the only girl who lacked this essential undergarment; while in the store, in a rare moment of rapprochement, she confided her fear that physical maturation had simply passed her by. Eager to find common ground and provide reassurance, her mother commented that she herself had matured rather late and that the daughter was likely to follow suit. After storming out of the store empty-handed with her bewildered mother in tow, the girl angrily muttered, "So *you* are the reason I'm embarrassed in gym class every day when all my friends show off their bras!"

Empirical work on preteen-parent relationships reveals significant increases in tension and reorganization of family structure. Some writers emphasize that true ruptures in the parent-child bond are not universal and that many dyads retain close and positive ties, but most agree that a general reworking and renegotiation of previously held roles are inevitable as the preadolescent struggles to achieve greater autonomy and self-definition. Loss of previously idealizing attitudes toward the parents, newfound resistance to the formerly deferential stance regarding parental authority, demands for greater power in making decisions, and growing negative and conflict-laden interactions are among the well-documented characteristics of this age group (Besser and Blatt 2007; Paikoff and Brooks-Gunn 1991). The mother-daughter bond, in particular, undergoes dramatic change, with both parties reporting deterioration of their previous relationship (Laursen et al. 2010). However, a history of secure attachment continues to provide a buffer during periods of upheaval, leading to somewhat milder disruption during the preadolescent phase; securely attached children suffer less loneliness, engage in less conflict, and enjoy more positive, reciprocal relationships with peers (Kerns et al. 1996).

The following vignette illustrates a painful but normative shift in a previously close mother-daughter relationship. A somewhat anxious 11-year-old girl, whose long-standing dependency on her mother and mild but enduring separation problems make it particularly difficult to achieve a sense of autonomy, enters the period of preadolescence with a notable set of strengths and vulnerabilities. Her latency capacities were very solid—good self-control, competence in an array of academic and extracurricular pursuits, and positive friendships—but the bodily and social stresses of preadolescence revive her earlier separation fears during a time when she feels unable to lean on her parents.

Zoe, a fifth grader, was a slightly anxious but sociable, well-adjusted latency youngster who excelled at academics and enjoyed a number of extracurricular activities. Her relationships with her parents were close, largely free of conflict, and mutually satisfying. As a preschooler, she had suffered intermittently from separation anxiety, often relying on her mother's patient coaxing and sometimes requiring her physical presence in order to attend birthday parties and kindergarten class trips. As far as parents and teachers could discern, Zoe's separation fears appeared to have largely disappeared by the time she entered grade school, and she participated enthusiastically in social events.

During the summer between fourth and fifth grades, two of Zoe's newer friends attended a sleep-away camp for the first time; now, as the summer before sixth grade approached, they persuaded her to sign up. As the time grew near, Zoe was plagued by doubts, some of which she expressed to her parents, such as fears of animals getting into the bunk, worries about mean campmates, and concerns about deep water in the middle of the lake. Her parents were surprised at the reemergence of her earlier anxieties and inhibitions, but encouraged her to give camp a try. To their surprise, Zoe erupted in anger at their attempted reassurances; at the same time, she seemed equally unsatisfied by their attempts to help her elaborate her fears. Both adults made it clear that she could opt out at any time, but this too seemed to elicit irritation. Privately, Zoe worried about the approach of her eleventh birthday, which would occur during camp season. She had learned about menarche in health class, knew that one or two of her classmates had already begun to menstruate, and was fearful about the possibility of her own period starting while she was at camp. Repeatedly, she reread the pamphlet she had been given by her health teacher, which listed the expected bodily changes signaling the imminent arrival of puberty. She sadly concluded that there was no way to precisely calculate when her period would arrive.

Her mother had observed a number of changes in Zoe over the course of the fifth-grade year. Zoe's impatient reactions were becoming more and more frequent and intense; often, she seemed unable to accept the maternal support that she had always needed and craved. Although she had previously spent most of her leisure time in the family living room, she now firmly closed the door to her bedroom and was vague about her activities. In the place of their former intimacy, shared conversations, and mutually pleasurable activities, Zoe evinced an increasing dissatisfaction with her mother, often audibly sighing when her mother entered the room. Zoe began to find fault with her mother's comments, even those not directed at her, and to poke fun at her mother's tastes and opinions. Eager to reestablish their former comradeship, her mother insisted that they spend time together on the weekends. Zoe would sometimes grudgingly agree, but she was so unpleasant that her mother wondered about the value of this idea.

At the same time, Zoe was spending more and more time in the company of a cadre of girls whose style and attitudes she mimicked closely. Often, they spent their time in small groups, roaming the main street of their neighborhood, passing by the ball fields where the boys congregated after school. These jaunts often left Zoe feeling overstimulated and brittle, and her behavior was particularly difficult when she got home afterwards. Her mother's exasperation led her to blame Zoe's new associates and to threaten to restrict her after-school freedoms. Initially relieved but also incensed, Zoe responded "You are ruining my life!"

This 11-year-old girl, wrestling with the early signs of bodily changes and mounting social pressures, can no longer rely exclusively on her mother for a sense of security and companionship. She is increasingly drawn to a popular peer group, yielding to the requirements of peer pressure, such as attending a popular sleep-away camp and engaging in contact with boys, but privately she is anxious and uncertain about these behaviors. Her mother, feeling bereft herself, hopes to soothe her daughter through restoring their formerly close, mutually gratifying ties. However, Zoe cannot give in to her dependent longings and struggles to maintain autonomy; her anxious tendencies and her history of reliance on her mother's presence for self-regulation create a particularly poignant preadolescent struggle, wherein she must forcefully renounce and reject her mother's help.

Friendships, Groups, and the Role of Peer Acceptance

The importance of friendships and social acceptance, which accelerates in the latency years, inclines sharply during preadolescence. Peer bonds serve multiple purposes, fulfilling the child's urgent need for companionship while helping to guard against regressive longings for parent-child intimacy. The idealization of friends, as well as their habits and behaviors, helps compensate for the loss of the previously venerated parental figures and their moral and behavioral guidance (Dalsimer 1979; Fischer 1991). Not surprisingly, failure to achieve peer approval and social connections during late childhood is empirically linked to deep feelings of loneliness and depression, as well as to aggressive and delinquent behaviors during later phases of development (Bagwell et al. 2000). The preadolescent's deeper understanding of others' opinions and heightened concern about group status make the plight of the bullied or otherwise rejected child particularly painful during this developmental period (Troop-Gordon and Ladd 2005).

In contrast to the latency child who seeks playmates and partners for activities and games, the preadolescent is increasingly drawn to peers for shared mental experience. Mutually validating conversations, often including avid discussion of other age-mates, acquire a more central role in friendships. Enhanced awareness of internal processes and psychological characteristics leads to greater focus on the less tangible dimensions of friends' personalities (Auerbach and Blatt 1996). Moreover, the preadolescent develops a capacity for sensitive, tactful, and sympathetic behavior during moments of personal disclosure (Buhrmester 1990; Westen 1990). Sharing private thoughts and opinions with peers provides an outlet for the multiple aspects of the self that can no longer be comfortably shared with the parents.

The quality of preteen friendships, however, is notably different from the deep, enduring nature of parent-child attachments or more mature love relationships. Normative preadolescent connections tend to be intense and exclusive but fleeting, often appearing interchangeable in nature (Sandler and Freud 1984). Best friends are eagerly sought, particularly by girls, but frequently exchanged; during the short-lived course of these relationships, there is active effort to solicit and copy each other's opinions and demeanor. Peer cliques are common and provide an important source of group socialization, deeply influencing the preadolescent's behavior, styles, and attitudes. Such mimicry of friends and groups serves a playful, experimental function reminiscent of the preschool child's attempts to try on numerous identities and roles.

Boys and Girls

In the years leading up to puberty, children must accomplish the sometimes contradictory tasks of maintaining gender boundaries while learning essential information about the opposite sex. The strict boy-girl divide of latency remains visible during preadolescence, but increasing interest in the other gender now finds expression. Teasing, playful conflicts, and even mildly aggressive boy-girl behaviors, testify to mounting excitement and curiosity. One sixth-grade girl reported the following experience with obvious enjoyment: "During recess the boys grab our backpacks and run away with them. So we have to chase them and grab back our stuff. Then they curse at us, and we scream at them. We hate them, really." According to Sroufe et al. (1993), "such high-energy contacts not only are generally brief, hit-and-run missions but are also accompanied by outspoken disavowal of interest" (p. 457).

At the same time, children's groups undergo a process of "gender intensification," which continues through mid-adolescence (McHale et al. 2004). As described in Chapter 6, "The Latency Phase," same-sex groups are an important source of socialization, feelings of belonging, and "gender-valued self-esteem" (Friedman and Downey 2008). During latency, girls' groups appear to tolerate a degree of gender ambiguity and a range of gender self-expression, such as "tomboy" behaviors. Within boys' groups, children are more likely to suffer rejection for perceived nonmasculine tendencies (Friedman 2001; Galatzer-Levy and Cohler 2002). However, with the arrival of puberty, both sexes gravitate toward greater conformity and stereotypic gender self-expression; for example, girls renounce perceived boyish styles and actions (Fischer 1991).

THE SHIFT TO MIDDLE SCHOOL

At the beginning of the fifth or sixth grade, preadolescents leave elementary school behind and enter middle school (or junior high school), where they must rapidly adjust to an unfamiliar environment, novel routines, and the presence of older adolescents. The sudden immersion in a surround of multiple teachers, large numbers of peers, and higher expectations for independent functioning can overwhelm the child despite a strengthened desire and capacity for autonomy. Many are unprepared for the required level of self-management; those who failed to consolidate latency-phase skills—industrious attitudes, tolerance for frustration, and solid organizational and planning abilities—are particularly vulnerable. As a result, a number of students suffer a decline in academic motivation, engagement, and performance, impairing their self-concept of academic and social competence. Such losses are particularly significant because middle school achievement is foundational for more consequential, academic successes in high school and beyond (McGill et al. 2012; Molloy et al. 2011).

Both external and psychological conditions contribute to the challenge of the middle school environment. Greater peer and curricular choices, the switching of classes during the school day, and diminished levels of supervision create a highly stimulating atmosphere during a time when preadolescent restlessness and motility are at their height. Contact with older students, who are in the midst of rapid physical development and adolescent culture, exposes the preteen to a number of novel, potentially risky behaviors, such as substance use and sexual activity. Anxieties about shifting cliques and friendships, and fears about the loss of these havens of security add to the child's burdens. Moreover, the former, highly personal bond between student and grade-school teacher shifts toward more distant student-teacher relationships with less individual support, harsher academic evaluations, and a sharper focus on performance. The preadolescent's increased capacity to consider others' opinions, use objective criteria for self-appraisal, and incorporate feedback into the self-concept intensifies the meaning of academic assessments. Negative evaluations or even constructive criticisms are more painfully felt.

The preadolescent's increased need for privacy, independence, and psychological distance from the parents means that the academic, social, and emotional trials of middle school are often managed alone, save for the guidance of equally confused peers. Indeed, parents are unlikely to be taken into their children's confidences and may be caught off guard by revelations of work or behavior problems. Often, adults instinctively react by attempting to reassert their own authority or by hastening to establish additional supervision or adult interventions, such as tutoring. Although parental actions tend to meet resentment and resistance from the child, certain types of adult-child interactions appear highly beneficial for the preadolescent. Discussions that communicate the parents' expectations, while enlisting the child's own thinking about learning strategies and complex situations, provide scaffolding for the preteen's autonomous decision-making and problem-solving abilities (Hill and Tyson 2009).

The following vignette illustrates an essentially well-functioning new sixth grader's difficult adjustment to the middle school environment. Like many parents, Joel's are caught by surprise when they learn, belatedly, of his academic decline.

A bright, charming child with mild organizational problems, Joel had always received extra support from his sympathetic elementary school teachers; their efforts had helped compensate for his own less than stellar self-management skills. Without being asked, they repeated instructions, checked to make sure he had correctly recorded his assignments, and evinced a generally forgiving attitude toward his occasional lapses in memory and planning. He always felt safe at school and took pride in his and his friends' small steps toward independence. For instance, since the beginning of the fifth-grade year, they gathered as a group every morning to walk to school together, without adult escort. Joel was small for his age, but his athleticism and good-natured demeanor had always assured him plenty of friends and a certain status among the boys of the grade. However, when Joel and his peers entered the middle school, which incorporated sixth graders from several elementary schools across the county, his social and academic life suffered a decline.

From the outset, Joel felt overwhelmed by the demands of middle school. He had trouble accommodating the distinctly different styles and expectations of his humanities and science/math teachers and frequently got lost as he navigated the large, unfamiliar building. None of his instructors provided the level of individual support to which he had grown accustomed; for example, none repeated their instructions or made sure that students correctly recorded the nightly homework assignment. As a result, Joel missed a number of homework deadlines and was unprepared for the more comprehensive exams. He did not know how to gauge the importance of these frequent but seemingly small mishaps, although he found them very upsetting. Joel was particularly nervous at the end of the school day, when older, much larger boys would gather in front of the building in noisy groups. On a number of occasions, Joel and his friends had been jostled by these intimidating crowds. Rumors circulated furiously throughout the sixth grade about the older kids, the bullies, and their delinquent feats; although almost entirely false, these tales were fueled by the teens themselves, who enjoyed their status in the minds of the younger children. The middle school basketball team was a source of additional anxiety. Slightly older but significantly taller and more muscular boys dominated the team. Most problematic for Joel was his sense that he no longer wished to share his daily experiences with his parents, and he suffered the combination of social anxiety and academic stress privately.

Joel's parents were unprepared for the initial teacher evaluations, which revealed an unprecedented decline in his academic performance. Moreover, when they attempted to implement a number of the teachers' suggestions, such as a math tutor and greater parental oversight of his daily work, he was uncharacteristically resistant. Luckily, his science/math teacher was a sensitive young man who emerged as an important source of support for Joel, tactfully offering extra help during after-school hours in a small group forum. By the middle of the sixth-grade year, Joel's academic performance stabilized; he was learning to employ strategies for better organization, and he and his friends were feeling less intimidated by the older adolescents.

The Family, Social, and Learning Environments of the Preadolescent

- The preteen's bodily changes and urgent need for autonomy lead to significant increases in parent-child conflict.
- A powerful turn toward the peer group helps compensate for the loss of mother-child bonding.

- Greater awareness of others' feelings, increased desire and capacity for reciprocity, and growing interest in friends' psychological qualities cause a gradual shift toward need for conversation and mutual validation of opinions and attitudes.
- The quality of preadolescent friendships and cliques is often fleeting and superficial. Brief, intense experimental connections are common, wherein peers imitate each other's attitudes and styles but then quickly move on to other affiliations.
- The shift from elementary to middle school marks a loss of previous teacher-provided structure and support, requiring vastly enhanced capacities for self-reliance and personal organization.
- As they adjust to middle school, many children suffer a decrease in perceived competence and self-confidence as well as an actual decline in academic success.

THE CHANGING PHYSIOLOGY OF PUBERTY: BOYS AND GIRLS

The Timing of Pubertal Onset

Puberty is not a singular event, but rather a multisystem process with neuroendocrine, psychosocial, nutritional, environmental, and numerous other components; all these systems are involved in an interactive cascade to effect preadolescent changes and pubertal transformation, even while each has its own development and proceeds at its own pace (Ellis et al. 2011; Navarro et al. 2007). The familiar signal events, the first menses and nocturnal emission, are visible markers of the ongoing evolution of two hormonal axes, the adrenal and the gonadal; the former creates conditions for the latter, although additional neural mechanisms seem to be responsible for the actual initiation of puberty. *Adrenarche,* the "awakening" of the adrenal glands responsible for axillary and pubic hair, actually begins early in latency, although it achieves its effect considerably later and extends its influence into the third decade of life. It is thought to be an essential precondition for the initiation of *gonadarche,* responsible for sexual organ growth.

There is new evidence of a crucial "brain event" (as opposed to an endocrine event) that is regulated by a group of peptides called *kisspeptins;* these are released in response to a variety of internal and external factors (e.g., size, body fat percentage, adequate nutrition) that indicate, from an evolutionary point of view, that reproduction is possible (Spear 2000). In response to the kisspeptin "gatekeeper," neurons secreting gonadotropin-releasing hormone are activated; this in turn acts on neural circuitry that is already sex-specific from infancy to produce secondary sexual characteristics, sexual behaviors, and further neural remodeling (Sisk and Zehr 2005).

Brains already differentiated into male- and female-typical patterns in the perinatal period are thus further remodeled by circulating sex hormones and are sexually dimorphic in overall size (boys>girls), regional size (boys' amygdalas>girls'; girls' hippocampi>boys'), and receptors.

Bodily Changes

The full attainment of physical and sexual maturity is a transformative bodily and psychological process, beginning in the preadolescent period (typically at around age 10 for girls and a year or two later for boys) and extending into late adolescence or, occasionally, into emerging adulthood. Despite sexually dimorphic brain development since birth and sex-linked differences in fat and muscle distribution demonstrable in latency-age children (girls' body fat>boys'; boys' paraspinous musculature>girls') (Arfai et al. 2002), grade-school boys and girls are relatively undifferentiated and rely on strict single-sex activities to reinforce their differences. During the preadolescent period, visibly dimorphic development is initiated. Preadolescence commences variably with early signs of secondary sexual characteristics (i.e., the appearance of darker body hair, breast buds, and increased penis and testicle size) and with general physical growth that affects boys and girls differently. Gains in height and weight and fat distribution in girls precede these changes in boys by up to 2 years. It is only when these pubertal changes commence that body dissatisfaction appears, especially among girls (Stice 2003).

The evolving mind of the preadolescent and pubescent child, while focused inward on bodily transformation, is simultaneously turned outward—toward peers, popular culture, fashions, and fads. Many aspects of personality functioning are affected by how the child "fits" into the present culture—that is, how well he or she meets standards of beauty (of face and form), popularity, athleticism, and academic achievement, as well as values of the family, peer group, and immediate cultural surround. Although all phases of development are influenced by the surround, the impact of culture is magnified as development proceeds and the child's own horizons expand to encompass the larger world. Examples abound regarding the multifaceted effect of society on adolescent bodily experience, but perhaps the most fundamental is its effect on the experience of the timing of puberty and the subsequent pace of secondary sexual development. There is a wide range of timing and outcome in all aspects of physical development during puberty and early adolescence, despite a relatively reliable sequence of events. As noted, asynchrony with the peer group can shake self-esteem and affect the teen in surprisingly lasting ways, particularly if the obvious markers of sexual development are precocious or delayed. The earlier onset of puberty poses a challenge for today's young adolescents, whose childhood is "shortened," on average, by 2 years relative to their parents' own experience (Mendle et al. 2010).

Moreover, the larger cultural context is nowhere more apparent than in regard to physical development, because youth culture is both a fount of and a sponge for shifting styles and fashions. For example, beginning in the 1960s, preteens and young adolescents have been bombarded with "thin imagery" by the media (Likierman 1997); in the 1970s, tattoos and body piercings, formerly prevalent only in marginalized groups, moved into the mainstream on the bodies of contemporary teen icons (Brown et al. 2000). Emulation of nearly impossible physical ideals as represented by supermodels or larger-than-life "cool" celebrities and sports heroes, as well as competition with the peer group, contributes to the favored types of body modifications (discussed in Chapters 8 and 9). Those who fall outside of the cultural ideal of the moment or who resist popular trends can be subject to painful self-doubts and social consequences, with potential long-term effects on self-image despite subsequent corrections.

Developmental Psychopathology: Emergence of Anxiety and Depressive Disorders

The timing and tempo of pubertal onset is consistently invoked as a risk factor; for example, early menarche is correlated with problematic outcomes in adulthood ranging from increased incidence of depression to increased risk of breast cancer (Ellis et al. 2011). Early maturation (by definition always relative to the contemporary peer group) has documented repercussions on psychology over the course of adolescence. Very early or unusually rapid physical maturation truncates the preadolescent period; premature exposure to sexual feelings, with limited time to consolidate latency-phase resources and capacities, creates self-regulatory vulnerabilities for these youngsters. Moreover, the distress of both appearing and feeling acutely out of sync with one's peers and the internal pressure toward early emotional separation from the parents can lead to painful isolation.

Precocious puberty and rapid pubertal tempo are well-documented risk factors for depressed mood, social anxiety, behavioral problems, and poor peer relationships (Blumenthal et al. 2011; Mendle et al. 2010). Puberty itself introduces a significant sexual differentiation in the incidence of certain forms of disorders, especially internalizing symptomatology, which is far more common in pubescent girls than boys; multiple factors, including vulnerability to sexual victimization, are recognized contributions (Hayward and Sanborn 2002). Early-developing girls and boys both show immediate perturbation in mood in the transitional moment, but it is the early-developing girls alone who show long-term vulnerability to low emotional tone, anxiety, clinical depression, and negative body image (Buchanan et al. 1992; Ge et al. 2003; Petersen et al. 1994). No doubt the more publicly obvious nature of their bodily changes and the associated premature tendency toward mother-daughter conflict add to this differential. Late-developing boys, who are also at risk, seem to "bounce back" from the low mood associated with their late onset (Ge et al. 2003, p. 438). As noted above, peak pubertal changes often coincide with a school change in many Western cultures—from elementary to middle school or junior high—and the sequence of these events can compound problems with adaptation (puberty preceding or simultaneous with school change having a relatively worse outcome) (Simmons and Blyth 1987). School transitions in general, especially to junior high school, elicit a dip in mood, more commonly in girls (Buchanan et al. 1992; Wichstrom 1999).

Key Concepts

Preadolescence, spanning the ages between 10 and 12, represents a brief but turbulent period of transition between latency and the advent of puberty. Children are buffeted by a subjective sense of change as well as by hormonal and physical maturation; under these pressures, urges and wishes from earlier developmental stages are revived. In contrast to the relatively calm and compliant attitude of the latency child, the preteen tends toward motoric restlessness and internal discomfort. The body feels out of control. Moreover, the increase in sexual and aggressive feelings, in the context of parent-child closeness, contributes to an urgently felt need for greater independence. The loss of the parental auxiliary ego support leaves the child feeling alone and confused. An accelerating drive toward autonomy, resistance to parent-child intimacy, and a decisive turn to the peer group are hallmarks of this developmental period.

The preadolescent's enhanced cognitive capacities lead to a deeper understanding of the self and others; more abstract, psychological qualities assume greater importance. Boys tend to seek safety and companionship in large groups, whereas girls often immerse themselves in brief but intense dyadic friendships. A shift from the safety and structure of elementary school to the increased social and academic pressures of middle school creates additional anxieties. Moreover, the timing and tempo of pubertal changes are associated with increased risk for a number of psychiatric disorders.

- The preadolescent must cope with the subjective sense that the body is starting to transform. Changes in weight and height, the beginnings of breast and testicular development, and increases in sexual and aggressive feelings must be integrated into the child's sense of self.

  · Fears about bodily exposure and the sense that the body is out of control are central to the preadolescent experience.

  · Under the pressure of increased sexual and aggressive urges, the preadolescent regresses to earlier phases of development. Oedipal, anal, and oral trends are evident in both boys' and girls' behavior and preoccupations.

- As preadolescents enter the period of formal operational thinking, their abstract and reflective cognitive capacities are expanded.

  · Enhanced self-observation and growing interest in one's own and others' psychological qualities stand in distinction to the younger latency child's more concrete cognition and focus on actions.

  · Preadolescents achieve a greater sense of abstract possibilities and a clearer understanding of consequences.

  · In addition, they possess a heightened and more accurate awareness of others' opinions and appraisals, leading to enhanced concern about status, achievement, and popularity.

- In an effort to escape bodily realities and pressures, two particular ego attitudes may emerge: *intellectuality,* whereby the child takes refuge in the noncorporeal world of ideas, and *asceticism,* in which self-denial represents a disavowal of bodily urges. In addition, preadolescents turn to action and technology in their attempts to avoid the bodily self.

- The preteen child is poised to enter adolescence, called the *second individuation phase,* and the relationship to parents is transformed.

  · Fears of dependency or passivity and of reengulfment in earlier attachments create an internal drive away from the parents, toward action and peer relations. The intimacy of earlier parent-child bonds is slowly loosened; roles and relationships are reorganized and renegotiated.

  · The preadolescent's loss of parental ego support during a time of increased inner confusion and vulnerability leads to deep feelings of separation and loneliness.

- As the child separates from parental ties, he or she turns powerfully toward the peer group.

  - Groups, cliques, and friendships become crucial sources of companionship, self-validation, and a sense of belonging.

  - As they approach puberty, children maintain a visible gender divide but manifest increasing interest and curiosity in the other sex.

- The transition to middle school, with its increased social and academic challenges, creates additional pressures during a vulnerable period of development. Many children experience a decline in their academic performance and a change in their previous sense of academic competence and mastery.

- Precocious puberty, delayed puberty, and a rapid developmental tempo are known risk factors for a range of mood and adjustment disorders.

REFERENCES

Arfai K, Pitukcheewanont PD, Goran MI, et al: Bone, muscle, fat: sex-related differences in prepubertal children. Radiology 224:338–344, 2002

Auerbach JS, Blatt SJ: Self-representation in severe psychopathology: the role of reflexive self-awareness. Psychoanal Psychol 13:297–341, 1996

Bagwell CL, Coie JD, Terry RA, et al: Peer cliques and social status in preadolescence. Merrill Palmer Q 46:280–305, 2000

Barkai AR, Hauser ST: Psychoanalytic and developmental perspectives on narratives of self-reflection in resilient adolescents: explorations and new contributions. Annual of Psychoanalysis 36:115–129, 2008

Barrett TF: Manic defenses against loneliness in adolescence. Psychoanal Study Child 63:111–136, 2008

Besser A, Blatt SJ: Identity consolidation and internalizing and externalizing problems in early adolescence. Psychoanal Psychol 24:126–149, 2007

Blos P: Preadolescent drive organization. J Am Psychoanal Assoc 6:47–56, 1958

Blos P: On Adolescence. New York, Free Press, 1962

Blos P: The initial stage of male adolescence. Psychoanal Study Child 20:145–164, 1965

Blos P: The second individuation process of adolescence. Psychoanal Study Child 22:162–186, 1967

Blumenthal H, Peen-Feldner EW, Babson KA, et al: Elevated social anxiety among early maturing girls. Dev Psychol 47:1133–1140, 2011

Brooks-Gunn J, Warren MP: The psychological significance of secondary sexual characteristics in nine- to eleven-year-old girls. Child Dev 59:1061–1069, 1988

Brown KM, Perlmutter P, McDermott RJ: Youth and tattoos: what school health personnel should know. J Sch Health 70:355–360, 2000

Buchanan CM, Eccles JS, Becker JB: Are adolescents the victims of raging hormones? Evidence for the activational effects of hormones on moods and behavior at adolescence. Psychol Bull 111:62–107, 1992

Buhrmester D: Intimacy of friendship, interpersonal competence, and adjustment during preadolescence and adolescence. Child Dev 61:1101–1111, 1990

Dahl EK: The impact of divorce on a preadolescent girl. Psychoanal Study Child 48:193–207, 1993

Dahl EK: Daughters and mothers: aspects of the representational world during adolescence. Psychoanal Study Child 50:187–204, 1995

Dalsimer K: From preadolescent tomboy to adolescent girl. Psychoanal Study Child 34:445–461, 1979

Ellis BJ, Shirtcliff EA, Boyce WT, et al: Quality of early family relationships and the timing and tempo of puberty: effects on biological sensitivity to context. Dev Psychopathol 23:85–89, 2011

Erikson EH: The concept of ego identity. J Am Psychoanal Assoc 4:56–121, 1956

Fischer RMS: Pubescence: a psychoanalytic study of one girl's experience of puberty. Psychoanalytic Inquiry 11:457–479, 1991

Fonagy P: A genuinely developmental theory of sexual enjoyment and its implications for psychoanalytic technique. J Am Psychoanal Assoc 56:11–36, 2008

Fonagy P, Gergely G, Jurist EL, et al: Affect Regulation, Mentalization, and the Development of the Self. New York, Other Press, 2002

Freud A: On certain difficulties in the preadolescent's relation to his parents, in The Writings of Anna Freud, Vol 4. New York, International Universities Press, 1949, pp 95–106

Friedman RC: Psychoanalysis and human sexuality. J Am Psychoanal Assoc 49:1115–1132, 2001

Friedman RC, Downey JI: Sexual differentiation of behavior: the foundation of a developmental model of psychosexuality. J Am Psychoanal Assoc 56:147–175, 2008

Galatzer-Levy R, Cohler BJ: Making a gay identity: coming out, social context and psychodynamics. Annual of Psychoanalysis 30:255–286, 2002

Ge X, Kim IJ, Conger RD, et al: It's about timing and change: pubertal transition effects on symptoms of major depression among African American youths. Dev Psychol 39:430–439, 2003

Granic I, Hollenstein T, Dishion TJ, et al: Longitudinal analysis of flexibility and reorganization in early adolescence: a dynamic systems study of family interactions. Dev Psychol 39:606–617, 2003

Hayward C, Sanborn K: Puberty and the emergence of gender differences in psychopathology. J Adolesc Health 30(suppl):49–58, 2002

Hill NE, Tyson DF: Parental involvement in middle school: a meta-analytic assessment of the strategies that promote achievement. Dev Psychol 45:740–763, 2009

Inhelder B, Piaget J: The Growth of Logical Thinking From Childhood to Adolescence: An Essay on the Construction of Formal Operational Structures. New York, Basic Books, 1958

Kerns KA, Klepac L, Cole A: Peer relationships and preadolescents' perceptions of security in the child-mother relationship. Dev Psychol 32:457–466, 1996

Knight R: The process of attachment and autonomy in latency. Psychoanal Study Child 60:178–210, 2005

Kuhn D: Do cognitive changes accompany developments in the adolescent brain? Perspect Psychol Sci 1:59–67, 2006

Laursen B, Delay D, Adams RE: Trajectories of perceived support in mother-adolescent relationships: the poor (quality) get poorer. Dev Psychol 46:1792–1798, 2010

Lemma A: An order of pure decision: growing up in a virtual world. J Am Psychoanal Assoc 58:691–714, 2010

Likierman M: On rejections: adolescent girls and anorexia. J Child Psychother 23:61–80, 1997

Marin KA, Bohanek JG, Fivush R: Positive effects of talking about the negative: family narratives of negative experience and preadolescents' perceived competence. J Res Adolesc 18:573–598, 2008

McCullers C: The Member of the Wedding. Boston, MA, Houghton Mifflin, 1946

McGill RK, Hughes D, Alicea S, et al: Academic adjustment across middle school: the role of public regard and parenting. Dev Psychol 48:1003–1018, 2012

McHale SM, Shanahan L, Updegraff KA, et al: Developmental and individual differences in girls' sex-typed activities in middle childhood and adolescence. Child Dev 75:157–193, 2004

Mendle J, Harden KP, Brooks-Gunn J, et al: Development's tortoise and hare: pubertal timing, pubertal tempo, and depressive symptoms in boys and girls. Dev Psychol 46:1341–1353, 2010

Molloy L, Ram N, Gest SD: The storm and stress (or calm) of early adolescent self-concepts: within- and between-subjects variability. Dev Psychol 47:1589–1607, 2011

Navarro VM, Castellano JM, Garcia-Galiano D, et al: Neuroendocrine factors in the initiation of puberty: the emergent role of kisspeptin. Rev Endocr Metab Disord 8:11–20, 2007

Paikoff RL, Brooks-Gunn J: Do parent-child relationships change during puberty? Psychol Bull 110:47–66, 1991

Petersen AC, Leffert N, Graham B, et al: Depression and body image disorders in adolescence. Womens Health Issues 4:98–108, 1994

Piaget J, Inhelder B: The Psychology of the Child. New York, Basic Books, 1969

Sandler J, Freud A: Discussions in the Hampstead Index on "The ego and the mechanisms of defense," XIII: instinctual anxiety during puberty. Bulletin of the Anna Freud Centre 7:79–104, 1984

Simmons RG, Blyth DA: Moving Into Adolescence: The Impact of Pubertal Change and the School Context. Hawthorne, NY, Aldine, 1987

Sisk CL, Zehr JL: Pubertal hormones organize the adolescent brain and behavior. Front Neuroendocrinol 26:163–174, 2005

Spear LP: The adolescent brain and age-related behavioral manifestations. Neurosci Biobehav Rev 24:417–463, 2000

Sroufe LA, Bennett C, Englund M, et al: The significance of gender boundaries in preadolescence: contemporary correlates and antecedents of boundary violations and maintenance. Child Dev 64:455–466, 1993

Stice EW: Puberty and body image, in Gender Differences at Puberty. Edited by Hayward C. Cambridge, UK, Cambridge University Press, 2003, pp 61–76

Troop-Gordon W, Ladd GW: Trajectories of peer victimization and perceptions of the self and schoolmates: precursors to internalizing and externalizing problems. Child Dev 76:1072–1091, 2005

Westen D: The relationship among narcissism, egocentricity, self-concept and self-esteem: experimental, clinical and theoretical considerations. Psychoanalysis and Contemporary Thought 13:183–239, 1990

Wichstrom L: The emergence of gender difference in depressed mood during adolescence: the role of intensified gender socialization. Dev Psychol 35:232–245, 1999

CHAPTER 8

Early and Mid-Adolescence

The Importance of the Body, Sexuality, and Individuation, the Role of Action, and the Special Problems of the Teen Years

INTRODUCTION TO ADOLESCENCE

Adolescence, divided here into early (ages 11–14 years), middle (ages 14–17), and late (ages 17–21, to be discussed in the following chapter), encompasses a phase of remarkable transformation, both internal and external. As the body undergoes the events of puberty and subsequent development to sexual maturity, the individual's mind grapples with the meanings of these changes and undergoes its own remodeling. This is a time of exquisite self-consciousness, as well as a new capacity for self-reflection, urgent interest in novel experience leading to risky and impulsive behaviors, and major reworking of relationships with family, peer group, and intimate friends. From the vantage point of the stable, well-regulated late latency child, puberty and adolescence appear to be a wild adventure certain to produce a person as yet unknown with a life as yet unimaginable. It is a much anticipated, exciting, but also fearful time of life.

Adolescence as a true developmental phase only achieved legitimacy at the turn of the twentieth century (Brooks 2007; Dahl and Hariri 2005; Shapiro 2008) and was still termed "a cultural invention" by mid-century contributors (Stone and Church 1955). In Western culture today, the status of the "adolescence" construct is secure among psychodynamic thinkers and observers from a range of disciplines in society at large; adolescents engage media attention, suffer very visible psychiatric disorders, engage in risky behavior with huge morbidity and mortality (Steinberg 2004), and have complex developmental trajectories that occupy parents, marketers, music and

Hollywood producers, and theorists alike. Puberty was always recognized as a powerful developmental moment. In 1905, Sigmund Freud dwelt at length on the role of puberty as an organizer of libido, sexual fantasy, and object choice in his *Three Essays on the Theory of Sexuality* (Freud 1905/1962). However, it was the publication one year earlier of G. Stanley Hall's groundbreaking two-volume tome, *Adolescence: Its Psychology and Its Relations to Physiology, Anthropology, Sociology, Sex, Crime, Religion, and Education* (Hall 1904) that conceptualized adolescence as a protracted period of developmental transformation, distinguished by "storm and stress": "Adolescence is a new birth, for the higher and more completely human traits are now born…new qualities of body and soul now emerge…suggestive of some ancient period of storm and stress when old moorings were broken and a higher level attained…." (Hall 1904, Vol. 1, p. xiii).

The notion of inevitable adolescent upheaval drew attention to this as yet unsung phase of development but also invoked controversy over the next century. It became linked to popular concepts such as "raging hormones" (Cauffman 2004; Dahl 2004) and was favored by many psychodynamic theorists, including Anna Freud (1958), Peter Blos (1968), and Erik Erikson (1968), each of whom offered theoretical conceptualizations that contributed to the complex picture of adolescence.

However, the notion of "storm and stress" or "adolescent turmoil," which certainly resonates with enduring popular images of adolescence, was simultaneously challenged by researchers and clinicians, most notably Daniel Offer (Offer 1965; Offer and Offer 1968), who surveyed adolescent behavior and subjective experience through psychological testing and serial interviews. His findings of relatively unruffled progression through early to late adolescence were repeated in subsequent research from a range of perspectives (Brooks-Gunn and Warren 1989; Doctors 2000; Flannery et al.1994; Offer and Schonert-Reichl 1992). Today, researchers and psychodynamic clinicians tend to embrace a middle ground, conceptualizing adolescence as a vulnerable period for manifestations of developmental conflict, risky behavior, and moodiness; there is also evidence that genetic predispositions toward psychopathology are "triggered" by adolescent hormonal events (Walker et al. 2004). Nonetheless, such vulnerabilities are powerfully mediated by psychosocial factors that modulate their impact on developmental progression (Arnett 1999; Rohner 2000; Rutter 2007). The overall experience of adolescence and the degree to which it constitutes an "interruption of peaceful growth" (A. Freud 1958, p. 267)—for adolescents themselves, their parents, and other involved adults—varies depending on individual, cultural, gender-based, familial, and other influences. Thus, the consensus in contemporary descriptive research appears to be that storm and stress are not always severe or universal, but manifestations of psychic upheaval are *more likely* to occur during adolescence (Arnett 1999). How else to explain the alarming 200% jump in morbidity and mortality "due to difficulties in the control of behavior and emotion" of this age group compared to school-age children (Dahl 2004, p. 3)?

The psychodynamic perspective takes a detailed look at the adolescent mind and highlights the profound upheaval, on a psychological level, that this phase entails. Whether or not the individual course involves outward disturbance, it inevitably traverses the most rapid and demanding transformational process yet experienced (Jacobson 1961); the preparatory growth spurt, the onset of puberty, the mysterious and unchartered process of secondary sexual development, the shifting self-representations, the reworking of defenses, the changing territory in terms of family life, and the interest in having an impact on the world all emerge within a compressed time period and then evolve through late adolescence into emerging adulthood. However calm the adolescent's demeanor may be, he or she has to manage an upsurge of drive—both sexual and aggressive—and develop a whole new array of defenses to deal with it. The law-abiding posture of the typical latency-age child—with its repressive attitudes toward sexuality and compliance in regard to parental rules and values—needs to adapt to the new reality of the sexual body, sexual and aggressive impulses, and the urge to establish autonomy from parents. The struggle to defend against the upsurge in drive can lead the young adolescent to renounce all bodily needs (the defense of *asceticism,* as described in Chapter 7, "Preadolescence") or take an oppositional stance and resist any containment of impulses (the "uncompromising" adolescent) (A. Freud 1958). The defenses against the childlike attachment to parents can result in withdrawal, rage, and defiance in some adolescents, and clinging and immature behavior in others. Adolescents are compelled by circumstances within and without to bring the authority and idealized images of their parents down to human size: parents have sex lives, make mistakes, and do not always practice what they preach. For thinkers like Anna Freud, some form of intrapsychic struggle, whether symptomatic or not, is necessary for the adolescent process to achieve its optimal result— that is, autonomous and productive emerging adulthood, with individually determined identity and values, including sexual identity, moral beliefs, and purpose.

Perhaps the most inclusive recent description of adolescence is offered by Dahl (2004): "that awkward period between sexual maturation and the attainment of adult roles and responsibilities" (p. 9). This definition, while relatively nonspecific, highlights the important fact that what begins with a biological event (puberty), discontinuous with prior development, ends with the attainment of a social status and enduring elements of identity. The end of adolescence is marked by psychosocial milestones that presumably denote the consolidation of personality that is the hallmark of adulthood. Yet as we discuss in Chapter 10, "The Odyssey Years," another developmental phase has been wedged into this transition, that of *emerging adulthood.*

THE PHASES

Following the defining moment of puberty, the early, middle, and late phase markers within the adolescent process are culturally determined and indistinct. They are often linked to school setting: middle school/junior high, high school, and college. *Tanner stages* (Tanner 1962), the sequence of physical changes introduced in the 1960s and still used today to chart the development of secondary sexual characteristics (see Table 8–1), are frequently out of sync with the chronological age and school situation for a given individual, creating potential tension in the adolescent who expects to progress according to standards set by peers and cultural trends. Such asynchrony between age and Tanner stage contributes yet another layer of complexity to what we suggest is a premier preoccupation of the young to mid-adolescent: the body, sexual desire, and gendered development.

Contemporary approaches to the adolescent process integrate the strands of brain development, biological maturation, genetic influences, effects of hormones, cognition, social-emotional regulation, and environment. These developmental forces operate in interaction, creating "practice grounds" for evolving capacities (Kupfer and Woodward 2004, p. 321); similarly, vulnerabilities associated with adolescence are understood to be the outcome of multiple interacting factors. Such a systems orientation informs and qualifies considerations of findings within each domain. A good example is the gender differentiation in the incidence of psychiatric illness that emerges during adolescence. For example, the robust finding that the prevalence of depression is far greater in girls than in boys has been linked to many variables, ranging from the role of hormones to body dissatisfaction fostered by media (Wichstrom 1999); most adolescent experts agree that there are likely multiple interacting sources and etiological factors. This is also true for the equally robust finding that in 17-year-olds, the prevalence of schizophrenia is much higher in boys than in girls; many factors, aside from genetic loading, contribute to variations in incidence, such as migration, urban environment, and ethnicity (Kirkbride et al. 2006).

In the following subsections, we briefly characterize the challenges of early and mid-adolescence, with the caveat that distinctions between the psychological tasks that dominate the two phases are fluid in the living sub-

TABLE 8–1. Tanner stages of sexual maturation

Stage 1	Prepubertal
Stage 2	Breast buds, changes in scrotal size and texture, sparse pubic hair
Stage 3	Breast and areolar growth, increased length and width of penis, coarsening, darkening and curling of pubic hair
Stage 4	Continued breast and areolar growth, darkening and further growth of penis and scrotum, pubic hair adult-like but not spread to medial thighs
Stage 5	Mature adult contours of breasts and genitalia in both genders, full adult complement of pubic hair

Source. Stang and Story 2005; Tanner 1962.

ject. Many themes ebb and flow through these stages and progress unevenly, by fits and starts. Following the overview of early and mid-adolescence, we describe the psychological impact of the bodily transformation, the central conflicts, and the resulting vulnerabilities of these two phases in greater depth. Late adolescence is explored in Chapter 9.

Early Adolescence (Ages 11–14)

In the wake of the relatively precise onset of pubertal changes, the early adolescent consciousness is dominated by momentous changes and the sense of disequilibrium in the bodily self. These changes occur whether the individual's actual physical development progresses gradually over the next decade or rapidly produces a mature sexual body. The growth spurt, which usually predates the signal events of puberty and lasts for up to 3 years (Neinstein 2002), proceeds from pre- through mid-adolescence at a velocity comparable to the rapid growth of infancy, but now occurs in a self-aware and highly self-conscious early teen. Despite individual differences, the pace of change is decidedly different from the relatively slow progression of bodily growth in latency and inevitably challenges the familiarity, reliability, and sense of ownership of the corporeal self. Each young adolescent grapples with the changing body, its rate of transformation, and new sensations, desires, thoughts, and feelings—all of which must be integrated into the metamorphosing self-representation. At the most fundamental level, then, the young adolescent's psychological challenge involves coming to terms with this whole new body and sense of self.

The variability in the progression of physical changes within a given cohort takes on significance commensurate with another aspect of early adolescence, one that has been gathering steam since latency: focus on the peer group. Although still dependent on parents, the young adolescent is none-theless increasingly interested in and absorbed by the social scene, which escalates in its complexity. Middle school (or junior high school) years often mark a rapid shuffling of peer hierarchies and dynamics into cliques and exclusionary "crowds," themes that are memorialized in coming-of-age books and recalled ruefully by the older adolescent. The relationship between physical changes and social status is painfully evident in the experience of the young adolescent and is corroborated by the finding that extremes in onset of pubertal changes, either "too early" or "too late," can pose significant challenges to social adaptation depending on the cultural surround. Onset of menarche before age 11 increases the risk for depression and substance abuse in girls; delayed menarche is associated with depressed mood (Stice et al. 2001). Some studies report similar risk for mood disturbance in early-developing boys, depending on the culture (e.g., especially in Norway; see Wichstrom 1999), whereas others demonstrate the risk for late developers, who suffer from low self-esteem and higher incidence of substance abuse (Biro and Dorn 2006). Thus, asynchronies with the peer group deeply affect the confidence, emerging sexuality, and loneliness of the early adolescent.

In addition to providing a yardstick for the concrete achievement of early sexual development and secondary sexual characteristics, the peer group engages the attention of the young adolescent by virtue of its new complexity and introduces intense social pressure, which extends well into mid-adolescence. Adolescents often remark that middle school is the worst time for social competition, exclusive cliques, bullying, and ostracism. Especially because developmental progression between ages 11 and 14 is so variable, the potential to feel left behind, out of the league, or like an outlier is often equivalent to a judgment on the self, most pointedly the physical self. Compounding the actual scrutiny of the peer group is the evolution of developmental egocentrism. In the early stages of formal operations, the new capacity to "think about thinking" creates the potential for a "cognitive flaw" (Rycek et al. 1998). Young adolescents assume that other people spend as much time thinking about them as they think about themselves; their self-consciousness plays to an "imaginary audience" of observers (Elkind and Bowen 1979).

Risky behaviors begin to emerge in this age group, as children counter-phobically embark on forbidden adult activities that defy parental rules and disavow their own fears. Early adolescents engage independently in social activities where they gain access to cigarette smoking, acts of violence to property and persons, drinking, marijuana, social media, and sexual contact (Rew et al. 2011). Fear of regressive, passive wishes makes aggression (and its inevitable enactment in the victimization of others) a pervasive aspect of the middle school experience; studies suggest that a significant majority of middle school students complain of memorable teasing (75%) and that only a small minority say that they committed no bullying in a given 30-day period (15% of boys and 23% of girls) (Espelage et al. 2000). The manifestations of interpersonal aggression assume gendered forms. Bullying predominates among boys; the pattern in girls is typically "relational aggression," defined as the intention to harm others by "attempts to damage another child's friendships or feelings of inclusion in the peer group" (Crick and Grotpeter 1995, p. 711). These behaviors are widespread in middle school and show correlations with physical attractiveness as well as broader contextual factors such as parental behaviors and neighborhood safety. Early teens increasingly engage in Internet activities that bring them into contact with peers, victims, and predators. Facebook opens its doors to users at age 13 and introduces an unprecedented level of awareness of the peer group. The excitement generated by this near-universal forum for social contact, showing off, and "stalking" is at the expense of personal privacy; such excitement can take a tragic turn when use of social media for hostile exposure and humiliation produces violence or suicides.

The absorbing spectacle of the peer group is increasingly unmitigated by the former protective shelter of family. Relationships with parents can become strained by the young teen's efforts to disengage from dependent childish feelings. There is an overall decline in the experience of "companionship and intimacy" with parents (Collins and Laursen 2006). Bodily changes introduce awkwardness as the boy or girl transitions into a mature form; parents and children alike struggle to position themselves on a different footing as sexuality intrudes on the domestic scene. There is usually an adjustment phase where parents either miss signs of excessive risk taking or misfire in their efforts to balance their interventions; it is no small task to simultaneously facilitate independence while monitoring access to overstimulating or dangerous situations. Moreover, parents lose their most significant allies in influencing their young teenager—that is, the child's own superego and lifelong desire to please them. The moral code of the latency-age child, based in part on an idealized view of parents, is shaken from within by both the upsurge of impulses and the shift in focus toward peers. The child who was formerly "good" and militantly opposed to teenage vices seems to transform overnight into someone who smokes and experiments with sex or substances. The abruptness of this change catches parents unawares, and they sometimes remain ignorant of their teens' risky behaviors for longer than they should.

Nonetheless, despite the popular idea that relationships with parents and peers may be inversely related (i.e., that conflicts with parents increase as peer relationships become central), evidence shows that these two domains usually show similarities, and that in cases where they diverge, positive relationships in one can modulate the other (Rubin et al. 2004; Sentse and Laird 2010). Overall positive relationships with both parents tend to improve social competence. Interestingly, parental use of behavioral controls (i.e., curfews and grounding) yields much better outcomes than psychological control (i.e., guilt or anxiety induction, name calling, or withdrawal of love); the latter increases externalizing symptoms in early adolescence (Rogers et al. 2003).

◆ **See the video "Early Adolescent Girl." This pubertal girl is still very close to her parents; she is highly responsible and not yet caught up in risky behaviors of adolescence. Nonetheless, she is fascinated and affected by the "drama of middle school." She is a good example of the variability of developmental progression, as well as its unevenness within a given individual.**

Siblings often respond strongly to the maturing teen; they are keenly aware of the developmental moment and respond with competitiveness, intrusiveness, or overexcitement to the transformation. Early and middle adolescents can be drawn into illicit activities by older siblings, especially those whose relationship to the parents is rebellious and conflictual. Early teens tend to lose both interest in and positivity about their relationship to their younger sibling playmates, especially if the latter take the whistle-blower role in regard to teen behavior. However, sibling relationships, especially those with a good foundation, tend to recover in late adolescence (McHale et al. 2006).

In the following vignette, the parents relied on their confidence that Ellie was a "law-abiding" and compliant latency-age child almost all the way through middle school, until her grades began to decline in eighth grade. Her excited interest in a "bad boy" is an example of the attractiveness of the cool and reckless kids for early teenagers, perhaps especially for those who dare not experiment themselves.

> At age 13, Ellie was still a slender, long-limbed girl, and could easily be mistaken for a sixth grader; she was beginning to develop but was definitely not precocious or sexy in an obvious way. She began menstruating at age 12. At her small multicultural school, a free-standing junior high, she gravitated toward girls from strict traditional families who were closely monitored and never allowed to attend parties. Her own professional parents were more permissive than her friends' and more preoccupied with their own careers. They nonetheless held high standards for Ellie's behavior and scholastic achievement. She had always been compliant and a "pleaser" and worked

hard to live up to her parents' expectations. However, in her eighth-grade year she seemed to lose her passion for school, and her grades dropped. She had enjoyed the attention of boys for several years and was now being courted by a classmate, Damian, a good-looking guy with a reputation for being "fast." "Everyone thought we were boyfriend and girlfriend, and they started giving us condoms as a joke. Rumors spread!" Ellie was clearly pleased by the notice she was getting. Eventually, Ellie and Damian began to "go out." As was typical in her school setting, this status consisted primarily of hanging out together at school. Nonetheless, as soon as the opportunity presented itself, she and Damian went to his empty house, and in their first sexual contact, had unprotected intercourse. Ellie was bursting with excitement and confided in her 11-year-old-sister, at best a fair-weather ally, who lost no time in telling their parents. Her parents were blindsided because they saw Ellie as risk-averse and even immature. They faulted themselves for their own naïveté but were equally angry at Ellie who, they felt, had betrayed their trust. Ellie explained her actions by the rather pat formulation that she was swept along by "peer pressure." She also offered a familiar self-observation: "I can't say no." Her parents cracked down, insisting she be chaperoned to and from school and working with the school administration to ensure she had no unsupervised access to Damian. Ellie complied but became increasingly distressed and lonely as rumors spread at school; she was subjected to a deluge of prank calls and postings on a youth-oriented blog site calling her "slut" and "whore." The entire family eagerly looked forward to high school because Ellie's classmates would be dispersed and be more likely themselves to become sexually active; perhaps then her reputation would recover.

This vignette illustrates a number of realities of early adolescent life: a quantum shift in terms of young teens' relationship to parental values and their own impulses can take parents unawares; teens' curiosity, excitement, and desires can takethe lead in decision making, despite their intellectual capacity to exercise good judgment; they have a shaky relationship to their wishes for autonomy and often invite parental intervention; and their actions are played out in a public forum, with painful results that can dog them for years.

Early Adolescent Challenges and Changes (Ages 11–14)

- Adaptation to the rapidly transforming body and integration of the sexual body into self-representation
- Shift in attention from parents to the increasingly complex peer group, associated with increased self-awareness and self-consciousness
- Reexternalization of the parentified superego of latency and reliance on the peer group for behavioral guidance
- Emergence of risky behaviors, including substance use, sexual experimentation, and aggression toward others, especially bullying

Mid-Adolescence (Ages 14–17)

The adolescent between ages 14 and 17 years approximates the typical teenager in high school as represented in the media and popular imagination. These are teens who have passed through the most revolutionary physical changes of puberty and are grappling with the realities of bodies that have been transformed, gendered, and sexualized. An action orientation predominates, expressing the urgent desire for experience and direct access to the world without the protective and limiting filter of parental supervision.

The dual processes of individuation (to be described in the next section, "The Second Individuation Process") and of establishing a new, more autonomous version of relatedness to parents are both in play as the power differential between parents and teens diminishes and conflict—often accompanied by anger—escalates (Collins and Laursen 2006; de Goede et al. 2009). Parents continue to feel at a loss to intervene, not only because they carry less authority but also because they are often woefully unfamiliar with the contemporary technology, music, bodily decorations/mutilations, substances, and venues that engage the teenager. For example, parents typically lag in their ability to navigate complex youth-oriented Internet networks that geometrically expand their adolescents' access to the world; as the teen becomes more savvy, parents are increasingly flummoxed. In most U.S. states, 15-year-olds can obtain a learner's permit which allows them to drive alone to school and work, further increasing their freedom from parental supervision. Increased purchasing power from allowances, credit card access, and jobs gives teens access to previously forbidden places, activities, and substances. The mid-adolescent is often keenly aware of feelings of loss and disillusionment with parents, whose own missteps and hypocrisy (or "phoniness," to use the favorite epithet of Holden Caulfield in J.D. Salinger's *The Catcher in the Rye*) are increasingly clear to their teenage child, adding to tension between them. Intergenerational conflict about everything from curfew to politics peaks during this phase.

As the following vignette demonstrates, the mid-adolescent transition to greater autonomy can be challenging for parents who are trying to adjust to their child's ability to sidestep their authority.

> Frankie at age 16 was generally a good kid according to his parents, but he regularly butted heads with them about driving to parties and school events. Letting him use a car was discretionary, because one was usually available, but his parents were worried about how much alcohol was being served at friends' houses and whether Frankie, who was among the first to drive, was always willing to abstain as the designated driver. Tension mounted amidst his ongoing resentment of restrictions, and after a stormy argument, he drove off without permission, did not tell his parents where he was going or

whom he planned to see, and did not reiterate his usual assurances that he would be careful. Both parents were upset and anxious; they spent the evening calling, e-mailing, and texting him. They tried to get onto his computer to see if anything could be gleaned from his Facebook page, but were surprised to learn that he had changed his password from Frankie50, the one his mother had given him in fifth grade. This complication added a new, more general concern that Frankie was having a life that he wanted to keep hidden from them. Trying to manage their fearful speculations, they began to call around to friends' homes and finally discovered that Frankie was watching a new horror movie in the basement entertainment center at the home of a classmate, someone they knew only peripherally. Unsure about whether to drive to that house, reprimand him, and insist he come home, or wait until the to discuss the matter when tempers had cooled, they finally decided to sit it out. At about 11 P.M., they received a text from Frankie saying he was sorry to have worried them, but he was fine and would be home by 1:30 A.M. While unhappy about this message, which clearly violated a long-standing 12:30 A.M. curfew, they reasoned that at least he was talking to them, he had always been trustworthy, and they could sort things out in the morning.

Frankie was cooperative during the next morning's conversation but drew the line at his parents' demand that he tell them his whereabouts at all times and give them access to his computer. Furthermore, he informed them that they should call him Frank, that 12:30 was a "ridiculous" curfew, and that he would just sleep over at the houses of friends with more reasonable parents if they insisted on that curfew. However, he assured them that he was more responsible than most kids and they should "just trust" him. His parents talked over accepting what felt like an ultimatum from Frank, and in the end they realized that they did trust him and preferred to keep their communication open. They told him that they wanted him to agree to their conditions: absolutely no drinking and driving, no unprotected sex, and no parties at their house without permission. They strictly forbade any illegal substances, although they knew marijuana use was common among Frank's friends. They felt that a firm rule was better than one that condoned illegal behavior, even if Frank was likely to violate it.

As demonstrated in this vignette, the goal of a mutually respectful relationship between parent and mid-adolescent is difficult to achieve, especially when the parent feels unsure of how to interpret some behavior. When to crack down and when to stand back and let the teenager figure it out is a quandary that renews itself at every turn during this transformational period. In this case, Frank's parents took a flexible stand, within limits that they made very clear. Frank kept his promises and continued to act responsibly; he did smoke marijuana eventually, but did it rarely and took what his friends considered to be extreme precautions.

During mid-adolescence, the peer group continues to increase in importance and exerts a degree of influence that eclipses parental judgment (Goodnight et al. 2006). These are the years during which the storied peer pressure exerts powerful sway; the peer group now can wield unopposed influence, and maladaptive and risky behaviors, such as substance abuse, aggression, bulimia, and unsafe sexual activity, proliferate while controls are still lagging. The search for new experience, the pressure of sexual and aggressive impulses, the anxieties that lead to attempts to rigidly control the changing body, and the hunger for acceptance and admiration are among the many factors that influence teenagers at this stage. The peer group also affects self-esteem in regard to the all-important measures of how one "fits in." Competitive pressure, both academic and social, escalates. For those who do not experience easy social or academic success, the feeling of alienation threatens on all sides and may heighten the predilection toward risk and aggression or isolation and depression. Conflict related to identity begins to occupy the inner and social life of many mid-adolescents, as they feel their way into peer groups and feel identified, willingly or not, with what they represent (e.g., popular "mean girls," outcasts, rappers, jocks, weirdos, stoners, Goths).

Gender differentiation deeply occupies the minds of teenagers in terms of self-definition and in regard to the emerging forms of their sexual fantasies and behaviors. Although early family life and childhood mental representations of adult relationships and gendered personas create idiosyncratic unconscious representations of what it means to be a man or a woman, the teenager, a major media target, is barraged by a steady stream of cultural input about masculinity, femininity, and sexuality that he or she must manage selectively. Media messages often introduce a degree of gender stereotypy that can override the complexity and nuance of gender roles within families. Can girls be great at math and also pretty and popular? Can boys be good athletes and nice guys? What kind of body must one have to be sexy and desirable? There are myriad versions of these enduring quandaries of high school students. Lying behind these can be more fundamental anxieties about sexual development, such as fears of sex and dread about adult responsibilities.

In regard to sexuality, mid-adolescence is typically the time for the internal clarification of sexual orientation and the idiosyncratic elements of arousing sexual fantasy. The psychodynamic concept of "the central masturbation fantasy" (Laufer 1976) refers to the configuration of unique elements that contribute to the adolescent's sexual preferences and requirements for excitement and orgasm, whether or not this is a conscious fantasy accompanying masturbation. This highly individualized, often unconscious personal fantasy is the product of multiple influences that include childhood experience, especially during the oedipal phase, trauma, family, and cultural input; it must gradually be adapted to an interpersonal context where it can be "normalized" (Shapiro 2008) and acted upon with another person.

• See the video "Mid-Adolescent Boy" for an example of a thoughtful boy whose peer environment was heavily immersed in risky behavior. His relationship with his girlfriend, attitudes toward love and sex, and management of his mother's interventions are good examples of an unusually self-reflective mid-adolescent.

As teens move through high school, their interest in developing guiding relationships with adults reemerges. Mentors, such as coaches, teachers, advisers, and trainers, can assume great importance in offering alternative adult role models who pull the teen forward instead of threatening a backward drag toward childhood, epitomized by parents. Moreover, the emergence of competence and better self-regulation diminishes the threat of dependency and supports confidence in an autonomous identity. The teenager who is about to leave home for college is usually able to achieve a reasonable rapprochement with parents, although some degree of "conflictual independence" facilitates adaptation to college (Lapsley and Edgerton 2002). Moreover, family relationships typically improve after the separation.

Contributing to these developments is the growing discrimination the adolescent brings to bear on the peer group. The cliques of high school often evaporate in senior year, and interesting individuals with their own identities appear in their place. High school seniors begin to appreciate their peers without stereotyping them and can reflect on their earlier perceptions with humor and forbearance. One graduating senior reported that a key assignment of ethics class in her final semester was to name the cliques and power gradients in her grade. To her surprise, the classroom reporting of everyone's formulation resulted in much laughter and a powerful bonding experience. This shift in perspective on the peer group often corresponds to the emergence of the capacity for romantic love. Intimate sexual relationships further facilitate the maturity of the mid- to late adolescent (see the section "The Importance of the Sexual Body" later in this chapter).

Mid-Adolescence (Ages 14–17)

- Heightened conflict with parents results as the mid-adolescent experiences autonomy and a greater capacity to assess and outsmart adults.

- Greater access to and interest in the pursuit of action and experience emerge, and risky behaviors increase.

- Gender role identity, central masturbation fantasy, and arousal requirements consolidate and gradually normalize to permit interpersonal sexual contact.

THE SECOND INDIVIDUATION PROCESS

Blos (1967) developed the paradigm of the "second individuation process of adolescence" to describe the overarching psychic process spanning the entire adolescent period. Although this term has drawn interest and criticism (e.g., see Ammaniti and Sergi 2003; Doctors 2000; Jacobs 2007; Kroger 2004) over the decades since its introduction, it remains a useful frame for understanding the adolescent experience, especially when integrated with newer thinking. It is important when considering this paradigm to recognize that the process is an internal one. The second individuation does not imply actual physical separation or intense conflict with parents, but rather the reworking of psychic structure that ultimately allows the adolescent to experience himself or herself as an autonomous individual with the freedom to seek new love objects and assume responsibility for life choices. In this way it dovetails with the process of identity formation to be discussed in Chapter 9, "Late Adolescence."

Because younger children's psychological well-being depends on parental approval, protection, and support to bolster ego capacities and compensate for areas of immaturity and ego weakness, adolescence, as a key phase in the transition to adulthood, requires that this parental scaffolding be relinquished, at least in part. The latency-age child, while interested in the peer group and the outside world, still experiences his or her primary focus to be the family in reality and in mental life. Parental values, parental love, rivalries for position in the family, and identifications with idealized images of parents must all be reworked so that the adolescent is free to discover his or her own ideals, goals, and standards and to find love and ultimately sexual gratification in the world of peers. For the early adolescent who is just beginning to grapple with the new equipment of a body capable of adult sexuality and reproduction, the pressure to disengage from the childhood preoccupation with parents is considerable. Parents are the first love objects; with physical development and sexual drive, the close physical relationship to parents can suddenly feel uncomfortable, and the young adolescent may try to establish privacy and some degree of distance. This distancing, which can be purely internal or overt and dramatic, is not infrequently experienced by teenagers as a loss, because both the internalized and the real parent had, in the past, supported aspects of their mental structure in the process of their evolution. The following vignette shows the interplay of these internal conflicts about parents with the many other influences shaping this process, such as idiosyncratic developmental pace and the opportunities provided by the peer group.

Lindsay had always been very attached to her parents and had an especially warm relationship with her handsome, youthful father. She was an avid equestrian and spent every Saturday at a barn in a neighboring town where, under her father's admiring eye, she perfected her riding. Early development and menarche at age 11 were surprising and uncomfortable for Lindsay, especially as her breast development advanced rapidly and drew considerable attention from peers. At home, she was uncomfortable with her father and felt embarrassed by his ongoing attentions. He continued to see her as naïve and innocent but now curiously distant and unwilling to engage in former easy exchanges of physical contact. At age 13, in seventh grade, Lindsay felt propelled into early sexual encounters not only by boys' assumptions that she was older than she actually was but by her need to deflect her arousal away from her father; she began to rely on "hookups" at parties to boost her self-esteem and to find an outlet for her desire for affection and her sexual tension. Lindsay's precocious maturity and her willingness to hook up with boys isolated her from other girls over the course of her seventh- and eighth-grade years. She was lonely, and despite a somewhat prickly relationship with her mother since preadolescence, she began to seek her company, especially before bed, for wordless comfort. By the beginning of high school, the girls in her grade had "caught up" in terms of development, and Lindsay was able to form a close relationship with another girl who had recently moved to the neighborhood. They became close confidantes and companions, reducing her reliance on her mother and her indiscriminant hookups. The two girls counseled each other on boys, clothing, and future aspirations and continued to be friends as they developed romantic relationships later in high school.

Attachment theorists object to Blos's (1967) term *the second individuation process of adolescence* because it invokes the separation-individuation process earlier in life and seems to underscore the presence of parent-child conflict; they prefer to call the process *attachment-individuation* (Ammaniti and Sergi 2003; Doctors 2000). They emphasize that in securely attached children, individuation need not result in physical or emotional separation. These theorists point out that a successful adolescent process does not require rupture of the actual attachment or an expulsion of the internalized parental presence; in regard to the latter, they would argue that the internalization of working models of attachment earlier in childhood is the basis for a "realignment and redefinition" (Steinberg 1990) of the relationship. The internal parental presence becomes perhaps more smoothly integrated, but not ejected. Many psychodynamic thinkers, however, observe that adolescent process shows evidence of a series of transitional states as the young person evolves from dependence on parents for love and guidance to a reliance on unique self-determined values and the capacity to give and receive mature love (Brandt 1977). There are signs along the way that adolescents experience some feelings of emptiness and loneliness as they progress from implicit acceptance of the parental worldview and need for parental support, both internal and external, toward self-determination and responsibility. This process inevitably involves a very specific form of structural developmental regression as the superego constraints are reexternalized (Blos 1968). For example, in mid-adolescence, typically the most conflictual period for children in relationship to parents, the internalized parental rules and limits are projected onto a range of authority figures that the teenager may experience as restrictive. Defiance toward these authorities is at least in part a struggle to disengage from childhood thralldom. As many of the vignettes in this chapter suggest, this struggle often involves the flagrant violation of parental values; parents' measured responses can make a crucial difference in the outcome. James, described in the following vignette, manifested a rebellion and then, by virtue of a timely intervention by his parents, found his way back to something similar to his parents' worldview.

> James was a raised by conservative professional parents, immigrants from a developing country with traditional values. Until middle school, he was considered a cooperative and engaging boy who patiently addressed his parents' "culture clash" with contemporary American society but never overtly rebelled. In many ways he was an ideal hybrid, conforming to standards of politeness and compliance with religious observances and yet also able to adapt to his progressive school environment. However, when James was in eighth grade his parents relaxed their careful monitoring of his activities. In the setting of greater autonomy, his flexible adaptation seemed to shatter and he became increasingly involved with a group of kids who were considered "wild" even by Western standards and, with them, began to experiment with alcohol, marijuana, and partying. Parental attempts to reassert control were met with outward compliance but, to the parents' dismay, more lying and sneaking. His defiance was never overt, but his oppositional behavior was increasingly poorly concealed. James's excellent grades declined and he definitely hurt his chances of getting into a competitive magnet high school. He began high school in a large public school where his access to the "fast crowd" skyrocketed. Despite their frustration with him, his parents' alarm and anger began to shift to concern for his mental state; they saw him as increasingly unhappy and yet unreachable. As the situation worsened, they decided to send him to a special summer program in their country of origin, intended to instill cultural and religious values under the guidance of a charismatic spiritual leader. This intervention had a remarkable effect: James became more religious and conservative than even his parents had hoped. He chose to go to a very traditional religious school for the remainder of high school and seemed to have no trouble giving up his middle school and early high school friends. He maintained a close Facebook connection with his summer group and the leader. Over the next few years, his conservatism softened and his views came more into line with his parents' relatively modern outlook, but he maintained his strong religious affiliation and planned his further education around his religious aspirations.

The task of individuating ebbs and flows throughout the adolescent experience and does not reach completion until its close. Ultimately, the adolescent recognizes the importance of determining one's own rules, neither relying on family culture and parental admonitions derived from childhood nor needing to reject them categorically. To aid this process, teenagers turn to the peer group as a substitute for parental guidance, with potential radical departure from past behavior and deviation from the family's ideals. Young adolescents, who are usually not concerned with lofty long-term goals, are nonetheless challenged to figure out how to conduct themselves through the immediate future. They are confronted with a youth culture that calls into question many cherished beliefs based on parents' implicit or explicit guidelines. The comfortable rules of the latency period no longer serve. Although many early adolescents are not put to the test during middle school, their confidence in parental values is shaken by their own fascination with high school legends regarding sexual activity, experimentation with drugs and alcohol, and other risky behaviors. There are many facets to this dilemma, but the second-individuation model underscores the psychological work of reorganizing the superego by loosening the reliance on identifications with parents. The ensuing regressive states and behavior are accompanied by a predilection for action and reactivation of old conflicts, overidealization of iconic figures (heartthrobs and cultural idols used to extricate oneself from former attitudes toward parents), and an intensification of the experience of ambivalence (Blos 1967). In Blos's formulation, this kind of regression, which produces the familiar picture of the preoccupied, sullen, exasperating, and disrespectful teen, is essential for forward movement. Although these features can persist through mid-adolescence, by the time of college enrollment young people are usually more firmly autonomous and more confident about making their own decisions; as a consequence, there is less need to quarrel with or defy parents, less need to adopt radical ideologies, and less need to supplant parents with false idols.

Previewing the discussion in Chapter 9 on identity as a concept that bridges psyche and culture, we suggest that in periods of social upheaval, the peaceful rapprochement with the older generation may be attenuated or disrupted. University and other youth environments in these circumstances become the vanguard of political and social change, as in the late 1960s and the 1970s in the United States. The shift toward a new order is grounded in pervasive societal discontent with inequities and injustices; the adolescent acts as a harbinger of the future (Esman 1990). This carries more gravitas for late adolescents, who are empowered to effect change by virtue of their adult privileges.

In mid-adolescence, however, there is typically a vacillation between positions—from argumentativeness and revolt to thoughtful disillusionment to regressive, unreflective reliance on parental guidance. Many high schoolers look forward to the concrete geographic distance from parents provided by college to consolidate their individuation. The following example of Peter shows the social price of clinging to parental values and the difficulty for some children of comfortably individuating. Often, it is only the prospect of the geographic separation that allows them to psychologically separate.

> Peter was a relatively shy and somewhat separation-anxious grade-school boy who was reluctant to sleep over at friends' houses and who much preferred overseeing his younger siblings like a third parent and hanging out with his family on weekends. Throughout most of middle school, he had little apparent interest in the parties and social gatherings of his grade. He was a superlative student who annoyed his peers with his air of intellectual precocity. He idolized his very successful self-made father, who was himself anxious about his children "getting into trouble." When Peter's eighth-grade science club friends cajoled him into attending a school dance, he professed shock at the realization that there was some "hooking up" and even signs of alcohol consumption among the larger group. After his increased isolation from the social events of his classmates over the next year, he broke through his inhibitions and attended a party where he experimented with beer and marijuana. For the next several months, he was an eager and enthusiastic partygoer, seemingly disengaged from academics and arousing considerable concern in his parents. However, as he contemplated his junior year in high school, he renounced his partying and buckled down to academic work. He wanted to find a happy medium, he said, but also feared disappointing his parents and felt more comfortable following their guidelines while "still living at home." When he went to college, "it would be a different story." Indeed, in his senior year, after early admission to his first-choice college, he engaged in a lengthy process of negotiation with his parents, where he argued persuasively that they needed to trust him to use his judgment and handle himself, because soon he would have to do so, and he began to socialize, experiment with alcohol, and approach a few girls while his parents fretted but did not interfere.

It is most frequently toward the end of the individuation process, in late adolescence, that the gradual transformation can be said to stabilize with the emergence of uniquely personal conscience, goals, and aspirations coexisting with an ongoing strong attachment to parents and a more knowing relationship to peers. The superego can then be seen as emancipated from the link to the parents, differentiated from the peer group, and fully autonomous; nonetheless, as a late-established mental structure that continues to evolve dynamically into adulthood, the superego remains vulnerable to corruption by external circumstances (e.g., extremes of financial circumstances or power) throughout life.

Blos (1968) considered individuation to be one of four central tasks of adolescence involved in the emergence of the adult personality organization or character. The three others are 1) the establishment of ego continuity (i.e., a personal narrative that provides self-coherence), 2) the integration of childhood trauma, and 3) the consolidation of sexual identity. These components are building blocks of identity, and their resolution into character formation is a late-adolescent event that will be described in Chapter 9.

THE IMPORTANCE OF THE SEXUAL BODY

Psychological Adjustment to the Transforming Body

Before addressing the powerful impact of emerging sexuality on mental life, we wish to underscore that the changing body itself is a major psychological challenge for the young to mid-adolescent. The rapid growth and bodily change that begin in preadolescence—including the emergence of secondary sexual characteristics; new and different demands for hygiene to deal with menstruation, acne, facial hair, and body odor; and the management of breast development, visible erections, and wet dreams—pose enormous psychological demands on the mind of the young teenager. Physical appearance is now a source of embarrassment, pride, shame, worry, pleasure, and countless other idiosyncratic emotions. This is compounded by the adolescent's awareness that he or she now possesses functional sexual and reproductive capacities (Laufer 1968). Whereas the young adolescent anticipates with anxiety and excitement the timing and progression of pubertal changes relative to the peer group, the mid-adolescent is over the shock of the physical transformations of the immediate postpubertal phase and on the way to managing the specific developmental task of "accommodat[ing] the reality of the changing body" (Lemma 2010, p. 691). Even though physical development has by no means come to a close, the pace of bodily change begins to slow by mid-adolescence, and the body of the average 15- to 17-year-old, especially of the average girl, is relatively stabilized; the boy can continue to show significant growth in height and strength, but with nothing like the velocity of growth of the early adolescent (Slap 2008; Tanner 1971). Despite the pleasure that many teenagers take in their bodies—in clothing, decorating, building up, and exhibiting this new object of status, competition, and desire—a significant number struggle with the challenge. Some teens experience their physical maturation with dread and fear, urgently wishing to remain children, whereas others plunge into a precocious embrace of adult activities. There is often a deep disappointment in the failure to live up to fantasized breast size, height, thinness, muscularity, weight, and beauty. Many of the conflicts and symptomatic disorders of early to mid-adolescence revolve around the complexity of coming to terms with and handling this new, very important aspect of the self; indeed, it is the rare individual who, settling into the transformed body, does not at least occasionally experience self-consciousness, doubt, and the painful question, "Is my body as hideously deformed as I think it is?" (Redd 2008, p. 17).

The body is at no time more present in the mind than during puberty and adolescence. Of course, the mind itself is part of the physiological transformation and is equally affected by the hormonal, cognitive, and relational shifts that are part of the adolescent experience. However, for the early to mid-adolescent, the body can *feel* like an alien presence that disappoints, excites, and elicits frightening impulses and desires from within the self and from others. The complexity of the mind-body relationship is evident in a number of arenas: attitudes toward gender and sexuality, eating and weight, appearance and deliberate alterations of appearance, virtual socialization, and, more broadly, risky behaviors that endanger health and well-being. The kaleidoscope of bodily transformations predisposes the early to mid-adolescent to disorders related to control of the body, such as eating disorders, nonsuicidal self-injury (cutting), and substance misuse, as well as promiscuity and violence.

Many other core issues, such as establishing an autonomous identity and the second individuation, are fundamentally linked to the process of coming to terms with the transformed physical self, because identity rests on a foundation of the body and its idiosyncratic and culturally determined meanings (Harris 2008). The body generates components of identity, which are, of course, filtered through the prism of culture, ethnicity, family, and peer subculture. The maturing body also propels the adolescent forward toward a new, more differentiated relationship to parents and to peers.

The Gendered Body and Body Image

Regardless of their direct effect on the mind, the hormonal events of puberty and adolescence result in transformation of the body from a relatively sexually undifferentiated prepubertal child to a gendered and reproductively competent adolescent. The changing body heightens the awareness of one's biological sex, gender, and sexuality and is a key component of identity. The new body carries gender-specific responsibilities, generates powerful urges, elicits responses in the environment, and thus alters the representation of the self. The body and bodily experience, in adolescence more than any previous time, is drawn into a close association with gender in terms of the idiosyncratic meanings of masculinity and femininity that have evolved in the child's mind over the course of development, emanating from family dynamics and fantasy (Harris 2008) plus the flood of highly gendered environmental input consumed by this age group. Inevitably, body image is also highly susceptible to the common stressors of adolescence: family conflict, school change, peer pressure, popularity, teasing, and media imagery (Hargreaves and Tiggemann 2004; Murray et al. 2011; Slater and Tiggemann 2011), as well as internal conflicts that work in dialectical relationship with these external factors (Lemma 2010).

Psychodynamic thinkers focus on the struggle in the mind of the young adolescent to come to terms with this newly altered, foundational core of identity which, while rooted in anatomical sex, is powerfully constructed by psychology and culture. However complex and individual the notions of masculinity and femininity and of sexual desire are for a given adolescent, he or she is faced with the concrete task of integrating the mature genitals and genital function, in addition to secondary sex characteristics, into the self-image (Laufer 1968), while also contending with a powerful upsurge in sexual interest, fantasy, and drive. Thus, the young adolescent must grapple with the complex mental tasks of making this changed body belong to the self and of tolerating and owning the associated desires and "lustful fantasies" (Friedman 1990) that emerge alongside the physical changes. The power of the body to influence the mind and the sense of self is dramatically increased in this age group, for better or for worse.

Moreover, sexual maturation introduces new tensions in the family, as mothers and fathers respond to their blossoming adolescents with their own complex views of masculinity, femininity, sexuality, and moral constraints, and also face their own waning sexual prime. Parents can struggle with a keen awareness of their child's attractiveness as a young man or woman; their own vicarious excitement about or defenses against forbidden sexuality can be expressed subtly or overtly in their attitudes and commentary. A father may view all boys interested in his teenage daughter as predators; a mother may demand to know all the gossip about her daughter's and her friends' sexual activities; a handsome teenage son may stir up intense competitive feelings in a father who is determined to outdo him; a mother may disapprove but inwardly relish her son's sexual escapades. A frequently cited outcome is the father who becomes so anxious about his daughter's maturation that he distances himself, leaving her to feel both sexually powerful and abandoned (Flaake 2005).

Masturbation, Sex, and Sexual Orientation

While clearly belonging to the category of the adolescent's relationship to the changing body, adolescent sexual activity has rightfully received considerable specific attention in recent developmental literature. In a review of the empirical findings from the first decade of the twenty-first century, a "sea change" in attitude was noted in the approach to sexuality in adolescence. No longer characterized as a risk behavior with pathogenic outcomes, adolescent "sexuality development" has been widely recognized by researchers as a "normative" developmental process with its own distinct progression and psychic reverberations (Tolman and McClelland 2011). Interestingly, this shift has occurred despite contradictory messages from political groups and a newly permissive media; the idea of abstinence is strongly promoted even while the media offers unprecedented access to sexual information and stimulation. Researchers have consistently broadened their approach beyond "risk behavior" to recognize that today's adolescents are faced with a range of choice in regard to sexual behaviors (including abstinence and virginity), a more self-aware sexual selfhood, and sexual socialization through peers and Internet access. Many scholars concur that an "abstinence-only" approach to sex education is problematic on both ethical and scientific grounds (Tolman and McClelland 2011).

Foundational for healthy adult sexuality, adolescent sexual development is yet another complex amalgam of multiple systems, including processes of gender identification, oedipal compromise formation, self-regulation, management of arousal and desire, and the specific adolescent tasks of individuation and identity formation. The adolescent's bodily transformation poses challenges in regard to body image and bodily control, but sexuality encompasses an aspect of the self that interfaces with many other important arenas: identity, sexual orientation, sexual fantasies, romantic longings, relationships with significant others, position in the family, religious beliefs, morality, guilt and shame, sense of responsibility, and more, depending on the individual. Sexuality that incorporates mature sexual capacity is a powerful and complicated self-experience that is, in the form that emerges after puberty, unprecedented in mental life and embedded in a "reticulum of motivational meanings" (G. Klein quoted in Person 1999, p. 38). In developmental research, this is studied as "sexual selfhood," a notion originating in the examination of young adolescent girls' experience of sexual desire, which has served to legitimize the evolving adolescent identity as a person with his or her own sexual agenda (Tolman and McClelland 2011).

As described in previous chapters, sexual feelings, fantasies, masturbation, and even sexual contact have their childhood versions. In fact, a number of studies document masturbatory activity and other evidence of sexual excitement in children that peak at age 4 (Leung and Robson 1993) or age 5 (Friedrich et al. 1998) and then ebb until puberty. After puberty these behaviors take on new dimensions, because sex preoccupies the mind of the young adolescent and carries new responsibilities and significance. The level of preoccupation is visible among boys, whose spontaneous erections and masturbatory urges are often the source of embarrassment as well as excitement. Cultural attitudes toward masturbation are nonetheless often harshly judgmental despite the clinical literature suggesting it is "normal," "healthy," and "almost universal" (Leung and Robson 1993, p. 238).

In the handful of surveys available, male adolescents acknowledge masturbation considerably more frequently than females, with up to 94% of boys and 60% of girls reporting at least one episode (Leung and Robson 1993). These numbers are all the more impressive because masturbation is typically underreported in adolescent surveys in comparison to retrospective reports by adults (Halpern et al. 2000). The reason for the gender divide has not been thoroughly researched, but psychodynamic theorists suggest that it may be related to specific female genital anxieties (Olesker 1998) and bodily shame established in early childhood (Gilmore 1998) that interfere with bodily exploration by manual touching. The responses of girls surveyed in an "exploratory" study ranged from enthusiastic endorsement to shame, uneasiness, and disgust (Hogarth and Ingham 2009).

Psychodynamic thinkers, in agreement with the surveys, consider masturbation to be an essential activity for the integration of the mature genitals and genital function into the self and body image. Masturbation acquaints the adolescent with the transformed body and facilitates his or her capacity to experience orgasmic pleasure. It is also an invaluable arena for learning the conditions and requirements for arousal ("the central masturbation fantasy" [Laufer 1976]) and integrating these into the sense of self. Over the course of adolescence, each individual's unique "sex print" (Person 1999, p. 44) is revealed; that is, the characteristic set of erotic stimuli that arouse and ultimately lead to orgasm emerges associated with genital maturity. This sex print is relatively stable but does show some degree of flexibility over the course of adulthood. It must be integrated into identity and ultimately must be modulated to bring these arousing elements into a relationship to another person. There is also, for the first time since infancy, the need for another person and his or her body for gratification (Ritvo 1971), creating considerable incentive for intimate relationships.

Many teens are frightened to discover what excites them; the most obvious example is homosexual orientation, which, although more widely accepted today, still poses challenges for the adolescent and his or her parents. The process of relatively healthy homosexual development is compromised by the conviction that one's parents disapprove or that it has to be hidden from peers. Moreover, homosexuality can require a massive reworking of identity, not only in the present but also in terms of the anticipated future. This is especially true for the teen growing up in an environment in which homosexuality is not well understood or easily tolerated, as in the following example.

> Matt grew up in a rural environment and was outgoing and gregarious throughout lower and middle school, popular with boys and girls alike. He had an array of talents that he demonstrated in school and in his many extracurricular activities; he was an excellent athlete, a good graphic artist, a leader in his church youth group, and a gifted actor. He went through puberty at age 13 and became aware of what had in retrospect "always been there": he was attracted to other boys. Although his parents were relatively forward thinking and "progressive," Matt was deeply concerned that this would disappoint them. He was equally worried about his highly valued religious peer group. He also struggled with what this might mean for his future because he was unacquainted with any homosexual men and homosexual lifestyles, and he had what he recognized were homophobic prejudices. In his view, these attitudes were both typical and widespread among his peers and, he believed, in his religious community. His attempts to get information about the gay world and the repercussions for his future were hampered by his concern that his parents periodically checked his Web-browser log and that the local bookstore was owned and operated by family friends. He was very frightened about the sex act itself because he had little knowledge and many misconceptions. Always a boy of decisive action, Matt decided that the best way to educate himself was to come to a big city, so he chose a New York acting program for the summer before his senior year of high school. This was initially very intimidating on many fronts because he was surrounded by a very forward gay community in the neighborhood of his dorm. Eventually, he met another inexperienced young man in the acting program and they developed a mutually supportive relationship in which they felt free to explore their sexuality. Nonetheless, Matt did not come out at home until after he left for college. He spent much of his senior year in high school subdued and slightly distanced from his prior close circle of friends, seeking individual relationships with a few artistic and idiosyncratic classmates with whom he previously had only passing contact. Although Matt believed that some of his friends, both old and new, intuited his orientation and would adapt to it, he felt bereft of his secure identity and his fantasy of a shared future lifestyle as a fraternity brother in a local college. He also became aware that he had romantic feelings for his closest friend, which was very painful for him. He chose a college in an urban setting where he hoped to feel more comfortable with his new identity.

Although the average age of first intercourse is notoriously unreliably reported (Upchurch et al. 2002), it appears to occur between 16 and 18 for girls and between 17 and 19 for boys (Pederson et al. 2003; Upchurch et al. 2002), so therefore toward the end of mid-adolescence. The timing of this event has been linked to many broad cultural factors, including ethnic and national attitudes, women's parity in employment and social status, access to birth control, and the availability of alcohol or other intoxicants, and also to the more idiosyncratic experience and near influences of the immediate peer group and family. For example, children of one-parent families and children from less well-off families tend to start having intercourse earlier (Pederson et al. 2003). Despite the trend in public policy and funding toward "abstinence-only" sex education (Santelli et al. 2006), there is considerable evidence that respectful sex education actually does more to delay intercourse and to prevent sexually transmitted diseases, unwanted pregnancies, and other unsafe sexual practices. Today's aware teens have the information and resources to be liberated in large part from the tight linkage of sexual activity with reproduction and even the risk of disease (Brockman and Russell 2005). This leaves them the complex job of applying what they know in moments of intense excitement and, on a deeper level, of integrating the sexual body into their mental lives and "normalizing" their sexual fantasies sufficiently to connect to another person and experience mutual pleasure (Shapiro 2008).

The achievement of a meaningful love relationship, with full measures of concern for the loved one and passionate sexual desire (Kernberg 1974), is increasingly sustained in late adolescence and will be further discussed in Chapter 9. For the early to mid-adolescent, sexual development and sexual contact exclusive of coitus are arenas in which the person comes to terms with aspects of himself or herself previously unformulated and singularly unremarked upon in childhood development (Fonagy 2008); despite the presence of earlier forms of masturbation and sexual excitement, these are not normally part of any real relationship with another person until postpuberty. As described earlier in this section in regard to homosexuality, the emergence, with maturation, of a specific arousing fantasy, whether conscious or unconscious, requires considerable psychological work to tolerate and to find an appropriate adaptation in order to engage in gratifying activities with others. Such fantasies, which may or may not require enactment, often have sadomasochistic elements that manage guilt about sexual pleasure or express the fusion of sexual and aggressive impulses. Prior to full capacity for romantic love, sexual experimentation is often driven by the opportunity for delineating the self and obtaining a highly valuable experience of self-affirmation and pleasure. Contemporary youth culture has been characterized as trending toward "hookups"—that is, brief coital or noncoital sexual contact without personal commitment. However, in a recent study of German and American teens, up to 50% described themselves as being in a romantic relationship at 16 years of age (Seiffge-Krenke et al. 2010). A growing literature suggests that the adolescent approach to romantic relationships, romantic experience, and sexual activity is linked to attachment style: people with avoidant styles have less and later experience, while those with anxious styles have more contact, often associated with risk taking (Jones and Furman 2011; Reis and Buhl 2008).

All sexual development in adolescence constitutes a new arena of personal experience that usually requires a qualitatively different kind of privacy and may distance the adolescent from parents, at least temporarily. For children who have relied on parents as confidants and guides, the navigation of this realignment with parents can also feel like loss. The evolution of a new, more equal relationship over the whole adolescent process involves shifts in identity in the teen's self-experience as a sexual person who must make his or her own decisions and seek intimacy in a different relational configuration. It also involves coming to terms with the disturbing recognition that parents "are people too" and engage in sexual activities with each other or, in the case of single parents, with other partners. Parents often struggle to adapt to the idea that their children have lives of their own and to trust them to manage challenging sexual encounters and ultimately forge deeply meaningful relationships.

CHANGING PHYSIOLOGY AND ANATOMICAL TRANSFORMATION: NEW CAPACITIES, PREOCCUPATIONS, AND PSYCHOPATHOLOGY

Brain and Cognitive Development

Changes in the adolescent brain and cognitive structure have been the focus of considerable attention from neuroscientists and developmental cognitive psychologists (Kuhn 2006), with an explosion of new information about brain plasticity in the second decade of life (Fields 2005; Hagmann et al. 2010; Rabinowicz et al. 2009). The dramatic brain remodeling that begins at puberty and extends over the next decade has eclipsed raging hormones in explanations of the biological basis of adolescent behavior, although researchers are quick to concur that it certainly cannot explain everything. Brain development during adolescence involves a remarkable process of *synaptic pruning*, with up to 50% loss in synaptic connections in the cortex (Spear 2007). Following peak gray matter volume achieved at age 10 (girls) or 12 (boys), the young adolescent undergoes considerable overall brain remodeling, especially in the frontoparietal cortical area, presumed to result from the wave of synaptic pruning that starts at puberty in the sensorimotor region of the frontal cortex and gradually spreads rostrally and caudally to include parietal and temporal areas. The implications of this surprising finding are not entirely understood, especially because all pruned synapses appear to have been functional in prior development, so presumably are not redundant. Pruning seems to be the targeted and specific "sculpting" of the adolescent brain into its adult form (Spear 2007, p. 13). The thinning of the cortex is accompanied by a decline in overall brain energy utilization, suggesting a more pared down, economic utilization of energy supplies. Broadly speaking, there is a correlation between intelligence and cortical plasticity during adolescent development; an accelerated and prolonged phase of cortical increase followed by vigorous pruning and cortical thinning is associated with higher IQ as measured by the Wechsler Intelligence Scales (Shaw et al. 2006).

In contrast to gray matter, white matter increases through adolescence into adulthood, suggesting new myelination and therefore selective increases in speed of information delivery. Researchers who emphasize the role of ongoing myelination during adolescence as a source of plasticity suggest that the gradual decrease in gray matter volume from puberty to adulthood may actually be a by-product of *late myelination* of frontoparietal cortical areas (Paus 2005). Still under active investigation, so-called late myelination, extending from adolescence through emerging adulthood, seems to be activity dependent—that is, to occur in the context of environmental requirements (Fields 2005)—and serves to optimize connectivity, neuronal synchronization, and integration (Hagmann et al. 2010).

In process, however, the radical remodeling of the brain is not necessarily coordinated or synchronous. The presence of "gaps" and "disjunction" in early adolescent brain development is linked to the oft-lamented disparity between arousal and motivation on the one hand and the emergence of regulatory competence on the other (Steinberg 2005, p. 69). The remarkable changes in brain structure especially affect regions and systems associated with overarching capacities described as *executive function:* response inhibition, calibration of risk and reward, emotion regulation, reading and interpretation of social cues, and integration of cognitive and emotion-related processes (Blakemore 2008; Paus 2005; Steinberg 2005). The typical environmental demand on high school students relies on the development of these mental capacities, because the students are expected to multitask, plan for the future, monitor their behavior, self-regulate, and empathize with others.

Most adolescents experience an upsurge in restlessness and in novelty and sensation seeking beginning at puberty, although their capacity to self-regulate through the exercise of executive function does not fully mature until much later (Chambers and Potenza 2003; Steinberg 2004). Powerful urges often override the emerging controls, "creat[ing] a situation in which one is starting an engine without yet having a skilled driver behind the wheel" (Steinberg 2005, p. 70; see also Dahl 2001; Dahl and Hariri 2005). These observations suggest a possible neurological contribution to the psychodynamic hypothesis that defensively driven removal from parents (frequently referred to as "object removal" in psychodynamic literature [e.g., Abrams 2003]) creates a vacuum in the mentation of adolescents because adolescents are unable (or not yet able) to assume the regulatory function that parents formerly performed.

Piaget's contributions (1958; 1972/2008) in regard to the emergence of formal operations, higher-level abstract thinking, and hypothetico-deductive reasoning in children ages 12–15 are closely related to executive capacities, and it is clear that this level of cognition, including symbolic thought, logic, planning, and thinking hypothetically, also does not emerge all at once, fully integrated, universal (Kuhn 2006), and without regard to context (Anthony 1982). As Piaget suggested, during adolescence, developmental pace in intellectual progression is uneven, and marked diversity in both interindividual and intraindividual capacities emerges. Teenagers differentiate in terms of their academic and extracurricular arenas of optimal formal operational thinking. Indeed, the impact of specific environmental stimulation on the adolescent brain rivals its influence in the first years of life (Feinstein and Bynner 2004), but now the young person self-selects the input. Adolescent cognitive development is understood in the context of the idiosyncratic interaction between individual aptitude, interests, opportunity, and "the internalization of 'tools' provided by a given culture" (Anthony 1982, p. 318); formal operations evolve in relation to environmental provision, guidance, and demand. Recent research on the effects of teaching young teenagers to understand poetry shows that a determined environment can inculcate some level of capacity in most normally developing teens; even the ability to understand the highly symbolic idiosyncratic meanings of poetry can be nurtured by instruction (Peskin and Wells-Jopling 2012). This observation supports the crucial role of education in the developmental emergence of learning how to think in a given arena.

Piaget (1958) noted that an especially important feature of formal operations is that "thought can take itself as its own object" (Kuhn 2006, p. 64). The adolescent mind is capable of reflecting on itself, thereby taking a giant step toward adult cognition. However, the twenty-first century understanding of adolescents' thinking is that this new capacity for metacognition is variable and inconsistent; blossoming reflective awareness is remarkably flexible, but it is highly context and meaning oriented (Kuhn 2006). Egocentricity continues to distort adolescent capacities through the college years, and the maturation of perspective-taking extends well into the 20s (Elkind 1996). As noted in regard to poetry, there are multiple arenas in which adolescent cognition can benefit from adult modeling and instruction. The increasingly important sphere of interpersonal relationships requires new or refined capacities, such as sensitivity to other points of view, internalized affective reactions (guilt), and self-reflective empathy. Although originating in the oedipal phase, these affects and cognitions mature erratically and can be eclipsed by "hedonistic reasoning" or the familiar egocentricity that shows a consistent uptick in youth ages 15–16 years (Eisenberg et al. 2012) and again in the early years of college (Rycek et al. 1998). Attachment/mentalization theorists suggest that the jump in the level of abstract thinking due to the emergence of formal operations creates "pressure for interpersonal understanding" (Fonagy et al. 2002, pp. 318–319) at a time when the adolescent's ancillary use of parents as cognitive supports is no longer tolerable. The inevitable decline in reliance on parents during this phase removes the scaffolding they formerly provided to bolster inadequate prior development of symbolization, which is as important for relationships as it is for poetry. Thus, for teens with problematic early development, the twin tasks of coming to terms with the dizzying new complexity of their social world and disengaging from parents create a potential "developmental hypersensitivity to mental states" without the means to comprehend them, thereby producing withdrawal, breakdown, and a predilection toward aggression (Fonagy et al. 2002, p. 319).

Hormonal Changes and Sex

Reviews of research concerning the reality of so-called raging hormones as a determinant of moods and behavior in adolescence conclude that the relationship is anything but simple and differs from the effects of hormones in adults (Buchanan et al. 1992; Walker et al. 2004). Some researchers suggest that the challenge for the adolescent is one of *adaptation,* not only to the overall increase in adrenal hormones and gonadotropins, but to the period of hormonal fluctuation that typically precedes the emergence of stable cyclical patterns and/or levels characteristic of the adult. These researchers also underscore the importance of mediating factors such as timing of puberty, family relationships, and prior personality.

Hormones are weakly correlated with a range of adolescent behaviors typically attributed to them, such as aggression, impulsivity, moodiness, sexual preferences, aggression in boys, depression in girls, increased need for sleep, and so on; these behaviors are heavily mediated by psychosocial factors (Ramirez 2003). In general, current data show a very complex relationship between hormone level and full-blown psychopathology, suggesting that many other factors interact with hormones to produce such complex outcomes. Hormone fluctuations and cumulative effects act on the body and mind throughout adolescence, and always in interaction with genetic predilection (Walker et al. 2004) and environmental factors (Susman 1997). Reported adolescent "stress sensitivity" may be associated with adrenarche and higher levels of circulating cortisol, but this remains to be verified (Walker et al. 2004).

Although the scientific focus on raging hormones as a primary biological shaper has undergone considerable modification (Dahl and Hariri 2005; Spear 2010), the physical manifestations of hormonal events—the emergence of secondary sexual characteristics and new functional capacities—remain hugely important in the mind of the young adolescent. The changes have repercussions in many arenas of psychological functioning, such as familial and peer relationships, identity, mood, and inner life. Whether or not hormonal changes directly affect the mental state of the young adolescent, he or she is observing the bodily events and transformations following puberty and reacting to them with a range of emotions: alienation, awe, excitement, and embarrassment (Brooks-Gunn and Warren 1989; Brooks-Gunn et al. 1994).

The Importance of the Body

- Adolescent bodily transformation encompasses changes on all levels of physiological development.
- The brain undergoes radical synaptic pruning with an increase in white matter, creating a leaner, more specialized brain.
- Secondary sexual development and the upsurge in drive demand the integration of the sexual self, conditions of arousal, and the mature genitals into self-representation.
- Bodily development is measured against the peer group and contemporary society.
- Physical development, the relationship to the maturing body, and the desire to own and control it are responsible for many early and mid-adolescent phenomena: dieting, strenuous workouts, body decorations, and use of the Internet to assume idealized physical attributes.

Preoccupation With Weight and Physical Development

The relationship to the body in adolescence is shaped by the culture-specific approaches, some mainstream and some unique to a given adolescent cohort, to taking control of an object that feels unreliable and alien. The remarkable pace of growth in height and especially in weight is a potent source of distress and bodily dissatisfaction from puberty onward. Although the diagnosable eating disorders (anorexia, bulimia, binge eating) have been historically characterized as having a bimodal onset, with increments at the entry into adolescence and into emerging adulthood (Petersen et al. 1994), epidemiological data suggest that the onset of eating disorders of all types is clustered in mid-adolescence (Coelho et al. 2006). The preoccupation with weight and food is a ubiquitous concern of most mid-adolescents, not only those identified as psychiatrically ill. This preoccupation reflects the struggle to accept the maturing body and/or to make it conform to idealized images promoted in the popular media and emulated with varying success by the peer group. In fact, the epidemic of eating disorders has been linked to the media flood of images of thinness and muscularity that appeal directly to teenagers. This media onslaught promulgates unattainable ideals and exacerbates vulnerability due to prior development, family dynamics, and current conflicts (Hargreaves and Tiggemann 2004).

Excessive preoccupation with weight and attempts to control size are more common in girls but increasingly evident in boys. Statistical accounts vary, but markers of dissatisfaction are widespread; for example, the Renfrew Center Foundation for Eating Disorders asserts that up to 50% of girls ages 11–13 and 80% of 13-year-olds, boys and girls alike, have tried to lose weight (Renfrew 2003). Subthreshold or partial eating disorders, which are of particular relevance to the "normally" developing young adolescent, are remarkably common. Interestingly, these subthreshold presentations, which share symptoms of full-blown eating disorders at a subclinical level, seem to be a specifically adolescent illness; using relatively inclusive criteria, such as occasional bingeing and purging and moderate restrictive dieting, it appears that subthreshold disorders are rampant among teenage girls but then remit after adolescence. At 10-year follow-up, most of these partial disorders have resolved, except those that approximate the actual diagnostic criteria (Chamay-Weber at al. 2005). Statistics in regard to boys have consistently demonstrated a lower incidence of weight dissatisfaction, but there is evidence that boys are underdiagnosed simply because there is a lower index of suspicion among their physicians. Boys, especially those with childhood obesity, may have an incidence of subthreshold disorders that approximates that of girls (Muise et al. 2003). For boys who are not overweight as they enter adolescence, the concern about muscularity dominates and evolves over the course of adolescence (Jones and Crawford 2005). Thus, although eating disorders are a pathological manifestation, they clearly lie on a continuum with varying degrees of preoccupation with weight that characterize most adolescents. Most teens today traverse these years with a consciousness of eating disorders and observe the minority who suffer real disturbance with a mixture of envy and pity.

The following vignette demonstrates a typical pattern of eating and weight preoccupation for female adolescents. Molly is similar to many teens whose focus on weight begins to mount with the transformations of early adolescence and continues with a waxing and waning course, but never crosses into a real disorder.

At age 13, Molly was feeling confident in her junior high school, where she was completing seventh grade. She reluctantly admitted that she held a leadership role among what she wryly acknowledged were the popular girls. She did pretty well in school but wasn't focused on excelling despite her good intelligence. She was preoccupied with Rafael, a new boy in her school, who was the clear favorite of many girls. Feeling rivalrous toward the many attractive girls who gravitated toward Rafael, she began to worry about her weight, which had been a concern of her mother's for several years. She restricted her intake and lost 15 pounds over the academic year. Her mother, initially approving of her new regimen, became alarmed but was afraid of getting into an eating battle with Molly because their relationship had been more argumentative recently. They had always been very close, but now Molly seemed moodier and uninterested in family life. Her mother took her to an adolescent medicine doctor, a specialist in eating disorders. At this point Molly herself became alarmed, because she did not want to identify herself as a "girl with a problem." She cooperated with her new doctor, and her weight stabilized. However, she did not confide in her mother when she began to hook up with Rafael at parties, and she felt chronically annoyed by her mother's monitoring, which she described as "controlling."

Other Bodily Modifications: Tattoos and Piercings

Although not limited to the adolescent population, most studies of self-determined tattooing and piercing practices—termed body modification, decorations, or mutilation—confirm that a significant majority of these behaviors originated in the teenage years, with piercing preceding tattooing and preference aggregating by gender (girls preferring piercing and boys tattooing). Recently, girls' interest in tattoos seems to have equaled or even surpassed boys' (Fischer 2002). Teens' access to professional services is limited because of cost and regulations governing vendors, so they frequently self-administer these body decorations or get a friend or unqualified "professional" to administer them (Brown et al. 2000). These behaviors have clear correlations with social trends; as they become increasingly mainstream, their links to other risk-taking behaviors (Deschesnes et al. 2006) and anger or aggression (Carroll and Anderson 2002) are weaker. Body modifications are done for a variety of conscious purposes: enhancing sexual attractiveness, demonstrating love, and marking individuality (Antoszewski et al. 2010). From a psychodynamic point of view, the self-selected body modification of the teenager reflects, at least in part, the age-specific struggle to come to terms with the bodily transformation over which he or she has no control. Body modifications are motivated by a desire to (re)claim a body that has transformed into an alien object by pubertal changes. They are the paradoxically public affirmation of personal privacy and serve to demarcate one's own uniqueness. Both tattoos and piercings can be understood as assertions about ownership of the body that so recently was the parents' domain; in fact, the skin can become the battleground with parents over control, serving to deflect the teenager's attention from internal conflicts and the meaning of his or her impulse to alter the body (Martin 2000).

Risk Behaviors

Impulsive and risky behaviors, including substance abuse, interpersonal violence, self-injury, gambling, carrying weapons, reckless driving, driving while intoxicated, unsafe sex, and a variety of culture-specific exciting and dangerous activities, can be grouped together as disorders of impulse control; these behaviors cluster together and show greater prevalence in adolescence and emerging adulthood than in adulthood (Chambers and Potenza 2003). Multiple systems contribute to this finding, including the neurophysiologically accelerated sensation-seeking (outstripping the evolution of self-regulatory capacities) and relative insensitivity of the adolescent brain to the negative effects of intoxicants (especially hangovers, disturbed sleep, and headaches from alcohol consumption) that often instigate these behaviors (Chambers et al. 2003; Spear and Varlinskaya 2005). From a psychodynamic perspective, the adolescent's urge toward action reflects a paradoxical willingness to risk the integrity and well-being of the physical self in order to "just do it." The predilection toward action derives from confluence of internal pressures of adolescence, especially the persistent desire to assert ego autonomy, resist passive regressive longings, and test one's mettle by engagement in the world (Chused 1990).

Action is also a way in which the adolescent asserts ownership of the newly transformed body. As with tattoos and piercings, aggressive or reckless activity is a powerful assertion of the right to determine one's own choices, especially for the adolescent who struggles to establish autonomy and manage parental involvement. Risk behavior has been described as "an adaptive, narcissistic response to the developmental challenge of separation-individuation" (Lapsley and Hill 2010, p. 848), allowing the adolescent to tackle the array of daunting tasks, more or less risky from an adult perspective, that are unavoidable for forward movement. The adolescent's fearlessness is fueled by fantasies of physical invulnerability and inviolable integrity in order to face a brutal world without parental support (Seidel 2006), sustaining an illusion of omnipotence and safety typical of the younger child. At the same time, he or she individuates by scoffing at parental anxiety (Altman 2007) and asserts ownership of the body by treating it cavalierly. Risk taking has also been understood as an attempt at self-regulation (Leather 2009) or as a maladaptive coping style in which counterphobic mechanisms and avoidance of precautions predominate (Zwaluw et al. 2011). Some thinkers have attributed the underlying attitude of invulnerability in these behaviors (i.e., an attitude of omnipotence and invincibility in regard to danger) to the developmental step toward formal operations; the temporary transitional egocentrism leads teens to overvalue their own uniqueness and immortality and to have difficulty acknowledging perspectives other than their own (Elkind 1967). After all, the adolescent capacity to think abstractly does not immediately bring with it a mature conception of death, which is, in itself, "an almost incomprehensible abstraction" (Noppe and Noppe 2004, p. 153). Risk behavior can be understood as an attempt to master the growing awareness of and experience with death that is typical of mid-adolescence.

Although the idiosyncratic cognition of the adolescent may figure into risk taking, ample evidence demonstrates that in a neutral setting, the mid-adolescent recognizes relative risks and benefits of certain behaviors, can consider alternative points of view at an adult level when presented hypothetical scenarios, and understands universal mortality. The mid-adolescent should be fully capable of *mentalization*, which inoculates him or her from wanton destructiveness and self-harm. Certainly, defects in that capacity, usually attributed to traumatic early development, are associated with problem behaviors in adolescence (Fonagy 2004). However, the normal adolescent with no trauma history acts, in certain situations, as if his or her capacity to think about other people's mental lives, to consider the consequences of choices, and to assess risk is compromised. It seems clear that issues other than cognition, including excitement, peer pressure, and underlying developmental tensions, make it well-nigh impossible to apply such higher-level reasoning in the decisive moment (Steinberg 2004).

Robust correlations exist between childhood signs of psychological disturbance and problematic behaviors, particularly behaviors that manifest in early adolescence and become patterned and persistent. The children who show difficulties beginning in preschool—including school maladjustment, impulsivity, hyperactivity and attentional problems, anxiety and depression, and conduct problems—tend to engage earlier and more regularly in substance abuse, sexual activity, thrill seeking, and violent antisocial behaviors (Fonagy 2004). These individual personality factors have been folded into a broader model of risk behaviors, called "problem behavior theory" (Jessor 1977, 1991, 2008; Schofield et al. 2008; Vazsonyi et al. 2008, 2010), which uses a systems approach to delineate a range of risk and protective factors in adolescent development. This model, which weighs deleterious environmental, internal, and familial elements against salutary ones, reliably predicts deviant behaviors across cultures, races, genders, and socioeconomic categories. Although a range of mediating factors have been cited in the vast literature of adolescent problem behaviors—including personality disorders (Leather 2009; Schofield et al. 2008), genetics and gene-environment interaction (Zwaluw et al. 2011), race, gender, and family (Fonagy 2004; Roche et al. 2008), social context (Kilpatrick et al. 2000), and the zeitgeist of a given generation—the robust cross-cultural predictive power from the application of problem behavior theory suggests that no one factor, but rather the balance between risk and protection in any social context for any given child, is key.

Problem behavior theory also applies to suicidal behavior (Phillips et al. 2002). Suicide is the second leading cause of death in people ages 10–24 years, and the majority of suicide completers are younger compared with half a century ago (Belfer 2011). Suicidal thoughts and behaviors in adolescents are positively associated with mental illness, but these thoughts and behaviors also appear in groups without known psychiatric disorders and are associated with personal and cultural factors such as exposure to inadequate resources, family violence, bullying, unwanted pregnancy, arranged marriage, shame, and humiliation (Belfer 2011, p. 54). In a suicide center run by psychodynamic clinicians in London, suicidal behavior during adolescence was understood to reflect a range of specific developmental conflicts directly related to the achievement of sexual maturity: a rejection of the sexual body (Laufer 1987), a renunciation of the shameful requirements of arousal (Laufer 1995), and a passive-to-active defense in which helplessness vis-à-vis the internalized parent is transformed into omnipotence (Friedman et al. 1972). These clinicians underscore that it is collective denial that leaves adolescent suicide attempters undiagnosed and untreated; most require intensive psychotherapeutic intervention to return to normal development (Laufer 1995).

We emphasize that the risk behaviors of most teens are not associated with severe psychopathology, sustained negative behaviors, or even, as noted earlier, the inability to recognize risk. Indeed, the complete absence of experimentation is worrisome; in the individual case, dedicated substance "experimenters" are more troubled, but, in general, those who have never tried any intoxicating substance by age 18 appear psychologically maladjusted (Wills et al. 1996). In this regard, researchers tend to emphasize common features of adolescent life, such as the impact of peer pressure, the uneven development of self-regulation, the lack of a sustained future orientation, diminished parental supervision, increased financial resources, and the pubertal-onset decrease in reward sensitivity that leads to boundary crossing and novelty-seeking behavior (Steinberg 2004).

Even with the recognition that adolescents with problem behaviors are outliers, distinguished by their histories and the extreme nature of their activities, statistics concerning the mid-adolescent population are alarming.

The jump in morbidity and mortality of this age group is not confined to disturbed youth. In a recent study, 25% of high school students reported drinking before age 13 (Rew et al. 2011); unfortunately, alcohol begets other problems, especially driving while intoxicated (or being a passenger with a drunken driver), unsafe sex, and other reckless behaviors. Nearly half of all deaths between ages 10 and 19 are due to accidents, and 70% of these are motor vehicle related (Sleet et al. 2010). Driving without a license is rampant—in one study, one-fifth of underage adolescents had already driven a motor vehicle (Bina et al. 2006)—and other unsafe driving practices are widespread. Equally problematic, however, are sports-related accidents that occur in psychologically healthy teens and frequently recur in the same individuals (Marcelli et al. 2010).

Addictions

For the same reasons that early to mid-adolescence is a period of experimentation with substances and behaviors, it is the peak time for the onset of chronic addictions (Volkow and Li 2005): 80% of adult smokers begin before age 18 years, 40% of alcoholics begin between ages 15 and 19 and 80% before age 30, and the median age at onset of illicit drug use is 16 years (Chambers et al. 2003). Researchers have also persuasively argued that excessive exposure to substances, such as cannabis, early in adolescence can have long-term deleterious effects due to age-specific neuroadaptations that predispose to cognitive impairments (Schneider 2008) and susceptibility to future addiction (Volkow and Li 2005).

Neurodevelopmental asynchrony, impulsivity, and lagging inhibitory controls are possible mechanisms behind the increased incidence of addictive disorders, both pharmacological and nonpharmacological, in adolescents beginning at age 12. The fact that adolescent neurocircuitry is more robustly impulse-promoting than inhibitory makes the adolescent brain particularly susceptible to novelty and pleasure seeking. Indeed, impulsivity is a central feature of addictive disorders. Some researchers consider it more fundamental than physical dependency and successfully sought to widen the DSM-5 diagnosis of addiction to include gambling disorder (Potenza 2006). In regard to other compulsive behaviors, further study has been mandated (O'Brien, personal communication) to determine their categorization.

Excessive Internet use, for example, did not earn the status of a true addiction in DSM-5 (Griffiths 2008). Recognizing the ubiquity of Internet use in contemporary youth and the need to establish proper criteria for psychopathology, proponents of the term *Internet addictions* apply it only to those who demonstrate the following: 1) *salience* (i.e., the activity in question is subjectively considered the most important activity in the teen's day and is associated with cravings and preoccupation, at the expense of socialized behavior); 2) *mood modification* (the activity has a stimulating or tranquilizing effect); 3) the phenomenon of *tolerance;* 4) *withdrawal symptoms* (e.g., irritability or other unpleasant states); 5) *conflict* on an interpersonal, occupational, or intrapsychic level; and 6) *relapse* after periods of abstinence (Griffiths 2008). The proposed Internet addictions, as defined by Young (1999), include 1) cybersexual addiction; 2) cyberrelationship addiction; 3) net compulsions (i.e., online gambling, shopping, or day trading); 4) information overload (surfing and searches); and 5) computer or video game addiction. These disorders have become the focus of attention as ownership of computers, access to the Internet, and gaming consoles have rapidly proliferated among teens everywhere in the last decade (Rehbein et al. 2010).

Risky Behaviors of Adolescence

- Risky behaviors reflect the action orientation of adolescents, who seek experience and novelty, struggle for independence and autonomy, and want to define themselves in the world.
- According to problem behavior theory, severity of risk can be predicted by the interaction of childhood disorders and other deleterious factors with supportive and salutary influences.
- Some experimentation during adolescence is almost inevitable, and its complete absence is associated with significant inhibition.
- Many addictions such as smoking, marijuana use, and alcoholism begin before age 18.

Key Concepts

The period between ages 11 and 17 encompasses a remarkably active phase of human development during which body, brain, and mental transformations occur at a rate comparable to the first years of life. The body is a continuous source of excitement and conflict in this age group and often is a battleground for struggles for autonomy and individuation from parents.

The line between phases of adolescence is not sharply demarcated, but the divisions underscore the shifting developmental agenda. Early adolescence is ushered in by puberty, and much of the mental work of this period is devoted to adaptation to the developing body and its implications. The young adolescent is preoccupied with his or her bodily changes and burgeoning sexuality; masturbation is a means of taking full possession of this newly equipped body, allowing the teenager the opportunity to discover and explore fantasies and desires that are uniquely his or her own. The relationship to the parents continues to diminish in importance in favor of the peer group, especially as the drama of peer relationships unfolds in middle school.

In mid-adolescence, the bodily transformation slows down, and the changing relationship to parents and peer group takes precedence. Conflict with parents peaks, and the importance of parents as guides and companions diminishes. Peer influence mushrooms. Risky behaviors increase at an alarming rate, well ahead of the capacity to control them, resulting in a huge jump in morbidity and mortality in this age group. Sexuality assumes its prominent role in organizing the mind; mid-adolescents become clearer about their sexual orientation, their preferred masturbation fantasy, and their sense of themselves as gendered and sexual people. The exploration of sexuality moves into relationships as this period comes to a close.

- Early adolescence extends from the time of the first menses or nocturnal emission, around age 11 or 12, to age 14.
    - This period roughly corresponds to the middle school years.
    - It is a time of remarkable and relatively rapid physical transformation. The growth spurt predates the markers of puberty by a year or more and proceeds at a rapid pace through mid-adolescence.
    - Individual onset and pace of pubertal changes is a potent source of the self-experience, especially in relation to the peer group.

- Mid-adolescence extends from ages 14 to 17.
    - This phase corresponds roughly to the high school years and ends as teenagers turn toward their futures as autonomous individuals.
    - The velocity of physical changes slows, but the body continues to pose a serious challenge to the mid-teen's mental life.

- The changing body is, in and of itself, the most profound challenge to early and mid-adolescents.
    - Brain and hormonal changes deliver unprecedented shifts that color and affect mood, interest in novelty seeking, judgment, impulses, desires, emotions, and interpersonal skills.

- Coming to understand the newly equipped sexual body and arousing fantasy is a major task. Masturbation serves to manage intense sexual urges and to integrate the transformed body into the self-representation.

- Interest in romance begins early in adolescence, and relationships are of interest to boys and girls alike. A majority of late high schoolers report significant romantic involvements, and fully 84% have their first experience of intercourse in a romantic relationship (as reported retrospectively by 19-year-olds [Tsui and Nicoladis 2004]).

- The *second individuation* process begins in early adolescence and becomes a major developmental task of early and mid-adolescence.
  - The shift in the direction of yearnings from parents to peers has been called *object removal;* it can create a sense of loss, emptiness, and gradual alienation from parents.
  - In turn, parents often struggle to adjust to their child's transformation into a sexual person and feel uncertain about how to calibrate their parenting. By mid-adolescence this can advance to significant overt conflict between parents and children.

- The marked uptick in risky behaviors accompanies focus on the peer group and is related to normally uneven maturation of the brain, sexual excitement, and heightened impulsivity.
  - Psychiatric disorders related to the body, such as eating disorders and substance use, can be understood as attempts to control sexual maturation or mental upheavals associated with this period.

- Cognitive development through these years is marked by a shift to formal operations, including abstract, logical thinking, perspective taking, and expansion of metacognitive processes known as executive functions.
  - Inhibitory capacities lag behind novelty seeking and the urge to act.
  - Theory of mind and perspective taking increase, but the emergence of formal operations is accompanied by an uptick in egocentrism and self-consciousness, especially in the young adolescent.

REFERENCES

Abrams S: Looking forwards and backwards. Psychoanal Study Child 58:172–186, 2003

Altman N: The children of the children of the sixties. J Infant Child Adolesc Psychother 6:5–23, 2007

Ammaniti M, Sergi G: Clinical dynamics during adolescence: psychoanalytic and attachment perspectives. Psychoanalytic Inquiry 23:54–80, 2003

Anthony J: Normal adolescent development from a cognitive viewpoint. J Am Acad Child Adolesc Psychiatry 21:318–327, 1982

Antoszewski B, Sitek A, Fijalkowska M, et al: Tattooing and body piercing—what motivates you to do it? Int J Soc Psychiatry 56:471–479, 2010

Arnett JJ: Adolescent storm and stress, reconsidered. Am Psychol 54:317–326, 1999

Belfer M: Suicide behavior in adolescence. Int J Soc Psychiatry 57:40–56, 2011

Bina M, Graziano F, Bonino S: Risky driving and lifestyles in adolescence. Accid Anal Prev 38:472–481, 2006

Biro FM, Dorn LD: Puberty and adolescent sexuality. Psychiatr Ann 36:685–690, 2006

Blakemore SJ: The social brain in adolescence. Nat Rev Neurosci 9:267–277, 2008

Blos P: The second individuation process in adolescence. Psychoanal Study Child 22:162–186, 1967

Blos P: Character formation in adolescence. Psychoanal Study Child 23:245–263, 1968

Brandt DE: Separation and identity in adolescence: Erikson and Mahler—some similarities. Contemp Psychoanal 13:507–518, 1977

Brockman MS, Russell ST: Abstinence in adolescence, in Encyclopedia of Applied Developmental Science, Vol 1. Edited by Fisher CB, Lerner RM. Thousand Oaks, CA, Sage, 2005, pp 1–4

Brooks D: The odyssey years. New York Times Opinion, October 9, 2007

Brooks-Gunn J, Warren MP: Biological and social contributions to negative affect in young adolescent girls. Child Dev 60:40–55, 1989

Brooks-Gunn J, Newman DL, Holderness C, et al: The experience of breast development and girls' stories about the purchase of a bra. J Youth Adolesc 23:539–565, 1994

Brown KM, Perlmutter P, McDermott RJ: Youth and tattoos: what school health personnel should know. School Health 70:355–360, 2000

Buchanan CM, Eccles JS, Becker JB: Are adolescents the victims of raging hormones: evidence for the activational effects of hormones on moods and behavior at adolescence. Psychol Bull 111:62–107, 1992

Carroll L, Anderson R: Body piercing, tattooing, self-esteem, and body investment in adolescent girls. Adolescence 37:627–637, 2002

Cauffman E: The adolescent brain: excuse versus explanation: comments on Part IV. Ann NY Acad Sci 1021:160–161, 2004

Chamay-Weber C, Narring F, Michaud PA: Partial eating disorders among adolescents: a review. J Adolesc Health 37:416–426, 2005

Chambers RA, Potenza MN: Neurodevelopment, impulsivity, and adolescent gambling. J Gambl Stud 19:53–84, 2003

Chambers RA, Taylor JR, Toensa MN: Developmental neurocircuitry of motivation in adolescence: a critical period of addiction vulnerability. Am J Psychiatry 160:1041–1052, 2003

Chused J: Neutrality in the analysis of action-prone adolescents. J Am Psychoanal Assoc 38:670–704, 1990

Coelho JS, Polivy J, Trottier K: Anorexia nervosa, in Encyclopedia of Human Development, Vol 1. Edited by Salkind NJ, Margolis L. Thousand Oaks, CA, Sage, 2006, pp 98–101

Collins WA, Laursen B: Parent-adolescent relationships, in Close Relationships: Functions, Forms, and Processes. Edited by Noller P, Feeney JA. New York, Psychology Press, 2006, pp 111–126

Crick NR, Grotpeter JK: Relational aggression, gender, and social-psychological adjustment. Child Dev 66:710–722, 1995

Dahl RE: Affect regulation, brain development, and behavioral-emotional health in adolescence. CNS Spectr 6:1–12, 2001

Dahl RE: Adolescent brain development: a period of vulnerabilities and opportunities. Keynote Address. Ann NY Acad Sci 1012:1–22, 2004

Dahl R, Hariri AR: Lessons from G. Stanley Hall: connecting new research in biological sciences to the study of adolescent development. J Res Adolesc 15:367–382, 2005

de Goede IH, Branje SJT, Meeus WHJ: Developmental changes in adolescents' perceptions of relationships with their parents. J Youth Adolesc 38:75–88, 2009

Deschesnes M, Fines P, Demers S, et al: Are tattooing and body piercing indicators of risk-taking behaviors in high school students? J Adolesc 29:379–393, 2006

Doctors SR: Attachment-individuation, I: clinical notes toward a reconsideration of "adolescent turmoil." Adolesc Psychiatry 25:3–17, 2000

Eisenberg N, Carlo G, Murphy B, et al: Prosocial development in late adolescence: a longitudinal study. Child Dev 66:1179–1197, 2012

Elkind D: Egocentrism in adolescence. Child Dev 38:1025–1034, 1967

Elkind D: Inhelder and Piaget on adolescence and adulthood: a post-modern appraisal. Psychol Sci 7:216–220, 1996

Elkind D, Bowen R: Imaginary audience behavior in children and adolescents. Dev Psychol 15:38–44, 1979

Erikson E: Identity: Youth and Crisis. New York, WW Norton, 1968

Esman A: Adolescence and Culture. New York, Columbia University Press, 1990

Espelage DL, Bosworth K, Simon TR: Examining the social context of bullying behaviors in early adolescence. Journal of Counseling and Development 78:326–333, 2000

Feinstein L, Bynner J: The importance of cognitive development in middle childhood for adulthood socioeconomic status, mental health, and problem behavior. Child Dev 75:1329–1339, 2004

Fields RD: Myelination: an overlooked mechanism of synaptic plasticity. Neuroscientist 11:528–531, 2005

Fischer J: Tattooing the body, marking culture. Body and Society 8:91–107, 2002

Flaake K: Girls, adolescence and the impact of bodily changes: family dynamics and social definitions of the female body. European Journal of Women's Studies 12:201–212, 2005

Flannery DJ, Torquati JC, Lindemeier L: The method and meaning of emotional expression and experience during adolescence. J Adolesc Res 9:8–27, 1994

Fonagy P: Early life trauma and the psychogenesis and prevention of violence. Ann
NY Acad Sci 1036:181–200, 2004

Fonagy P: A genuinely developmental theory of sexual enjoyment and its implications for psychoanalytic technique. J Am Psychoanal Assoc 56:11–36, 2008

Fonagy P, Gergely G, Jurist E, et al: Affect regulation, mentalization, and the development of the self. New York, Other Press, 2002

Freud A: Adolescence. Psychoanal Study Child 12:255–278, 1958

Freud S: Three essays on the theory of sexuality (1905), in The Standard Edition of
the Complete Psychological Works of Sigmund Freud, Vol 7. Edited by Strachey
J. London, Hogarth Press, 1962, pp 123–246

Friedman M, Glasser M, Laufer E, et al: Attempted suicide in adolescence: some observations from a psychoanalytic research project. Int J Psychoanal 53:179–183,
1972

Friedman R: Homosexuality: A Contemporary Psychoanalytic Perspective. New Haven, CT, Yale University Press, 1990

Friedrich WN, Fisher J, Broughton D, et al: Normative sexual behavior in children:
a contemporary sample. Pediatrics 101:e9, 1998

Gilmore K: Cloacal anxiety in female development. J Am Psychoanal Assoc 46:443–
470, 1998

Goodnight JA, Bates JE, Newman JP, et al: The interactive influences of friend devi-
ance and reward dominance on the development of externalizing behavior during middle adolescence. J Abnorm Child Psychol 34:573–583, 2006

Griffiths M: Internet and video-game addiction, in Adolescent Addiction: Epidemiology, Assessment and Treatment. San Diego, CA, Elsevier, 2008, pp 231–267

Hagmann P, Sporns O, Madan N, et al: White matter maturation reshapes structural
connectivity in the late developing human brain. Proc Natl Acad Sci USA
107:19067–19072, 2010

Hall GS: Adolescence: Its Psychology and Its Relations to Physiology, Anthropology,
Sociology, Sex, Crime, Religion, and Education. New York, D Appleton, 1904

Halpern CJT, Udry JR, Suchindran C, et al: Adolescent males' willingness to report
masturbation. J Sex Res 37:327–332, 2000

Hargreaves DA, Tiggemann M: Idealized media images and adolescent body image:
"comparing" boys and girls. Body Image 1:351–361, 2004

Harris A: Gender as Soft Assembly. London, Routledge, 2008

Hogarth H, Ingham R: Masturbation among young women and associations with
sexual health: an exploratory study. J Sex Res 46:558–567, 2009

Jacobs T: On the adolescent neurosis. Psychoanal Q 76:487–513, 2007

Jacobson E: Adolescent moods and the remodeling of psychic structures in adolescence. Psychoanal Study Child 16:164–183, 1961

Jessor R: Problem Behavior and Psychosocial Development: A Longitudinal Study of
Youth. New York, Academic Press, 1977

Jessor R: Risk behavior in adolescence: a psychosocial framework for understanding
and action. J Adolesc Health 12:597–605, 1991

Jessor R: Description versus explanation in cross-national research on adolescence
(editorial). J Adolesc Health 43:527–528, 2008

Jones DC, Crawford JK: Adolescent boys and body image: weight and muscularity concerns as dual pathways to body dissatisfaction. J Youth Adolesc 34:629–636, 2005

Jones MC, Furman W: Representations of romantic relationships, romantic experiences, and sexual behavioral in adolescence. Pers Relatsh 18:144–164, 2011

Kernberg O: Mature love: prerequisites and characteristics. Int J Psychoanal 92:1501–1515, 1974

Kilpatrick DG, Acierno R, Saunders B, et al: Risk factors for adolescence substance abuse and dependence: data from a national sample. J Consult Clin Psychol 68:19–30, 2000

Kirkbride JB, Fearon P, Morgan C, et al: Heterogeneity in incidence rates of schizophrenia and other psychotic syndromes. Arch Gen Psychiatry 63:250–258, 2006

Kroger J: Identity in Adolescence: The Balance Between Self and Other, 3rd Edition. Hove, UK, Routledge, 2004

Kuhn D: Do cognitive changes accompany developments in the adolescent brain? Perspect Psychol Sci 1:59–67, 2006

Kupfer DJ, Woodward HR: Adolescent development and the regulation of behavior and emotion: comments on part VIII. Ann NY Acad Sci 1021:320–322, 2004

Lapsley DK, Edgerton J: Separation-individuation, adult attachment style and college adjustment. Journal of Counseling and Development 80:484–493, 2002

Lapsley DK, Hill PL: Subjective invulnerability, optimism bias and adjustment in emerging adulthood. J Youth Adolesc 39:847–857, 2010

Laufer E: Suicide in adolescence. Psychoanal Psychother 2:1–10, 1987

Laufer M: The body image, the function of masturbation, and adolescence: problems of the ownership of the sexual body. Psychoanal Study Child 23:114–137, 1968

Laufer M: The central masturbation fantasy, the final sexual organization, and adolescence. Psychoanal Study Child 31:297–316, 1976

Laufer M (ed) and The Brent Adolescent Centre for Research Into Adolescent Breakdown: The Suicidal Adolescent. London, Karnac Books, 1995

Leather NC: Risk taking behavior in adolescence: a literature review. J Child Health Care 13:295–304, 2009

Lemma A: An order of pure decision: growing up in a virtual world and the adolescent's experience of being-in-a-body. J Am Psychoanal Assoc 58:691–714, 2010

Leung AK, Robson WL: Childhood masturbation. Clin Pediatr 32:238–241, 1993

Marcelli D, Ingrand P, Delamour M, et al: Accidents in a population of 350 adolescents and young adults: circumstances, risk factors, and prediction of recurrence. Bull Acad Natl Med 194:953–964, 2010

Martin A: On teenagers and tattoos. Reclaiming Children and Youth 9:143–145, 2000

McHale SM, Kim JY, Whiteman SD: Sibling relationships in childhood and adolescence, in Close Relationships: Functions, Forms, and Processes. Edited by Noller P, Feeney JA. New York, Psychology Press, 2006, pp 127–150

Muise AE, Stein DG, Arbess G: Eating disorders in adolescent boys: a review of the adolescent and young adult literature. J Adolesc Health 33:427–435, 2003

Murray KM, Byrne DG, Rieger E: Investigating adolescent stress and body image. J Adolesc 34:269–278, 2011

Neinstein LS: Adolescent Health Care: A Practical Guide, 4th Edition. Philadelphia, PA, Lippincott Williams & Wilkins, 2002

Noppe IC, Noppe LD: Adolescent experiences with death: letting go of immortality. Journal of Mental Health Counseling 26:146–167, 2004

Offer D: Normal adolescents: interview strategy and selected results. Arch Gen Psychiatry 17:285–289, 1965

Offer D, Offer JL: Profiles of normal adolescent girls. Arch Gen Psychiatry 19:513–522, 1968

Offer D, Schonert-Reichl KA: Debunking the myths of adolescence: findings from recent research. J Am Acad Child Adolesc Psychiatry 31:1003–1014, 1992

Olesker W: Female genital anxieties: views from the nursery and the couch. Psychoanal Q 67:276–294, 1998

Paus T: Mapping brain maturation and cognitive development during adolescence. Trends Cogn Sci 9:60–68, 2005

Pederson W, Samuelson SO, Wichstrom L: Intercourse debut age: poor resources, problem behavior, or romantic appeal? A population-based longitudinal study. J Sex Res 40:333–345, 2003

Person E: The Sexual Century. New Haven, CT, Yale University Press, 1999

Peskin J, Wells-Jopling R: Fostering symbolic interpretation during adolescence. J Appl Dev Psychol 33:13–23, 2012

Petersen AC, Leffert N, Graham B, et al: Depression and body image disorders in adolescence. Womens Health Issues 4:98–108, 1994

Phillips MR, Yang G, Zhang Y, et al: Risk factors for suicide in China: a national case-control psychological autopsy study. Lancet 360:1728–1736, 2002

Piaget J: Intellectual evolution from adolescence to adulthood (reprint of Human Development 15:1–12, 1972). Human Development 51: 40–47, 2008

Piaget J, Inhelder B: The Growth of Logical Thinking From Childhood to Adolescence. Translated by Milgram S. London, Routledge & Kegan Paul, 1958

Potenza MN: Should addictive disorders include non-substance-related conditions? Addiction 101 (suppl 1):142–151, 2006

Rabinowicz T, Petetot JM, Khoury JC, et al: Neocortical maturation during adolescence: change in neuronal soma dimensions. Brain Cogn 69:328–336, 2009

Ramirez JM: Hormones and aggression in childhood and adolescence. Aggress Violent Behav 8:621–644, 2003

Redd NA: Body drama. New York, Gotham Books, 2008

Rehbein F, Kleimann M, Mossie T: Prevalence and risk factors of video game dependency in adolescence: results of a German nationwide survey. Cyberpsychol Behav Soc Netw 13:269–277, 2010

Reis O, Buhl HM: Individuation in adolescence and emerging adulthood. Int J Behav Dev 32:369–371, 2008

Renfrew Center Foundation for Eating Disorders: Eating Disorders 101 Guide: A Summary of Issues, Statistics and Resources. September 2002, revised October 2003.

Rew L, Horner S, Brown A: Health-risk behaviors in early adolescence. Issues Compr Pediatr Nurs 34:79–96, 2011

Ritvo S: Late adolescence: developmental and clinical considerations. Psychoanal Study Child 26:241–263, 1971

Roche KM, Ahmed S, Blum RW: Enduring consequences of parenting for risk behaviors from adolescence into early adulthood. Soc Sci Med 66:2023–2034, 2008

Rogers KN, Buchanan CM, Winchell ME: Psychological control during adolescence: links to adjustment in differing parent/adolescent dyads. J Early Adolesc 23:349–383, 2003

Rohner RP: Enculturative continuity and adolescent stress. Am Psychol 54:278, 2000

Rubin KH, Dwyer KM, Booth-LaForce C, et al: Attachment, friendship and psychosocial functioning in early adolescence. J Early Adolesc 24:326–356, 2004

Rutter M: Psychopathological development across adolescence. J Youth Adolesc 36:101–110, 2007

Rycek RF, Stuhr SL, McDermott J, et al: Adolescent egocentrism and cognitive functioning during late adolescence. Adolescence 33:745–749, 1998

Santelli J, Ott MA, Lyon M, et al: Abstinence and abstinence-only education: a review of U.S. policies and programs. J Adolesc Health 38:72–81, 2006

Schneider M: Puberty as a highly vulnerable developmental period for the consequences of cannabis exposure. Addict Biol 13:253–263, 2008

Schofield JL, Bierman KL, Heinrichs B, et al: Predicting early sexual activity with behavior problems exhibited at school entry and in early adolescence. J Abnorm Child Psychol 36:1175–1186, 2008

Seidel RG: Anna, leaving home—an adolescent girl's journey. Psychoanal Study Child 61:101–120, 2006

Seiffge-Krenke I, Overbeek G, Vermulst A: Parent-child relationship trajectories during adolescence: longitudinal associations with romantic outcomes in emerging adulthood. J Adolesc 33:159–171, 2010

Sentse M, Laird RD: Parent-child relationships and dyadic friendship experiences as predictors of behavior problems in early adolescence. J Clin Child Adolesc Psychol 39:873–884, 2010

Shapiro T: Masturbation, sexuality, and adaptation: normalization in adolescence. J Am Psychoanal Assoc 56:123–146, 2008

Shaw P, Greenstein D, Lerch J, et al: Intellectual ability and cortical development in children and adolescents. Nature 440:676–679, 2006

Slap GB: Adolescent Medicine: The Requisites in Pediatrics. Philadelphia, PA, Mosby Elsevier, 2008

Slater A, Tiggemann M: Gender differences in adolescent sport participation, teasing, self-objectification, and body image concerns. J Adolesc 34:455–463, 2011

Sleet DA, Ballesteros MF, Borse NN: A review of unintentional injuries in adolescents. Annu Rev Public Health 31:195–212, 2010

Spear LP: The developing brain and adolescent-typical behavior patterns: an evolutionary approach, in Adolescent Psychopathology and the Developing Brain. Edited by Romer D, Walker EF. New York, Oxford, 2007, pp 9–30

Spear LP: The Behavioral Neuroscience of Adolescence. New York, WW Norton, 2010

Spear LP, Varlinskaya EI: Adolescence: alcohol sensitivity, tolerance, and intake. Recent Dev Alcohol 17:143–159, 2005

Stang J, Story M: Adolescent growth and development, in Guidelines for Adolescent Nutrition Services. Edited by Stang J, Story M. Minneapolis, Center for Leadership, Education and Training in Maternal and Child Nutrition, Division of Epidemiology and Community Health, School of Public Health, University of Minnesota, 2005, pp 1–8

Steinberg L: Autonomy, conflict, and harmony in the family relationship, in At the Threshold: The Developing Adolescent. Edited by Feldman SS, Elliot GR. Cambridge, MA, Harvard University Press, 1990, pp 255–276

Steinberg L: Risk taking in adolescence: what changes, and why? Ann NY Acad Sci 1021:51–58, 2004

Steinberg L: Cognitive and affective development in adolescence. Trends Cogn Sci 9:69–74, 2005

Stice E, Prenell K, Bearna SK: Relation of early menarche to depression, eating disorders, substance abuse and co-morbid psychopathology among adolescent girls. Dev Psychol 17:608–619, 2001

Stone LJ, Church J: Childhood and Adolescence. New York, Random House, 1955

Susman EJ: Modeling developmental complexity in adolescence: hormones and behavior in context. J Res Adolesc 7:283–306, 1997

Tanner JM: Growth in Adolescence. Springfield IL, CC Thomas, 1962

Tanner JM: Sequence, tempo, and individual variation in the growth and development of boys and girls aged twelve to sixteen. Daedalus 100:907–930, 1971

Tolman D, McClelland SI: Normative sexuality development in adolescence: a decade in review, 2000–2009. J Res Adolesc 21:242–255, 2011

Tsui L, Nicoladis E: Losing it: similarities and differences in first intercourse experiences of men and women. Can J Hum Sex 13:95–106, 2004

Upchurch DM, Lillard LA, Anesthenal CS, et al: Inconsistencies in reporting the occurrence and timing of first intercourse among adolescents. J Sex Res 39:197–206, 2002

Vazsonyi AT, Chen P, Young M, et al: A test of Jessor's problem behavior theory in a Eurasian and western European developmental context. J Adolesc Health 43:555–564, 2008

Vazsonyi AT, Chen P, Jenkins DD, et al: Jessor's problem behavior theory: cross-national evidence from Hungary, the Netherlands, Slovenia, Spain, Switzerland, Taiwan, Turkey, and the United States. Dev Psychol 46:1779–1791, 2010

Volkow N, Li TK: The neuroscience of addiction. Nat Neurosci 8:1429–1430, 2005

Walker EF, Sabuwalla Z, Huor E: Neuromaturation, stress sensitivity, and psychopathology. Dev Psychopathol 16:807–824, 2004

Wichstrom L: The emergence of gender difference in depressed mood during adolescence: the role of intensified gender socialization. Dev Psychol 35:232–245, 1999

Wills TA, McNamara G, Vaccaro D, et al: Escalated substance use: a longitudinal grouping analysis from early to middle adolescence. J Abnorm Psychol 105:166–180, 1996

Young K: Internet addiction: evaluation and treatment. Student British Medical Journal 7:351–352, 1999

Zwaluw CS, Kuntsche E, Engels RC: Alcohol use in adolescence: the role of genetics (DRD2, SLC6A4) and coping motives. Alcohol Clin Exp Res 35:756–764, 2011

CHAPTER 9

Late Adolescence

Identity, Sexuality, Autonomy, and Superego
Formation in the Late Teens and Early Twenties

INTRODUCTION TO LATE ADOLESCENCE

The broadening of the time frame for the adolescent process affects the notion of adolescent resolution, a process viewed as the central intrapsychic task of late adolescence by psychodynamic thinkers such as Peter Blos and Erik Erikson. The term *adolescent resolution* implies a gradual consolidation of the many transformations of adolescence, a process arguably extending into the late 20s. Late adolescents, between ages 17 and 21 or 22 years, experience a significant shift in their maturity and in their confidence in their own values and ideals. Optimally, late adolescents fully inhabit the new body and take responsibility for functional sexual and reproductive capacity; with this comes a deeper interest in love and intimacy. They are looking expectantly forward to the future with a mental picture of who they want to be. A sense of secure personal identity—a complex entity that we discuss at length later in this chapter— is growing, at least in some domains. The integration of the childhood self is part of this process; childhood is viewed from a new perspective and incorporated into the emerging sense of who one is. Although adulthood is not fully achieved by the end of this period, these individuals are teenagers no longer; their concerns focus predominantly on their personal vision of adulthood.

Many contemporary theorists and researchers suggest that the deepening of love relationships, the consolidation of the superego, and the intrapsychic achievements of individuation and identity formation in multiple domains, such as sexual identity and ethnic identity, can be traced from early adolescence well into the third decade of life. Nonetheless, late adolescence is still recognized as a developmental phase with its own challenges and opportunities, as well as its own problematic outcomes. Despite the contemporary predilection among recent high school graduates, whether in college or employed, to assume that there is plenty of time to make adult commitments, late adolescents gradually focus on their entry into the adult world. For college students, who comprised 68.3% of all U.S. high school graduates in 2010 (U.S. Department of Labor 2012), this process is formalized in the passage through the college years, with the hierarchical sequence of demands to explore a broad array of interests and then narrow them down as graduation approaches. This process is reinforced by expectations from parents and society at large that these youth emerge from college with a clear sense of direction.

From a psychodynamic point of view, late adolescence is marked by stabilization of ego capacities and interests, consolidation of sexual preferences, and the establishment of a relatively well-functioning and individualized set of defenses and sublimatory channels that ultimately become the foundation for the adult personality: "[I]t defines that period at the end of adolescence when the last major spontaneous integration and structuring of the personality take place as the adolescent enters upon the psychological and reality tasks of adult life" (Ritvo 1971, p. 242). The appropriate experience of guilt and concern, the capacity to sustain meaningful relationships, and the evolution of personal values are important prerequisites for engagement in intimate relationships that emerge during late adolescence (Kernberg 1974); in contemporary society the first such relationships do not typically lead to permanent commitment, but they pave the way for increasingly discerning object choices. With cognitive maturation and the new perspective offered by the college experience, the late adolescent is able to think deeply about the course of his or her own life, forms a sense of personal history, and contemplates a life plan. As graduation looms, the young person also looks toward the future and imagines a life. Future-oriented ideas involve the anticipation of concrete achievements such as marriage and career, which in turn reflect internal psychological shifts. More broadly, such ideas forming within each individual young person bear on what kind of life—what values and personal qualities— are worth striving for (Esman 1972; Ritvo 1971; Seton 1974). The commencement ceremony is the institutionalized recognition of the importance of late adolescence as a stepping-stone into adulthood. Whether or not there follows a period of further searching (see Chapter 10, "The Odyssey Years"), the well-functioning late adolescent has done some major psychological work to "connect the dots" of the past (Steve Jobs, 2005 Stanford University commencement speech) and set his or her future course.

If the developmental process rests on a faulty foundation, the adolescent period often reveals its impairment; management of the body transformation, sexual and aggressive impulses, and family and peer relations is impeded, and late adolescent consolidation is impossible. Late adolescence is the period when severe psychiatric disturbances, including psychotic illness and personality disorders, make their appearance (Ritvo 1971) (see section "Maturation, Physical and Mental Health" later in this chapter). Although most psychopathology is understood dynamically as rooted in past maladaptation with complex etiology (genetic, environmental, constitutional, etc.), contemporaneous environmental impingements and specific internal limitations (e.g., impaired and unremediated executive function) may contribute to pathological responses to the developmental challenges of late adolescence (Blum 1985). The period of late adolescence in postindustrial Western society is arguably extended into the 20s to blend into emerging adulthood; nonetheless, the young person who has foundered in the resolution of developmental tasks is unable to achieve the internal integration and personality stabilization that are hallmarks of the successful negotiation of this period. Intrapsychically, these achievements arise from the extension of conflict-free ego functioning and a consolidation of the subjective experience of identity and personal agency. The sense of continuity, personality cohesion, and psychological stabilization persists and sustains the individual even in the face of setbacks and unexpected adversity, provided these do not rise to a traumatic level (Blum 2010). The inconsistency and unpredictability of the earlier phases give way to relatively reliable and patterned adaptive responses. Ideally, late adolescents are also capable of a deeper level of self-reflection and perspective taking, which equips them with a sustaining autobiographical narrative, a sense of unique individuality, and the capacity to discern meaning in choices and events.

Tasks of Late Adolescence (Ages 17–21 or 22)

- Consolidation of identity
- Reworking of the superego
- Integration of love and sex in intimate relationships
- Stabilization of personality, defenses, sublimatory channels, and sense of self
- Integration of childhood trauma
- Self-continuity

TO COLLEGE OR NOT?

There is no question that the college-age adolescent is palpably different from his or her high school self and that an evolution occurs over the course of the college years. Subjectively, the break with the life of childhood, concretely represented by leaving home for college, is often both liberating and disorienting. The child's relationship to parents shifts abruptly into a paradigm wherein the supervisory role is dissolved and both parents and child must grope toward a new basis for their relationship. Successful negotiation of this transition has been connected to childhood attachment style; interestingly, it appears that some degree of "conflictual independence" (found with secure and dismissing attachment styles) predicts "positive separation feelings," which augur success in adaptation and peer relationships in college (Lapsley and Edgerton 2002). The benefits of "positive separation" feelings, without excessive guilt, resentment, or anxiety, seem to provide the freedom to move forward to this next stage of life without being hampered by looking backward. Indirectly supporting these findings is the fact that greater geographic distance and less contact seem to correlate with initial improvement in relations and the experience of greater mutuality between parents and their late adolescent (Lefkowitz 2005).

College provides a unique opportunity for identity exploration in all its domains, such as sexual identity, career commitment, political orientation, religious observation, and ethnicity. The adolescent can embrace these arenas as self-determined and deliberately chosen. The process of identity exploration is consistently placed, by psychodynamic thinkers and developmental researchers, in the college time frame of the 18- to 22-year-old (Erikson 1956; Meeus et al. 1999). The young person entering college must navigate a world full of possibilities—interests, ambitions, communal life, fraternities, sororities, teams, clubs, friends, sexuality, mentors, substance use, responsibility, and self-control—without the guidance of proprietary adults. Unless serious trouble occurs, the adults that the young person encounters in the college or employment setting will approximate a parental role only if actively sought out.

Even for those late adolescents who complete high school with confidence and sense of purpose, entry as novice into the new world of college can pose destabilizing challenges. In some cases, of course, the opportunities far outweigh any negative effect; many late adolescents thrive in a setting where they can focus on their academic and extracurricular strengths without concern for the weaknesses that plagued their high school careers. However, many individuals who enter college intending to pursue a field of study become derailed by the unexpected difficulties encountered when faced with college-level course work. Long-standing fantasies of "what I am going to be" crumble, and the student who has depended on them must now embark on a relatively unguided search for what interests him or her and what foundation it provides for the future. For those who have no clear agenda, the college experience, initially so liberating, becomes painfully reality oriented when a major must be chosen and even then can feel "just for now" because liberal arts majors are not always career pathways. The choice of major *can* represent a commitment to a professional goal, but often it defies such a pragmatic purpose. Majors chosen at the end of the sophomore year may reflect passionate interests with a long history or a recent, fortuitous discovery, but they are not solely dictated by the reality of life after college. Indeed, poor educational guidance can transform the institutionalized moratorium of college into a dead-end in terms of future employment (Cote 2006).

• **See the video "Late Adolescent Boy." This young man, interviewed on the last day of his senior year in high school, reminisces about his school experience and the college process. He anticipates the identity dilemmas of a "new beginning" that college brings.**

The four years of college have their own trajectory in terms of individual development, based on the widened horizon of interests and capacities followed by the incremental expectation of more focused commitments central to identity formation. College begins with the preoccupation about how to "make it" in campus life—that is, how to negotiate the proliferation of social options, intimate relationships, academic responsibilities, and extracurricular opportunities without the security or the constraints of one's established role in high school and often without pragmatic concerns about earning a living. Studies of late adolescent cognition suggest that the egocentrism of early adolescence seems to recur in the early college years as a response to the transition to a new environmental context; self-consciousness and loss of perspective taking may hamper the adjustment to the college milieu (Schwartz et al. 2008). Over the course of college life, the upsurge in egocentrism remits and late adolescents engage in a process of self-discovery and self-definition, learning what interests them, whom they like, and where their talents lie. As the college student settles into more committed interests and stable social networks, personality maturation is increasingly evident. The upperclassman is ideally deeply engaged in college life, both intellectually and socially. As graduation approaches, these advances must be adapted to the "real world." The opportunities available in the larger society can seem rich and exciting or potentially deflating, because graduation and the end of the "psychosocial moratorium" (Erikson 1968) reinforce the consequences of college choices and their impact on lifestyle.

Certainly, some adolescents emerge from the college experience with a strong sense of direction and a well-developed, autonomous identity. For example, the contemporary notion of "noble purpose" usually consolidates in late adolescence and is a developmental asset that organizes the college journey and projections into the future (Bronk 2011). Although the groundwork for such goals is usually laid in childhood, some graduates require further exploration to develop a sense of purpose that will sustain them going forward. Even for these young people who require the decade between ages 20 and 30 to step into their adult roles, the college experience has served by providing the psychosocial moratorium that Erikson (1968) recognized as a facilitator of identity. College provides the space to consolidate the individuation process, grapple with identity commitments by experimentation and exploration, develop the capacity for intimacy, learn to think with a full appreciation of psychic reality, and move forward into self-responsibility.

The high school graduates who do not head to college are a clear minority due to the contemporary "college-for-all" mandate of high school counselors, following a presidential initiative whose impact has been revolutionary and controversial (Rosenbaum 2011). The shift in the counseling approach from the much-criticized role of "gatekeeping" to the current posture of facilitation, in addition to the much greater availability of open admissions in community colleges, has greatly increased the number of high school graduates who are college bound, regardless of their likelihood of success. There has been a huge jump in the number of high school students who report that they are being counseled for or have their own intentions to attend college (depending on the report and the grade of the student, up from 32% in 1982 [Rosenbaum and Person 2003] to 85% in 2011 [Domina et al. 2011]). Despite this increment, the number of high school graduates who actually get a college degree within the 6 years following high school graduation ranges, depending on ethnic and gender differences, from 57% to 40% (National Center for Education Statistics 2011). The confidence of these college dropouts is often additionally eroded by their lack of alternative vocational training. Moreover, the absence of institutional structure for the transition to work in this and other Western countries has created an underclass of youth, "losers in a globalizing world"; even in those Western nations that divide students into college-bound or work-bound programs as early as fourth grade, job preparation paths in the form of apprenticeships are shrinking (Haase et al. 2008, pp. 671–672). In the United States, the push toward "college for all" is accompanied by declining vocational preparation in high school. This is especially unfortunate in the light of current research suggesting that the trajectory of young people toward work, college, or unemployment is predictable based on occupational and, especially, academic aspirations as early as eighth grade (Rojewski and Kim 2003). The decline in opportunities for training leaves the work-bound young person without institutional support.

Many dropouts and most late adolescents who go straight from high school into the workforce have lower occupational aspirations and lower socioeconomic status than college-bound youth (Rojewski and Kim 2003). Occasionally, they have the good fortune to find themselves in engaging fields chosen on the basis of "specific" career exploration that aligns the world of work with personal attributes and interests; this is contrasted with "diversive" career exploration that involves broad learning about careers based on their glamour or prestige without correlating them to personal aptitude, which some researchers believe is more typical of college-bound youth, at least in the early years of college (Porteli and Skorikov 2010). Thus, structured preparation and the vision of a future career pathway are central to the success of employed youth, as are job continuity, general satisfaction, and absence of interpersonal conflict in the workplace. Increased alcohol consumption is associated with dissatisfaction in both employment and college life (Aseltine and Gore 2005).

IDENTITY

Identity is a complex construction popularized by Erikson over half a century ago (Erikson 1950, 1956). Erikson's original epigenetic sequence of eight stages of human development and developmental crises placed *identity* versus *identity diffusion* at the heart of adolescence and stressed the importance of the institutional *psychosocial moratorium* (typically in the form of the college experience) for identity exploration and resolution. Erikson's ideas were operationalized to become the focus of a vast body of psychosocial research into *identity status* (Kroger 2000; Marcia 1966, 1993) that continues to this day. However, because the identity concept is uniquely situated in the interface between self and society, it has not been consistently incorporated into psychodynamic thinking. Its conceptual breadth and its psychosocial orientation have been criticized by some as linear and lockstep; sexist; too culture specific (Strenger 2003); too vague (Kroger 2004); and insufficiently intrapsychic (Kernberg 1966). With the rise of interest in the self among many psychodynamic schools, the general notion of identity has been somewhat eclipsed, although interest in some of its component domains, such as sexual and ethnic identity, continues (Lachmann 2004).

From our point of view, the identity concept remains immensely useful in understanding adolescent experience, both as a general phenomenon and in regard to its multiple domains. Erikson's (1968) emphasis on societal context is nowhere more fitting in development than in regard to adolescence, because this period is so profoundly influenced by the environment and historical era. The interface is most evident in its effect on the multiple domains of personal identity, such as gender, race, ethnicity, object relations, sexuality, beliefs, morals, ambitions, and so on. For example, changing societal attitudes toward sexuality and sexual orientation over the last quarter century have had demonstrable impact on identity formation among late teens of all sexual stripes. Shifting views of race and ethnicity over the last half century have similarly altered the perception and self-definition of many minorities in the United States for better or worse. In our view, these culturally embedded facets of identity contribute to the relatively integrated subjective experience of "who I am in the world," the hallmark of committed identity, that accompanies the late adolescent process.

Moreover, the identity concept refers to an ongoing, largely unconscious mental process integrating self-representations and subjective sense of self as a continuous, thinking, and feeling agent. Intrapsychically, the formation of identity involves the reworking of childhood identifications that served important functions in development, contributing to defenses that are essential for frustration tolerance and for managing deprivations (Jacobson 1961). Identifications with parents bolster the child's vulnerable ego and shape the superego and ego ideals throughout childhood. In adolescence, the ongoing presence of parents paradoxically permits a temporary disavowal of similarities and the reprojection of superego elements, as the teenager "rebels" and provokes discipline or punishment. The adolescent process optimally results in the reintegration of these elements, modified by events and the increased capacity for self-reflection and self-determination. Childhood identifications are thus selectively incorporated into the autonomous individual identity and the maturing self-representations. Identity includes an "integrated self-concept, an investment in standards and goals that make life meaningful, a weighting of the importance to oneself of various aspects of self, meaningful efforts to actualize one's ideal self-representations, a commitment to a worldview, and some recognition by the social milieu that 'one is indeed who one thinks one is'" (Westen 1992, p. 11). By definition, identity encompasses the active interface between the environment, both within and beyond the family, and a psyche equipped with the capacity to introspect, the striving for autonomy and individuality, and an urgent need to find a place in the world.

In our view, Erikson's conceptualization of identity is not neatly staged and linear despite its frequent visual presentation as a grid; he clearly emphasizes that identity formation is a lifelong process that is revisited and reconfigured throughout the life cycle and incorporates the multiple editions of self that begin in infancy (Lachmann 2004). The sense of self originating in relation to caretakers in the first months of life accrues throughout development; the adolescent period is a crucial moment in this process wherein a normative *identity crisis* occurs (Erikson 1956; Kernberg 1974). The adolescent is in transition from the childhood self to a viable adult personal identity firmly situated in the world; the search for identity is achieved through both an intrapsychic integration of component self-representations and a more or less conscious exploration and experimentation in the moratorium that society provides, such as the college experience, until *identity commitment* emerges. This dynamic understanding can lend itself to a more complex systems view, as suggested in Erikson's formulation:

> *Identity formation,* finally, begins where the usefulness of identification ends. It arises from the selective repudiation and mutual assimilation of childhood identifications, and their absorption in a new configuration, which, in turn, is dependent on the process by which a *society* (often through subsocieties) *identifies the young individual,* recognizing him as somebody who had to become the way he is, and who, being the way he is, is taken for granted. (Erikson 1956, p. 68)

Erikson's ideas resonate with Blos's (1968) description of the four components of character formation that "close" the adolescent process: the establishment of individuation, self-definition and self-continuity, sexual identity, and the integration of past trauma. Although Erikson focuses on the dialectic between the self and society in adolescence, highlighting the importance of *context* in the transformation of childhood identifications into true "identity formation," he does acknowledge the importance of the intrapsychic process that Blos addresses. The concept of identity contextualizes the unique individuation process in its specific cultural milieu, incorporates sexual identity and other domain-specific self-representations, marks the development of values and self-standards, establishes continuity with the past, and looks to the future (Wilkinson-Ryan and Westen 2000). It is the achievement of knowing who you are, what you want, and where you are going in the world you live in, reflected back and acknowledged by the people around you who matter.

Identity Achievement (Erikson)

- Identity achievement is a lifelong process, with many component elements, including relational identity and ethnic identity. It reaches a crisis in late adolescence, when it interfaces meaningfully with the environment.
- Identity achievement is facilitated by the psychosocial moratorium provided by college.
- Identity achievement requires coherent self-concept, personal standards, commitments to a worldview, and achievement of environmental recognition.
- Its alternative, *identity diffusion,* is a core symptom in severe personality disorders.

Identity exploration, which is not intrinsically stormy, is nonetheless typically associated with internal struggle and with a temporary weakening of the ego. As in the individuation process, the loosening of reliance on parental identifications creates inevitable instability and disorientation. Moreover, contemporary postmodern society thrusts the adolescent into a world in which identity exploration is complicated by the disappearance of prescribed and linear pathways to approved identities, but simultaneously offers access to self-invention and reinvention through technology and "makeovers." The rising dominance of the Internet as the social arena of contemporary youth has created new possibilities for identity manipulation whose impact is only beginning to be examined. Much of the individual's leisure time during mid- and late adolescence is conducted in cyberspace, where self-creation of identity is often the point of entry, especially in chat rooms and online gaming sites. The facts of identity can be crafted in a plastic alternative reality; for example, a hyperdesirable body can be inhabited through avatars, and basic facts regarding the self can be altered by deliberate online misrepresentation. Social networking sites such as Facebook also facilitate conscious and public manipulation of self-image and heighten the experience of playing to an audience, invisible but also all too real. Moreover, the contemporary romance with body transformation—by boot camp workouts, cosmetic alterations, and body decorations and adornments such as tattoos and piercings—encourage physical self-invention. These twenty-first century realities concretize the process of experimentation with alternative identities and can further decenter vulnerable adolescents.

The late adolescent's step into college provides a unique opportunity to transform, reinvent, or discover untapped aspects of the self. This is especially welcome if the teenager is struggling to throw over an unwanted identity established in high school. A liberal arts college experience is by definition the playground of identity exploration; it provides the freedom to try out different academic areas and offers infinite choices for extracurricular identity examinations, including fraternity life, teams, theater, newspaper reporting, and so on. As college students approach their senior year, such exploration takes on a new significance. Graduation marks the transition to adulthood and the entry into "real life." Like identities established and abandoned in high school, identities formed in college may or may not provide a sustaining self-scaffold in the years following; psychological stability, endowment, and, most crucially, social opportunity all play a part in whether these undergraduate identities go the distance.

The following vignette describes a young man who turned his direction around while in high school and then took advantage of opportunities to discover a path while an undergraduate at a liberal arts college.

Henry described himself as a clown until he got serious in his junior year in high school and took a second look at his way of presenting himself. The youngest of three boys of politician parents, he was comfortable in the "baby" role, which was useful to safeguard his status in the family and to avoid competition with his very ambitious and competitive twin brothers, who are 5 years older. Henry ingratiated himself by being funny, boyish, and cute, but "not a contender." He was in fact quite athletically gifted but avoided team sports and ran track indifferently. As he got swept up in the "college insanity" of junior year, he realized this was "serious business." He described a "lightbulb" revelation that he wanted to go to an excellent college, like his Ivy League brothers, after "not caring" at all for the first two years of high school. He began to apply himself academically and got more involved with the track team. He spent considerable time improving his fitness, and by senior year he even impressed himself with his altered appearance; he looked like a young *man*. He was gratified with his performance in academics and sports and even showed some real intellectual heft. Recruited for track by several good small liberal arts colleges, Henry arrived at his first-choice college without a clear idea of what interested him. In short order, he realized he just was not as dedicated to running as he thought he should be for the team, nor was he taken with the rather confining and hard-drinking "brotherhood" of sports teams at his college. After freshman year and much soul searching, he withdrew from the team, although he continued to run for pleasure. Leaving the track team meant a change in his living, eating, and socializing arrangements, and at the start of sophomore year he found himself in a dorm with other unmatched sophomores and a lot of freshmen. Disheartened, he spent that semester feeling painfully lonely.

However, Henry was able to invoke some of his valued outgoing childhood characteristics to rescue himself. He sought new opportunities to socialize and stumbled upon the department of Russian studies in his college while sampling language courses to fulfill requirements. Russian and Ukrainian ancestry was a valued aspect of his family's identity, and Henry had been included in several trips to Kiev, Moscow, and St. Petersburg when, in retrospect, he "was too young to appreciate them." The department of Russian studies was very warm and welcoming and encouraged students to hang out, eat, and study together to improve their language skills. Henry became increasingly interested in the politics of the region, which were very dynamic at that time. He developed close friendships with other students in the department and was part of a cadre that went to St. Petersburg for junior semester abroad. During that experience, he seemed to blossom and his extroverted personality became a real asset. He took naturally to the culture and rapidly developed fluency because he was willing to talk to anyone; he networked and made lasting contacts in all walks of life. At the same time, he became seriously involved in a relationship with another visiting student from a different small liberal arts school who was similarly smitten with Russian culture. When his parents visited, he made use of their political connections to get introductions and meetings with local political figures and served as interpreter. Although not sure whether he would approach the field through journalism, academics, or policymaking, he was committed to studying and understanding Russia; he was confident he would be able to do something serious and important with his knowledge and his expanding network.

Despite detractors, the notions of identity and identity diffusion, or confusion, are enduring constructs in the field of development and in psychodynamic theory. The research into identity status, conducted primarily using self-reports (e.g., Marcia's Objective Measure of Ego Identity Status) and structured interviews, identified two broad categories of identity achievement: committed and noncommitted, and two styles within each: *foreclosed* and *achieved* within the committed group and *moratorium* and *diffuse* within the noncommitted group. Of these, the achieved and moratorium styles both showed evidence of past or present active exploration and in general are associated with more mature object relations, moral reasoning, and ego development (Kroger 2000). Research into identity status has borne out the observation that the process of identity formation is most active between ages 18 and 22, thus in the college years. In addition, although individuals maintain a degree of consistency in personality characteristics over time, the prevalence of *achieved identity* increases (representing optimal identity formation) as adolescence advances (Kumru and Thompson 2003). Marcia's paradigm can be understood to illuminate personality configurations that show progression from greater confusion to greater clarity over the course of late adolescence, but nonetheless reflect enduring identity features within a given individual (Meeus et al. 1999).

This latter finding touches on the significance of identity diffusion, a concept that is the cornerstone of psychodynamic theorizing about borderline personality, especially in Kernberg's important contributions (Kernberg 1966, 2006) and in Westen's empirical research (Westen 2011). Identity diffusion, or identity confusion, is considered the core disturbance in severe personality disorders that typically make their appearance in mid- to late adolescence (Chanen et al. 2004). As suggested by the findings from identity status research, identity diffusion reflects enduring personality traits that are observable from early childhood. In Kernberg's thinking, the failure to successfully traverse the normative adolescent identity crisis is predetermined by prior developmental disturbance, due to temperamental predispositions (toward negative affects and impulsivity), a history of disorganized attachment, and, especially, childhood trauma or chaotic family environment. In these circumstances, the integration of positive and negative self- and object representations cannot be accomplished. Notably, Kernberg's idea is concordant with Blos's (1968) idea about the central task of coming to terms with childhood trauma in adolescence.

For many psychodynamic thinkers, then, the establishment of a well-integrated committed identity, neither prematurely foreclosed by absence of choice and/or intrapsychic rigidity nor diffuse by virtue of temperamental vulnerability, unsecure attachment, and trauma, reflects adequate prior development and is intrinsic to the successful entry into adulthood, as in the previous vignette about Henry and in the following example.

Susannah grew up in an affluent suburb, the older of two daughters of an engineer father and a stay-at-home mother. She was early identified as a talented singer and was groomed to become the opera star that her mother had always wanted to be. During high school, she focused on the drama department; her performances received kudos from family, the school community, and her entire hometown. She felt her future was set and therefore applied and was accepted at a prestigious conservatory specializing in opera and musical theater. This success consolidated her identity as a local celebrity. Her mother hovered in the background as Susannah attempted to position herself in her program, auditioning for parts both within and outside the conservatory. Meanwhile, her social immaturity became abundantly clear to her as she observed her classmates managing their newfound freedom and access to alcohol, casual sex, and romantic relationships. Her dependency on her mother, involving multiple daily phone calls, began to feel onerous and unnecessary, especially as she experienced recurrent rejections in her auditions and felt she had to manage her mother's disappointment in addition to her own. Confidence in her mother's judgment and guidance declined, and the contact diminished. Susannah began to party and to drink to excess, which in turn led to impulsive and regretted sexual encounters.

After a particularly humiliating sexual experience with a very successful, haughty actor in her program, Susannah became alarmed by what she viewed as the dissolution of her own values and "guiding principles," and she sought counseling within the larger university that housed her conservatory. This proved to be a very satisfying connection, and she was able to make good use of her 10 allotted sessions without requiring her parents' financial support. She became aware that her path had been heavily determined by her mother's career disappointment and her own childhood talents, which she now recognized as modest in comparison to those of her conservatory peers. With this new perspective, she grappled with her confusion about her ambitions; she spent her sophomore conservatory year sampling classes in the university and "realized" that she wanted to become a doctor. This led to her transfer to the university to begin a rigorous premed program. Her fellow premed students were highly competitive and serious; partying inevitably declined. Her academic success in the sciences initially "shocked" Susannah, but she soon assumed a leadership role, organizing a study group and community service activities.

Paradoxically, her sense of relief from competitive pressure related to singing was enormous, despite the competition among premed students; she felt less need to escape to alcohol and parties, less worry about her appearance, and less concern about disappointing her entire hometown. Her mother, whose brother was a physician, reconciled herself to Susannah's changed course and focused her artistic yearning on Susannah's younger sister Beth. Her father could hardly contain his pleasure at this turn of events.

Susannah pursued her premed courses with great enthusiasm but was dismayed to find that she was troubled by envy of her sister's artistic progress. Beth had entered the same conservatory program and achieved considerable success there. Susannah struggled with her feelings of competition and even ill will toward Beth, recognizing the situation as a new chapter in their "sibling rivalry" in which she had formerly been the winner. Nonetheless, her conviction about her career path was steadfast. Her feelings about Beth's success seemed to be mollified following two signal events: 1) Susannah developed a serious relationship with a fellow premed student in her senior year and 2) she was admitted to an excellent medical school. After these developments, she found that she was able to attend Beth's performances with equanimity and take pride in her sister's accomplishments.

Contemporary research into the importance of autobiographical narrative and memory telling highlights another facet of identity formation in late adolescence and links it to the growing importance of intimate relationships, to be discussed in the next section, "The Capacity for Intimate Relationships." The late adolescent's cognitive capacities for meaning making and perspective taking are fundamental to the subjective experience of identity. A history of supportive listening to personal narratives by parents (especially mothers as "family historians") facilitates identity development and subsequent capacity to engage peers in similarly productive dialogues (Fivush et al. 2011; Weeks and Pasupathi 2011). These capacities are exercised in the deepening connection with peers as late adolescence progresses and cognition matures. As is true for many identity tasks, peer relationships gradually eclipse parental relationships as the central context for integration of the past via autobiographical narratives. Even though the extent of parental knowledge is inevitably greater, the memories and myths within families can sometimes constrain the late adolescent's autonomous identity formation. Telling one's past in the new peer-relational context of college or employment allows for a new perspective on the self and enriches the complexity of self-representation (Weeks and Pasupathi 2010). Especially in the college context, which creates an institutionalized "object removal" (separating the late adolescent from the old love objects—i.e., family members), there is an opportunity to redefine and reconfigure identity through reconsideration of the historical self. The past and the present are woven into the evolving consolidation of identity as a coherent narrative, facilitated by the cognitive expansion of self-insight and awareness of others (McLean 2005; McLean and Thorne 2003).

• **See the video "Late Adolescent Girl."** This young woman, who just completed her sophomore year in college, speaks eloquently about her struggle to individuate and develop her own identity. Her close relationship to her parents, especially her mother, has undergone a difficult transition to a less dependent and more adult form, allowing her greater freedom to discover her own interests and requirements in a romantic partner. She seems ruefully aware that the choice of her high school boyfriend was bound to provoke her parents' disapproval.

THE CAPACITY FOR INTIMATE RELATIONSHIPS

Romantic fantasies and longings are observable in children of all ages, but in latency the universal phenomenon of gender segregation reduces opportunities for relaxed contact; interest is expressed primarily in "borderwork" behaviors, such as teasing and chase games. With puberty, interest and excitement mounts and venues for more romantic and sexually arousing contact proliferate; however, in early adolescence these are often consigned to fantasy or so-called dating relationships that involve almost no contact, in school or out of it. However, romantic fantasies, real romantic relationships, and sexual encounters become more common in middle adolescence. Interestingly, research on the widespread public perception that experimental hooking-up (sexual contact outside a romantic relational context) is the norm in the twenty-first century has shown that it is not as prevalent as anticipated, tends to be with familiar partners, and, in one-third of those surveyed, was connected to hopes for a more enduring relationship (Tolman and McClelland 2011). Romantic yearnings and intense love feelings for a specific individual can certainly emerge in middle adolescence, sometimes developing into a disruptive preoccupation. As mentioned in Chapter 8, "Early and Mid-Adolescence," a recent survey showed that a full 50% of 16-year-olds consider themselves to be in a romantic relationship (Seiffge-Krenke et al. 2010), although this is often retrospectively modified as the teen matures. Middle adolescent love is typically characterized by passion and idealization, but rarely includes thoughts of long-term commitment and interdependence (Beyers and Seiffge-Krenke 2010).

Beginning at the threshold of late adolescence, many teens experience their first intercourse and first real love affair, one that meaningfully endures in their minds as their "first love." These graduating seniors in high school and young college students may still have considerable intrapsychic work to do in regard to identity and superego maturation, but the first relationship is vital for the integration of sexual and tender feelings and the experience of the self as a desirable gendered person. Although Erikson's model (1950) suggests that identity must be achieved before intimacy is possible, the bidi-rectional facilitation of late adolescent tasks is supported by contemporary studies, which also note their roots in earlier childhood and their extensions into adulthood (Beyers and Seiffge-Krenke 2010; Montgomery 2005). Thus, while intimate relationships require a degree of identity formation, identity in turn requires relationships with important others, including romantic partners, to reach its mature form (Beyers and Seiffge-Krenke 2010).

The capacity to develop a meaningful romantic relationship is a signifi-cant psychological accomplishment. Increasingly, psychodynamic thinkers recognize that such signal events of adolescence are powerful shapers of adult personality. The first love experience has the potential to color future romantic relationships, creating both a standard of intensity and a dynamic relational template. Of course, subsequent experience in relationships can modulate the impact of the first passion, but the latter remains unique in its mobilization of fantasy (Glick 2008; Kulish 1998), its strong vein of idealiza-tion of the love object (Kernberg 1974), and, especially, its first fusion of sex-ual passion and dependency longings in the individual's experience. It is also the first time since infancy, where the nursing baby is comforted, sustained, and gratified, that the individual becomes dependent on the body of the loved person, not only for sexual pleasure but also for self-esteem regulation (Ritvo 1971).

The experience of falling in love is a "nearly universal phenomenon" (Yovell 2008, p. 124) with palpable neurobiological underpinnings and state alterations, including "extreme energy, hyperactivity, sleeplessness, impul-sivity, euphoria, and mood swings" (Yovell 2008, p. 126); in addition, it has its own unique set of priorities, anxieties, and motivations. It involves the melding of key intrapsychic "systems," including attachment, sexuality, and object choice.

In the adolescent first love experience, the individual may be aware of two other elements, prominent by virtue of the developmental moment, that have been elucidated by Otto Kernberg, a major contributor to psychody-namic thinking about adolescent love. First is a "sense of mourning":

> [T]he mourning processes involved in being in love are those of growing up and becoming independent, the experience of leaving behind the real objects of childhood at a time when the most intimate and fulfilling kind of love re-lation with another human being is established. In this process of separation from the real objects of the past, there is also a reconfirmation of the good relations with internalized objects of the past, as the individual becomes confident of his capacity to give and receive love and sexual gratification si-multaneously—with a growth-promoting mutual reinforcement of both—in contrast to the conflict between love and sex in childhood. (Kernberg 1974, pp. 748–749)

Second is a sense of "transcendence," a feeling of kinship with the environment—both the cultural surround and the inanimate world (Kernberg 1974, p. 755). Falling in love deepens the connection with things and places and enhances their importance, embedding them in an interpersonal network of meaning and affect. This concept highlights the close link between love and the experience of a safe, valued, and enhanced external world. The relatively sturdy adolescent who is capable of falling in love finds, in loving, an answer to residual feelings of alienation and ennui that are the by-products of the individuation process. Objects and events are newly invested with meaning as the late adolescent builds bridges to the future: "As the adolescent goes out to meet the world, the people he or she meets, studies with, works with, and makes love with become lifelong friends, comrades, and often mates, never to be forgotten. All of this is experienced with perhaps the deepest intensity and emotion of one's life" (Kulish 1998, p. 541).

This transcendent feeling of the first passionate love affairs can be understood as a composite of idealization, merger, and narcissistic identification with the love object that elevates the couple and creates a sense of unity and specialness (Sklansky 1977). The endowment of the loved person with unique and extraordinary qualities actually improves self-esteem by identification and by reciprocity, such that self-representation and self-feeling are enhanced. Love relationships of this type, if mutual and gratifying, can restore the late adolescent's optimism and investment in his or her own life. The sexual experience serves a vital function in consolidating the sexual self and in integrating sexual excitement and orgasm into the self-representation. It can also make more self-evident the individual's sexual role identity and sexual orientation. Especially for those teens worried and unsure about the latter, the gender of the first love partner is not necessarily conclusive. Nonetheless, for both heterosexual and homosexual first loves, the course and outcome of the first meaningful relationship can affect the individual's future direction. In general, first loves can greatly enhance self-esteem and feel subjectively like a maturing experience.

The following vignette illustrates both maladaptive and adaptive experiences of adolescent love. Liam's self-esteem was affected by both, but the second—a mutually satisfying, tender, and consummated love affair—contributed significantly to the consolidation of this young man's self-representation, his reflectiveness, his sexuality, his willingness to take responsibility, and his identity as an artist.

> Liam had been a separation-anxious child with very busy parents who were both in finance and traveled extensively. He developed close relationships with live-in sitters/homework helpers whom his parents employed until he

was in seventh grade. At school he was an indifferent student except in regard to art. He was never in the popular crowd and felt alienated from his schoolmates; his best friends were the children of family friends and neighbors he had known "forever." He had two romances in high school. The first was with Renee, a girl who had considerable popularity and prestige in his school and kept him "on a string," refusing to spend time with him on the school's suburban campus and often breaking dates on the weekend. Sexual encounters were limited to nongenital contact, which Liam found increasingly frustrating. The relationship with the second girl, Joann, began at the end of his senior year and persisted for a year into college. Joann was two years younger and was a newcomer to the school. They began a friendship based on their common interest in art and what Liam felt was their shared experience of "difference" from their suburban environment. Asked to describe her, Liam said, "We are the same person. Well, anyway, we're a lot alike: she's nothing like the usual girls at school. She's an artist and she's not a follower." Liam was awestruck and moved by her willingness to have intercourse with him and felt his love for her deepen with their increasing intimacy. He was concerned that her family was conservative about premarital sex and he therefore insisted on an active role in regard to precautions about pregnancy. He had confidence in the emotional support he could offer Joann. He recognized the significance of her going against her family's values and was able to buoy her up by his sensitivity and attentiveness. During the prior relationship with Renee, he had been distracted and unhappy at school, felt belittled, and was still dependent on his parents. The relationship with Joann boosted his confidence and his investment in his "own life." He was noticeably less ruffled by his parents' comings and goings and was able to see himself as quite different from them in terms of his aspirations. He identified himself as an artist and devoted himself to developing an impressive portfolio and a much greater fund of knowledge about art. He decided to apply to an arts-related college close to home so that he could continue to see Joann. The relationship ended in the summer following his freshman college year, in part due to his growing recognition that he was not fully present at college because his mind was occupied with Joann. He knew this recreated his high school career and his anxious preoccupation with his parents' whereabouts. The breakup was very painful for both but without rancor. Liam's artistic identity continued to unfold over the years of college, and he went on to apply to a prestigious graduate art school.

THE EVOLUTION OF THE SUPEREGO
THROUGH ADOLESCENCE

As adolescence comes to a close, young people undergo a fundamental internal shift in the way they think about their choices, actions, and responsibilities. The upheavals of the early phases have settled; the new body and new sense of autonomous agency are presumably integrated into the sense of self. The quality of relationships with friends, family, and sexual partners has matured. In regard to family, there may be rocky times ahead, especially if the late adolescent is returning home after college, but there is an expectation that the power differential, control over behavior, and maintenance of appropriate values are no longer heavily weighted toward parents. What do these changes reflect in regard to the mental organization of the late adolescent?

The concept of the superego focuses attention on components of personality that coalesce into a relatively stable configuration during the course of late adolescence. Whether these components comprise a discrete mental structure or a complex amalgam of ego capacities, defenses, identifications, and ideals is a subject of considerable controversy among psychodynamic thinkers; in our view, the idea of mental structure is useful because it emphasizes the organizing function that the superego provides for personality development from the oedipal phase through adulthood. Included within the superego concept are the standards of moral conduct; the regulation of self-esteem, especially as it pertains to these moral concerns; the specific emotions of guilt and sense of goodness; and the hierarchy of values. The idea of structure does not imply fixity; the superego is notoriously undependable and uneven in its role as policeman and judge (Arlow 1982). Moreover, in regard to development over the lifespan, the superego undergoes continuous maturation, revision, modification, slippage, and recovery.

During the early phases of adolescence, the young person struggles with the legacy of latency: a superego that was, at least initially, experienced as an unintegrated and minimally nuanced voice of parents and other influential adults. Ideally, by late latency this superego is more modulated and seamlessly integrated into personality by the natural process of ego maturation. Nonetheless, with the rapidly changing internal landscape of puberty and early to mid-adolescence, the child is unmoored, not only by the flood of impulses but also by the need to disengage from this inner outpost of parental influence. However softened the late latency superego was, it now comes into conflict with new feelings, fantasies, desires, and the drive toward action. Its former, relatively straightforward prohibitions were based on a child's idealized view of parental constraint, moral integrity, and purity, a view that crumbles under the combined influence of new sexual desires, a body that insists on their gratification, and the recognition that parents are neither perfect nor asexual. Pressure from sexual and aggressive impulses and the need for distance from parents thus profoundly dislodges the complacent superego of late latency, with its origins in wholesale identification with the parents and ongoing compliance with rules and regulations.

Superego vicissitudes during adolescence illustrate the normal fluctuations of the superego in an extreme form. The early mid-adolescent reprojects its prohibitive functions onto parents and other authorities and comes un-der the spell of peer influence and "group-think"; gradually, by late adoles-cence, a modified and self-determined set of moral standards and values is internalized. The superego's relatively late appearance in development as a stable mental structure is reflected in its greater vulnerability to disruption and corruption compared to other ego capacities. The superego can be swayed throughout life by the force of groups and under duress; it can be deeply altered by excesses of power, fame, and wealth.

The evolving cognitive capacities of the adolescent make it inevitable that adults are seen more clearly and ambivalently than before, especially compared to the child's idealized images of adults. As the perception of par-ents shifts and sexual urges propel the adolescent outside the family, he or she struggles with the feelings of loss and of being lost. In extreme cases or desperate times, parents and their entire generation become the paradoxical embodiment of prohibition and corruption, as illustrated by the attitudes of youth toward the "establishment" in the 1960s and 1970s. In its more path-ological incarnations, it is as if the strict latency superego is re-externalized at the same time that the adolescent's own illicit desires and behaviors are attributed to parents and other representations of authority. This form of teen rebellion invokes the moral corruption of the adults as justification for defiance, bolstering the vulnerable mid- to late adolescent by a measure of self-righteousness.

Nonetheless, middle adolescents are subject to an array of self-doubts as they violate sacrosanct prohibitions, often unconsciously arranging for dis-covery and punishment. Moreover, the alternative idealized figures that these high schoolers sometimes rely on—including sports stars, musicians, models, cult leaders, and idolized peers—often elicit feelings of inferiority and shame, which can be confused with guilty feelings. A common example is the tenth grader who idolizes the latest superthin celebrity and feels "guilty" when she eats too much. The mingling of the narcissistic with the moralistic and the blending of shame with guilt contribute to some of the in-tense mood states of this period (Jacobson 1961).

It is the work of the subsequent late adolescent process to reinternalize a superego that is selectively individuated from family values, distinguished from narcissistic gratification, more personalized, more tolerant of ambigu-ity, and capable of sustaining a more autonomous path. In this context, the geographic remove from home is helpful because it leaves the adolescent without the easy choice of resistance to disappointing parents and their val-ues. Access to other respected adults who represent positive role models is invaluable in providing the late adolescent with "mentors." Such adults, serv-ing as coach, college adviser, or employer, are psychologically offering alternative examples that can be partially and selectively internalized, thereby bolstering the evolving superego and value system without threatening it with the regressive pull of the parent-child relationship (Chused 1982). This mentoring person is most useful if "interested, yet disinterested" (Chused 1982, p. 843). To successfully remodel the superego, late adolescents must rely on their own choices, values, and moral decisions, partaking of adult advice only if it is offered without pressure or coercion.

The developmental challenges outlined in this chapter are all reliant on the process of developing a personal worldview and set of values. The multifaceted consolidation of identity and the establishment of intimate relationships rest on a foundation of morality and the self-enhancement that comes with implementation of one's own inner convictions about human interactions, the value of action in the world, and the kind of life one wishes to live. The adolescent process can thus be viewed through the lens of superego development, because it plays a leading role in the conflicts of each subphase. This process is demonstrated in the following vignette.

> Jan was considered a polite and well-mannered girl and was proud of her parents, both of whom were religious leaders and community activists. In grade school, she was idealistic and excited by the idea of a life dedicated to causes and moral beliefs. She was well liked by everyone and was a fair team player, a responsible student, and an enthusiastic participant in church activities. However, from middle school through high school, she fell in with a group of girls who were popular, sexually precocious, and prone to risky behaviors. While her participation in her family's religious activities and her excellent school performance continued, Jan was also engaging in drinking, hookups, and partying on the sly. She thought at that time that her parents' apparent obliviousness to these behaviors was due to her capacity to seamlessly shift between her "good" and "bad" girl personas. She herself felt untroubled by her "double life." However, when her parents separated in her sophomore year of high school, she was profoundly disappointed, especially when she became aware of her father's infidelities. She no longer worried about hiding her partying, especially considering that her parents seemed too preoccupied with their marital troubles to notice. When they reconciled a year later, she was resistant to their authority, sarcastic with both of them, and bitterly disillusioned about their piety and beliefs. She nonetheless maintained her school performance and cleaned up her Facebook page in preparation for college applications.
>
> Jan chose to attend a historic college abroad, where she hoped she could start over. Reflecting on her high school self, she became aware of a degree of self-loathing and an unconscious identification with her father, whose moral transgressions were, in retrospect, detectable all along. Indeed, she was immediately enamored of her college culture, where intellectual and socially conscious accomplishments were highly valued and partying was modest compared to the scene at colleges she had considered in the United States. At

first, she remained somewhat emotionally distant from her parents. Jan became devoted to promoting women's rights in repressive countries and participated actively in programs supporting women's education and self-determination. She developed a close relationship with a woman professor in the field and, to Jan's great joy, was invited to help with the woman's forthcoming book. As Jan's expertise and nuanced understanding of her field expanded, she felt increasingly able to tolerate and even enjoy her time with her parents. She realized that their interests had many points of correspondence and that she could respect their social commitments. Jan did not altogether trust her father but felt he was trying. Her anger at her mother for "just taking him back" softened as she recognized the depth of their relationship and her mother's reliance on him. In regard to her own values, she understood her high school bad girl persona as an overreaction to her family. After a phase of relative sexual abstinence, which she felt was somehow connected to her new feminism, she began dating and had a number of brief lesbian relationships. Finally, she developed a lengthy relationship with a young man who shared her specific interests during her last years of college.

Jan's evolution illustrates the late adolescent's capacity to tolerate flaws in the self and others, to reflect on extenuating circumstances, and to nonetheless maintain optimism and hope. Such capacities inform the more flexible and yet stable superego appropriate to this age group. Although never fully immune to the sway of group pressure, the seduction of excessive narcissistic gratification, and the idolization of celebrities, the young person seems better grounded in a reasonable belief system shaped by the desire to be productive as well as successful. Such a belief system provides the internal guidelines that help in selecting from the infinite number of daily events and choices that require the individual to know what he or she thinks, believes in, and upholds. In optimal circumstances, the mature superego operates silently and blends into ego functions. It continues to recognize and reward good acts and can imbue the life choices that present in late adolescence with meaning and honor.

Superego Development

- The superego undergoes marked transformation over the course of the adolescent process.

- The superego can be externalized in early to mid-adolescence, but is reintegrated by adolescent resolution, often with the help of mentors and opportunities to craft an individuated life course.

- Development of the superego involves the establishment of self-selected values, beliefs, and goals that are autonomous, although not necessarily different from parents' standards.

PHYSICAL AND COGNITIVE CHANGES

Physical Changes in Late Adolescence

Although physical changes during late adolescence are insignificant relative to the prior transformations of puberty, the bodily and mental changes of late adolescence can alter the teenager both subjectively and in the eyes of others. The fully mature sexual body, Tanner's stage 5, is usually achieved between ages 18 and 22, as are adult body mass and height (Neinstein 2002). These final steps in physical growth are significant in that late adolescents often have the sense that they only assumed their adult forms in the several years *after* high school; they sometimes look backward at their high school selves with embarrassment and a burning desire to exhibit their subsequent evolution. For example, the boy who graduated from high school feeling childish, smooth faced, and puny triumphantly returns for the second-year reunion transformed into a taller, buffer, fully bearded man. Even in the more typical cases of modest changes, the feeling and appearance of greater physical maturity inform the experience of most late adolescents. Certainly, the initiation into sexual life and romantic love can *feel* physically transforming even if full sexual maturation involves relatively minor changes.

For some individuals, however, some hopes for the outcome of development in terms of physical transformation are inevitably not achieved and must be renounced with the leveling off of the growth curve. For example, a very petite young woman recalled her childhood yearning for a voluptuous body and her disdain for her mother's small stature and "insignificant" breasts. She was deeply disappointed when she failed to surpass her mother, and in her own mind she remained a prepubescent child. Similarly, some hopes that awkward or painful aspects of puberty and early adolescence will fade away over time are decisively dashed. For example, severe acne, often attributed to the onset of adolescent "hormones" (Tan et al. 2001), peaks for males in late adolescence (Goodman 2006); it is not uncommon for acne to have been left untreated prior to this point, in expectation of natural remission. Also, the onset of dysmenorrhea is usually delayed until consistent ovulatory menstrual cycles are established, and thus it can become more pronounced in late adolescence (Coco 1999).

Brain and Cognitive Development

The structural development of the brain described in Chapter 8 continues through the late teens and early 20s. Brain remodeling includes ongoing myelination of white matter and pruning of the cerebral cortex, especially the frontal and parietal regions (Choudhury et al. 2006). The resulting increased connectivity has been hypothesized to bear a relationship to the late adolescent's capacity to specialize his or her interests and develop expertise. Moreover, during the period between preadolescence and late adolescence, areas of the brain that bear directly on the maturity of "social cognitive development"—that is, the capacity to mentalize, understand the minds of others, and take another's perspective—undergo a predictable age-related shift from frontal to posterior brain regions and from bilateral to unilateral left inferior parietal cortex; this shift is associated with improved efficiency in the processing of perspective-taking tasks (Dosch et al. 2010). These demonstrable brain changes underscore the complexity of the evolution of social cognition during adolescence by highlighting the role of neural maturation in a process in which environmental, interpersonal, and emotional systems are undergoing parallel development (Choudhury et al. 2006).

As noted in Chapter 8, the advent of formal operations and executive function in early adolescence marks a significant cognitive milestone that is nonetheless a graduated process responsive to environmental input and is relatively variable within and between individuals. Similarly, prosocial moral reasoning advances unevenly and is especially vulnerable when assessed in contexts where the cost of helping others is high. So-called hedonistic thinking appears to increase from mid-adolescence through the early college years, perhaps because young people are preferentially focused on "responsibility to self" (Eisenberg et al. 2012, p. 1194). This can be understood in part as a decline in unrealistic idealism and more pressing concerns about personal success as the future bears down on the developing teenager.

Continuation of Risky Behaviors

Risky behaviors jeopardizing physical health take on new forms in late adolescence without the constraints of parental monitoring, despite presumed enhanced self-regulation. The college-bound teen is likely to be impacted by the "college effect" on alcohol consumption—namely, a significant increase in binge alcohol abuse that well exceeds that of age-matched youth not attending college (Osberg et al. 2011). Other forms of substance abuse vary with contemporary trends; a slight uptick in marijuana use, a significant increase in (unprescribed) amphetamine use, and a notable increase in cocaine abuse were all observed in the first decade of the twenty-first century. Similarly, unwanted sexual advances, assault, drunk driving, suicide, and unsafe sex are alarmingly prevalent in colleges (College Parents of America 2012; Neinstein et al. 2009); for example, only one-third of students who are active sexually report using condoms (Scott-Sheldon et al. 2008). These behaviors, experienced directly or vicariously through the peer group, infiltrate the college environment and have the potential to spread by contagion. "Greek life" (i.e., fraternities and sororities) can be an important source of community but also is documented to increase a number of risky behaviors, including marijuana and alcohol use, sex under the influence of alcohol, sex with multiple partners, and cigarette smoking (Scott-Sheldon et al. 2008). As one college junior said ruefully, "College—and especially my fraternity— is like summer camp without the counselors." The absence of parents and the stated refusal of most colleges to serve in loco parentis leave some late adolescents stranded, as it were, with a dizzying array of opportunities for excitement and potentially risky activities. Although some late adolescents have sowed their wild oats in high school and arrive at college with an evolved personal agenda, others, especially those who were relatively inhibited while living with their parents, can come unraveled in this permissive atmosphere. These dynamic issues can be augmented by the emergence of more serious psychiatric illness during these years, as discussed in the following section. It is often difficult to differentiate developmental adjustments from more ominous psychopathology. This is also true of diagnosable substance abuse, sometimes masked at colleges awash in alcohol or other drugs, where serious problems can be mistaken for "typical" behavior on campus.

ONSET OF PSYCHIATRIC ILLNESS

Many psychiatric illnesses, such as schizophrenia, affective diatheses, substance abuse, and severe personality disorders, become manifest or are first diagnosed in late adolescence. The National Comorbidity Survey Replication (Kessler et al. 2005) showed that three-fourths of all cases of psychiatric illnesses other than schizophrenia start by age 24. Median age at onset of substance abuse is 20. An earlier review noted that substance abuse is associated with significant psychiatric comorbidity (Kessler et al. 1994). The median age at onset of schizophrenia, while difficult to establish precisely due to delays in treatment seeking, is generally understood to be late adolescence through the early 20s (Kessler et al. 2007).

DSM-5 criteria for personality disorders place the onset "before adulthood," with symptoms usually appearing sometime in adolescence (American Psychiatric Association 2013); thus, the diagnosis of personality disorders in children and adolescents under 18 is not customary, except in unusual cases. Similarly, psychodynamic thinkers have historically resisted diagnosing personality disorders, with their implication of stability and chronicity, earlier in development; by definition, a personality disorder is not susceptible to developmental transformation. In addition, late adolescence is considered a phase of active personality remodeling or consolidation, with positive or negative outcomes; the internal loosening of object ties, reworking of defenses, revamping of superego, and resolution of identity that characterize this phase are seen as providing an opportunity for a reconfiguration of prior development (Jacobson 1961). Indeed, as the upheavals of the prior phases diminish, some late adolescents can achieve a higher level of personality organization than predicted by their histories.

Nonetheless, official classification of childhood personality disorders has been urged by some psychodynamic thinkers (see Kernberg et al. 2000), who argue that the problem is primarily one of recognition, because the characteristic distinctive pattern of the adult disorder is obscured by high comorbidity in children. Some childhood traits are clear precursors to personality disorder Clusters A (odd), B (dramatic/impulsive), and C (anxious) (Paris 2003; Weston and Riolo 2007). Traits resembling these adult clusters can be identified in childhood and have been conclusively linked to later illness (Paris 2003, 2004). The internalizing and externalizing distinction in regard to childhood presentations may also forecast the cluster into which the personality disorder emerging in late adolescence will fall. However, many influential researchers point out that these earlier behaviors do not predict *whether* the later disorder will emerge, because the latter depends on environmental issues and the elusive factor of resilience (Paris 2003, 2004; Rutter 1987). Therefore, although environmental stressors are typically implicated in the adolescent outbreak of illness, childhood variables color the form of the disorder and also impart a remarkable righting capacity, even to those exposed to chronic adversity (Paris 2003, p. 11).

In addition to personality disorders, schizophrenia and related disorders most often have an onset in late adolescence; these disorders can appear earlier in childhood but are rarely diagnosed. Schizophrenia over the lifespan is slightly more common in males; this preponderance emerges at age 17 (Kleinhaus et al. 2011). Onset in males is consistently earlier than in females and shows a unimodal onset of positive symptoms (hallucinations and delusions) with peaks between ages 18 and 25, whereas females show a bimodal onset with peaks between ages 20 and 30 and after age 40 (Buchanan and Carpenter 2005). The early manifestations of serious disorder are often nonspecific and do not readily distinguish schizophrenic from affective disorders (Hodgman 2006). In populations over age 18, earlier onset of schizophrenia has been shown to be strongly correlated with cannabis use, panic disorder, and age at onset of psychosis in relatives (Hall et al. 2008; Hare et al. 2010). Many common childhood disorders, including attention-deficit/hyperactivity disorder, separation anxiety disorder, and posttraumatic stress disorder, increase the risk for psychotic disorders by up to sevenfold, with externalizing disorders associated with schizophrenia and internalizing with mood disorders (Rubin et al. 2009). In addition, subtle developmental abnormalities, including perinatal complications and early deviant neuromotor and neurocognitive development, are associated with an increased risk of psychotic illness (Isohanni et al. 2004). Researchers generally agree that neurobiological underpinnings achieve full expression under the influence of unique adolescent stressors (Paris 2004; Spear 2010). Like contemporary psychodynamic theory, the neuroscientific view suggests that adolescent breakdown is primed by genetic loading and/or extremely early adversity, but that the events of adolescence, both intrapsychic and environmental, can affect outcome.

Psychiatric Disorders of Late Adolescence

- Three-fourths of all psychiatric illnesses are diagnosed by age 24 years.
- Serious substance abuse can be confused with "normal" risky behavior; average age at onset of substance abuse is 20 years.
- Personality disorders are more evident and more readily diagnosed in late adolescents.
- Schizophrenia and related psychotic disorders generally emerge in men between ages 18 and 25 and in women between ages 20 and 30.

Key Concepts

Late adolescence, which we define as the years between 17 and 21 or 22, corresponds to the end of high school and the post–high school experience of college or early employment. Called the *psychosocial moratorium* by Erikson (1968) in regard to the ubiquitous college experience provided by Western society, it comprises an active intrapsychic phase of consolidation—of identity, personality traits, and superego—in the context of advancing individuation and the changing power differential in the parent-child relationship.

For college students, there is an opportunity for active exploration of identity in a relatively sheltered environment unburdened by preconceptions. The college campus offers many alternative paths to future commitments; career, sexual identity, race, religion, and political belief systems are available to try on and to discard, usually with little real consequence. These component elements of identity are the more visible manifestations of the internal process of consolidation and are deeply embedded in the specific culture—both the immediate college culture and the larger cultural surround.

The environment either affirms or denies adolescents' search for identity by its response to them. In this process, the late adolescent comes to terms with the rapidly shifting self-representations that were an inevitable part of earlier adolescent phases and develops patterned and reliable ego organization and defenses that will carry forward into adulthood.

The other crucial intrapsychic tasks of this phase concern the capacity for intimate relationships and the establishment of an internal value and moral system that feels like one's own. These tasks are mutually facilitating, because intimate relationships promote consolidation of values and sense of self; one's moral credo guides the search for a meaningful life; and a well-developed identity supports the capacity to love another and dedicate oneself to the future.

The late adolescent has yet to traverse emerging adulthood and, in contemporary culture, does not usually emerge from college "full grown" at age 22. Indeed, most students attending college (who can range in age from 18 to 29) do not consider themselves adults (Nelson et al. 2007). Among late adolescents who do not attend college, the career or work identity question may be resolved more quickly if they find a good job fit, with growth opportunities, that imparts a consolidated experience of self-in-the-world. However, for many non–college-bound late adolescents, as for contemporary recent college graduates (to be discussed in Chapter 10, "The Odyssey Years"), the search for a meaningful occupational path is tortuous, adding to the internal quandaries of identity consolidation. As we discuss in Chapter 10, the trend toward postponing the concrete commitments associated with adulthood has contributed to a new phase of development: emerging adulthood.

Key developmental achievements of late adolescence are not identically timed for all individuals. Some begin earlier in adolescence and come to fruition in the late adolescent period. Certainly, by the end of late adolescence, the milestones are met.

- Late adolescent development typically occurs in the context of the psychosocial moratorium.

- Consolidation of personality traits, defensive organization, and sublimatory channels (i.e., interests and abiding belief systems) occurs during the late adolescent period.

- Identity crisis is a normative experience.
  - This crisis results in the sense of self as a unique individual.
  - Resolution of the identity crisis requires affirmation from the environment.
  - The multiple domains of personal identity include race, sexuality, gender, and political and religious affiliations.
- Full sexual relationships and the first intimate love affair contribute to but also rely on progress in regard to the integration of the sexual body and "sex print" (see Chapter 8) into identity.
- The integration of superego, as the reservoir of self-monitoring, self-esteem regulation, value system, and personal ideals, occurs. This process of superego reworking in late adolescence establishes internal autonomy from parents.

REFERENCES

American Psychiatric Association: Diagnostic and Statistical Manual of Mental Disorders, 5th Edition. Arlington, VA, American Psychiatric Association, 2013

Arlow A: Problems of the superego concept. Psychoanal Study Child 37:229–244, 1982

Aseltine RH, Gore S: Work, postsecondary education and psychosocial functioning following the transition from high school. J Adolesc Res 20:615–639, 2005

Beyers W, Seiffge-Krenke I: Does identity precede intimacy? Testing Erikson's theory on romantic development in emerging adults of the 21st century. J Adolesc Res 25:387–416, 2010

Blos P: Character formation in adolescence. Psychoanal Study Child 23:245–263, 1968

Blum H: Superego formation, adolescent transformation, and the adult neurosis. J Am Psychoanal Assoc 33:887–909, 1985

Blum H: Adolescent trauma and the Oedipus complex. Psychoanalytic Inquiry 30:548–556, 2010

Bronk KC: The role of purpose in life in healthy identity formation: a grounded model. New Dir Youth Dev 2011:31–44, 2011

Buchanan RW, Carpenter WT Jr: Schizophrenia and other psychotic disorders: concept of schizophrenia, in Kaplan and Sadock's Comprehensive Textbook of Psychiatry, 8th Edition. New York, Lippincott Williams & Wilkins, 2005

Chanen AW, Jackson HJ, McGorry PD, et al: Two-year stability of personality disorder in older adolescent outpatients. J Pers Disord 18:526–541, 2004

Choudhury S, Blakemore, SJ, Charman T: Social cognitive development during adolescence. Soc Cogn Affect Neurosci 1:165–174, 2006

Chused J: The idealization of the analyst by the young adult. J Am Psychoanal Assoc 35:839–859, 1982

Coco AS: Primary dysmenorrhea. Am Fam Physician 60:489–496, 1999

College Parents of America: Student statistics on alcohol consumption and abuse. Available at: http://www.collegeparents.org/members/resources/articles/student-statistics-alcohol-consumption-and-abuse. Accessed June 2012.

Cote JE: Emerging adulthood as an institutionalized moratorium: risks and benefits to identity formation, in Emerging Adults in America: Coming of Age in the 21st Century. Edited by Arnett JJ, Tanner L. Washington, DC, American Psychological Association, 2006, pp 85–116

Domina T, Conley AM, Farkas G: The link between educational expectations and effort in the college-for-all era. Sociology of Education 84:93–112, 2011

Dosch M, Loenneker T, Bucher K, et al: Learning to appreciate others: neural development of cognitive perspective taking. Neuroimage 50:837–846, 2010

Eisenberg N, Carlo G, Murphy B, et al: Prosocial development in late adolescence: a longitudinal study. Child Dev 66:1179–1197, 2012

Erikson E: Identity and the Life Cycle. New York, International Universities Press, 1950

Erikson E: The problem of ego identity. J Am Psychoanal Assoc 4:56–121, 1956

Erikson E: Identity: Youth and Crisis. New York, WW Norton, 1968

Esman AH: Adolescence and the consolidation of values, in Moral Values and the Superego Concept in Psychoanalysis. Edited by Post SC. New York, International Universities Press, 1972, pp 87–100

Fivush R, Bohanek JG, Zaman W: Personal and intergenerational narratives in relation to adolescents' well-being (Special Issue: The Development of Autobiographical Reasoning in Adolescence and Beyond. Edited by Habermas T.) New Dir Child Adolesc Dev 131: 45-57, 2011

Glick R: Commentary: is there a drive to love? Neuropsychoanalysis 10:145–148, 2008

Goodman G: Acne: natural history, facts and myths. Aust Fam Physician 35:613–615, 2006

Haase CM, Heckhausen J, Koller O: Goal engagement during the school-work transition: beneficial for all, particularly for girls. J Res Adolesc 18:671–698, 2008

Hall W, Degenhardt L, Patton G: Cannabis abuse and dependence, in Adolescent Addiction: Epidemiology, Assessment and Treatment. Edited by Essau CA. Oxford, UK, Elsevier, 2008, pp 117–148

Hare E, Glahn DC, Dassori A, et al.: Heritability of age of onset of psychosis in schizophrenia. Am J Med Genet B Neuropsychiatr Genet 153B:298–302, 2010

Hodgman CH: Psychosis in adolescence. Adolesc Med Clin 17:131–146, 2006

Isohanni M, Isohanni I, Koponen H, et al: Developmental precursors of psychosis. Curr Psychiatry Rep 6:168–175, 2004

Jacobson E: Adolescent moods and the remodeling of psychic structure in adolescence. Psychoanal Study Child 16:164–183, 1961

Jobs S: Commencement address, Stanford University. June 14, 2005. Available at: http://news.stanford.edu/news/2005/june15/jobs-061505.html. Accessed October 13, 2012.

Kernberg O: Structural derivatives of object relationships. Int J Psychoanal 47:236–252, 1966

Kernberg O: Mature love: prerequisites and characteristics. J Am Psychoanal Assoc 22:743–768, 1974

Kernberg O: Identity: recent findings and clinical implications. Psychoanal Q 75:969–1003, 2006

Kernberg PF, Weiner AS, Bardenstein KK: Personality Disorders in Children and Adolescents. New York, Basic Books, 2000

Kessler RC, McGonagle KA, Zhao S, et al: Lifetime and 12-month prevalence of DSM-III-R psychiatric disorders in the United States: results from the National Cormorbidity Survey. Arch Gen Psychiatry 51:8–19, 1994

Kessler RC, Berglund P, Demler O, et al: Lifetime prevalence of age-of-onset distributions of DSM-IV disorders in the National Comorbidity Survey Replication. Arch Gen Psychiatry 62:593–602, 2005

Kessler RC, Amminger GP, Aguilar-Gaxiola S, et al: Age of onset of mental disorders: a review of recent literature. Curr Opin Psychiatry 20:359–364, 2007

Kleinhaus K, Harlap S, Perrin M, et al: Age, sex and first treatment of schizophrenia in a population cohort. J Psychiatr Res 45:136–141, 2011

Kroger J: Ego identity status research in the new millennium. Int J Behav Dev 24:145–148, 2000

Kroger J: Identity in Adolescence: The Balance Between Self and Other, 3rd Edition (Adolescence and Society Series). East Sussex, UK, Routledge, Taylor & Francis, 2004

Kulish N: First loves and prime adventures: adolescent expressions in adult analyses. Psychoanal Q 67:539–565, 1998

Kumru A, Thompson RA: Ego identity status and self-monitoring behavior in adolescents. J Adolesc Res 18:481–495, 2003

Lachmann FM: Identity and self: historical antecedents and developmental precursors. International Forum on Psychoanalysis 13:246–253, 2004

Lapsley DK, Edgerton J: Separation-individuation, adult attachment style and college adjustment. J Couns Dev 80:484–493, 2002

Lefkowitz ES: "Things have gotten better": developmental changes among emerging adults after the transition to university. J Adolesc Res 20:40–63, 2005

Marcia JE: Development and validation of ego-identity status. J Pers Soc Psychol 3:551–558, 1966

Marcia JE: The ego identity status approach to ego identity, in Ego Identity: A Handbook for Psychosocial Research. Edited by JE Marcia, AS Waterman, DR Matteson, et al. New York, Springer-Verlag, 1993, pp 3–21

McLean K: Late adolescent identity development: narrative meaning making and memory telling. Dev Psychol 42:685–691, 2005

McLean K, Thorne A: Late adolescents' self-defining memories about relationships. Dev Psychol 39:635–645, 2003

Meeus W, Iedema J, Helsen M, et al: Patterns of adolescent identity development: review of the literature and longitudinal analysis. Dev Rev 19:419–461, 1999

Montgomery MJ: Psychosocial intimacy and identity: from early adolescence to emerging adulthood. J Adolesc Res 20:346–374, 2005

National Center for Education Statistics: Fast facts: enrollment. 2011. Available at: http://nces.ed.gov/fastfacts/display.asp?id=98. Accessed June 2012.

Neinstein L: Adolescent Health Care: A Practical Guide, 4th Edition. Baltimore, MD, Lippincott Williams & Wilkins, 2002

Neinstein LS, Gordon CM, Katzman DK, et al: Handbook of Adolescent Health Care. Philadelphia, PA, Lippincott Williams & Wilkins, 2009

Nelson LJ, Padilla-Walker LM, Carroll JS, et al: "If you want me to treat you like an adult, start acting like one!" Comparing the criteria that emerging adults and their parents have for adulthood. J Fam Psychol 21:665–674, 2007

Osberg TM, Insana M, Eggert M, et al: Incremental validity of college alcohol beliefs in the prediction of freshman drinking and its consequences: a prospective study. Addict Behav 36:333–340, 2011

Paris J: Personality Disorders Over Time: Precursors, Course, and Outcome. Washington, DC, American Psychiatric Publishing, 2003

Paris J: Personality disorders over time: implications for psychotherapy. Am J Psychother 58:420–430, 2004

Porteli EJ, Skorikov VB: Specific and diversive career exploration during late adolescence. Journal of Career Assessment 18:46–58, 2010

Ritvo S: Late adolescence: developmental and clinical considerations. Psychoanal Study Child 26:241–263, 1971

Rojewski JW, Kim H: Career choice patterns and behavior of work-bound youth during early adolescence. J Career Dev 30:89–108, 2003

Rosenbaum J: The complexities of college for all: beyond the fairy-tale dreams. Sociol Educ 84:113–117, 2011

Rosenbaum JE, Person AE: Beyond college for all: policies and practices to improve transitions into college and jobs. Professional School Counseling 6:252–260, 2003

Rubin KH, Coplan RJ, Bowker J: Social withdrawal in childhood. Annu Rev Psychol 60:141–171, 2009

Rutter M: Psychosocial resilience and protective mechanisms. Am J Orthopsychiatry 57:316–331, 1987

Schwartz P, Maynard AM, Uzelac SM: Adolescent egocentrism: a contemporary view. Adolescence 43:441–448, 2008

Scott-Sheldon LA, Carey KB, Carey MP: Health behavior and college students: does Greek affiliation matter? J Behav Med 31:61–70, 2008

Seiffge-Krenke I, Overbeek G, Vermulst A: Parent-child relationship trajectories during adolescence: longitudinal associations with romantic outcomes in emerging adulthood. J Adolesc 33:159–171, 2010

Seton P: The psychotemporal adaptation of the late adolescent. J Am Psychoanal Assoc 22:795–819, 1974

Sklansky MA: The alchemy of love: transmutation of the elements in adolescents and young adults. Ann Psychoanal 5:76–103, 1977

Spear L: The Behavioral Neuroscience of Adolescence. New York, WW Norton, 2010

Strenger C: The self as perpetual experiment: psychodynamic comments on some aspects of contemporary urban culture. Psychoanal Psychol 20:435–440, 2003

Tan JKL, Vasey K, Fung KY: Beliefs and perceptions of patients with acne. J Am Acad Dermatol 44:439–445, 2001

Tolman DL, McClelland SL: Normative sexuality development in adolescence: a decade in review, 2000–2009. J Res Adolesc 21:242–255, 2011

U.S. Department of Labor, Bureau of Labor Statistics: Economic news release: college enrollment and work activity of 2011 high school graduates. April 29, 2012. Available at: http://www.bls.gov/news.release/hsgec.nr0.htm. Accessed June 2012.

Weeks TL, Pasupathi M: Autonomy, identity, and narrative construction with parents and friends, in Narrative Development in Adolescence: Creating the Storied Self. Edited by McLean KC, Pasupathi M. New York, Springer, 2011, pp 65–92

Westen D: The cognitive self and the psychoanalytic self: can we put our selves together? Psychol Inq 3:1–13, 1992

Westen D: Identity disturbance in adolescence: associations with borderline personality disorder. Dev Psychopathol 23:305–313, 2011

Weston CG, Riolo SA: Childhood and adolescent precursors to adult personality disorders. Psychiatr Ann 37:114–121, 2007

Wilkinson-Ryan T, Westen D: Identity disturbance in borderline personality disorder: an empirical investigation. Am J Psychiatry 157:528–541, 2000

Yovell Y: Is there a drive to love? Neuropsychoanalysis 10:117–144, 2008

CHAPTER 10

The Odyssey Years

Emerging Adults on the Path to Adulthood

In an opinion piece titled "The Odyssey Years" that appeared in the *New York Times,* David Brooks (2007) endorsed the recognition of this generational phenomenon, also called *emerging adulthood,* which has been proposed as the new developmental phase of the twenty-first century, much as adolescence had been for the twentieth century. This is "the decade of wandering" in which "fluidity" is the unifying theme: fluidity in jobs, love relationships, domiciles, and long-term aspirations. Adulthood, traditionally defined through the achievement of concrete markers—completion of education, financial independence, living away from home, marriage, and parenthood—has been pushed forward to the 30s. The 20s have become a period of uncertainty and searching in all these domains. In contemporary Western society, 20- to 30-year-olds typically feel very far from adult commitments; they are worried but nonetheless relatively comfortable with an extended trajectory and the mystery of how it will all turn out.

INTRODUCTION TO EMERGING ADULTHOOD

The phase of life following late adolescence—itself imprecise in its boundaries—is specific to Western postindustrial culture. Forecast in Blos's (1962) prescient conceptualization of "postadolescence," this phase was officially designated "emerging adulthood" by James Arnett in 2000 (Arnett 2000, 2007). This phase has also been called "contestable adulthood" (Horowitz and Bromnick 2007), "youthhood" (Cote 2006), and young adulthood. The term *emerging adulthood* and its theoretical elaboration have been quickly integrated into developmental studies, seeming to answer a felt need to characterize this period. A close look at the growing body of theory and research about this age group underscores its indistinct borders; some observers, like Arnett, consider its range to be ages 18–24, whereas others suggest that late adolescence extends as late as age 25 (Adatto 1958), that emerging adulthood extends to age 30 (Cote 2006), or that young adulthood is best captured by the age range of 20–40 years (Colarusso 1991). Based on our own observations, and recognizing the absence of biological indicators, we believe that the age range of 21–30 best encompasses emerging adulthood. This range uses familiar social markers for its beginning: the last year or two of college, the end of being a teenager, reaching legal drinking age, and entry into the adult world. Concluding at age 30 reflects the commonly observed pressure to make commitments across numerous domains as this milestone approaches. Placing emerging adulthood solidly in the 20s minimizes the muddying effect of late adolescent conflicts or at least identifies their extension into a new phase with its own distinct features. Most significantly, the 20s are usually accompanied by a potent shift in the contextualization of experience that ensues when confronted with the "rest of one's life."

In many ways, emerging adulthood seems to recapitulate the same developmental challenges described in late adolescence: the consolidation of identity, the commitment to an intimate relationship, the clarification of personal goals and values. The reality that these tasks are incomplete or subject to reconsideration is, at least in part, a reflection of the diminished societal expectations that the graduating college student or young employee be clear about what he or she intends to "become." The subjective experience of people in their early 20s attests to the idea that they are not quite adults and not quite ready to make adult commitments. As we discuss in this chapter, emerging adulthood is a product of the intersection of many societal and psychological factors in our culture and has its own set of concerns and conflicts. Whether it is a true developmental phase or a transient epiphenomenon of societal change remains a subject of debate.

The Generational Shift

Despite the discrepancies in the range of ages for emerging adulthood employed by scholars and researchers, there is a discernible epidemiological shift in the time frame of the "adult transition" over the last century. As noted in Chapter 8, "Early and Mid-Adolescence," adolescence was ushered into the general scientific awareness by the publication of G. Stanley Hall's (1904) two-volume work *Adolescence: Its Psychology and Its Relation to*

Physiology, Anthropology, Sociology, Sex, Crime, Religion and Education. In Hall's formulation, adolescence was the decade between ages 14 and 24 years. His time frame, which he did not fully explain, seems to span the years between the median age of menarche at that time, which was 15 years old, and the typical age of marriage and parenthood (Arnett 2000). The current trend in social science research is to place the adolescent phase in the second decade of life, or from ages 10 or 11 to 20 or 21 years. The shift to a younger onset no doubt reflects the significant change in the rate of biological development in Western society, where the median age of menarche is now 12.5 years. However, the significant differences in contemporary placement of the end point are less well justified. In Chapter 9, "Late Adolescence," we set late adolescence solidly in the college period, because the majority of American youth enter college and thus take part in the experience of psychosocial moratorium that serves to delay the confrontation with adulthood. From the vantage point of our clinical experience and our understanding of the developmental tasks of late adolescence, it makes sense to assign the college-age population to late adolescence and to place emerging adulthood in the decade between ages 21 and 30.

Indeed, the last half-century witnessed another wave of societal change, and in its wake, the developmental trajectory of the 20s has been radically altered. In a word, the emblematic achievements of adulthood have been postponed. In 1960, all the traditional indicators of adulthood (employment, marriage, parenthood, financial independence) had been accomplished by 44% of males and 68% of females by age 25, whereas in 2000, they had been accomplished by only 13% of males and 25% of females by this age (Furstenberg 2010). A more detailed look shows that in 1950, the median age for marriage was 20 years for women and 23 years for men, compared to the medians of 25 and 27 years, respectively, at the turn of the twenty-first century (Arnett 2005). Moreover, Arnett (2000) documented that the 20s show trends that were formerly attributed to the teen years, such as peak levels of alcohol consumption and high-risk behaviors, including unprotected sex, high-speed driving, and driving under the influence. Although some of these behaviors can be "explained" by various societal changes, such as the legal drinking age and increased college attendance, they do imply that many behaviors we formerly saw as manifestations of adolescent psychology extend into and even peak in the 20s and must be understood in that context. Some theorists believe that this change reflects the reality that development is not monolithic and that certain domains mature while others may extend deep into adulthood without the expected transformation. Although unevenness is present throughout development, it is nowhere more visible than in the transition to adulthood.

Is It a New Developmental Phase?

The notion of emerging adulthood as a developmental phase, derived from these findings, has been widely promulgated among sociologists, developmental psychologists, and youth theorists, but it remains controversial. Proponents argue that this phase represents a discrete period along the path to adulthood, one that is replete with its own conflicts and challenges. Arnett, who made reference to the idea of emerging adulthood as early as 1994 (Arnett and Taber 1994), offers five criteria for this stage: identity (role) explorations, instability, self-focus, feeling in-between, and a widening of possibilities (Arnett 2004, p. 55). He emphasizes the centrality of role exploration as "the heart of emerging adulthood" (Arnett 2000). It is his contention that in Western societies, the cognitive, emotional, and behavioral transformations accompanying the 20s are sufficiently pronounced to qualify for their recognition as a discrete developmental phase. The dynamic interface of culture, society, and development is indeed far more significant in emerging adulthood than in any other phase; it is a culture-specific phenomenon related to the impact of broad socialization. Broad socialization, for which a liberal arts education is emblematic, relies on "independence, individualism, and self-expression" for the transition to adulthood, in contrast to narrow socialization, which occurs in societies in which prescribed pathways are the rule (Arnett and Taber 1994, p. 519).

There are several arguments against a developmental (as opposed to a sociological) designation for the phase of emerging adulthood. Many of Arnett's (2004) criteria have of course been applied to adolescence and would seem to simply extend the adolescent process into the 20s, long after the dramatic events of puberty and physical transformation have ebbed. Some important developmental psychodynamic thinkers insist that developmental phases are to be distinguished from other periods of life by their "maturationally determined program" and the "emergence of novelties" (Abrams 1990, p. 664). Emerging adulthood fails to meet criteria because it is arguably not associated with a significant transformation physically or cognitively (see section "Physical and Cognitive Development" later in this chapter). From a sociological viewpoint, dissenters point to the societal changes that have served to "delay adulthood." For these thinkers, a developmental conceptualization minimizes the structural constraints imposed on youth in Western societies, thereby misidentifying a phenomenon as developmental when in fact it is attributable to educational, economic, and institutional factors and varies across industrialized countries (Bynner 2005). Unlike narrowly socialized cultures, where adulthood is strictly defined and individuals are prepared and then channeled into adult roles, Western society no longer provides such clear-cut signposts: the official attainment of adulthood is highly "contestable" (Horowitz and Bromnick 2007). That is, the initiation markers of adulthood are "intangible, gradual, psychological and individualistic" (Arnett 1997, p. 15), and its achievement fluctuates in both self-experience and the eyes of the world. The notion of contestability rests on the observation that preadults (i.e., emerging adults) expend considerable time and energy "arguing... [their] way into adulthood" (Horowitz and Bromnick 2007), because the subjective sense of the self as adult fluctuates so dramatically. Moreover, some influential sociologists such as James Cote (2006) assert that very little role exploration is accomplished in what Arnett designates as the time frame for emerging adulthood, and that the fragmentation of structural supports for concrete identity formation leaves a significant percentage of this age group arrested in an unresolved identity crisis.

Cote (2006) and others suggest that the late modern delay in adulthood is the result of widespread changes in Western societies: changes in economic opportunities, educational requirements for the current job market, lack of strong ideological commitments, advances in pregnancy prevention linked to delays in the pressure to marry and a shift in sexual attitudes, high divorce rates and social tolerance of cohabitation, and other contemporary social realities (Bynner 2005). It is argued that these twenty-somethings are not in their own developmental phase but rather are living "divided lives"—simultaneously youth and adult—but also that they are "nowhere" because they cannot rely on societal regulation to make the transition (Shulman et al. 2005, pp. 578–579). Today's emerging adults are less psychologically equipped to consolidate their identities and less privileged in terms of real opportunities; a significant number lapse into an unresolved state that shows no natural developmental progression (Cote 2006; also see section "Prolonged Adolescence?" later in this chapter). Calling this contemporary crisis a "developmental phase" obscures the reality that with further societal transformation, such a phase might disappear. What Arnett is designating as developmental is simply today's version of early adulthood, a complex dynamic interaction of multiple systems, including "structural factors, individual agency and experience, encounters with social institutions, and cultural imperatives" (Hendry and Kloep 2007, p. 78).

As noted earlier, the counterargument points out that adolescence was once also a new developmental phenomenon and an outgrowth of a cultural transformation of the twentieth century. One could make the case that what today seems undeniable about the internal transformation during adolescence only came into focus with the moratorium provided by Western culture. Erik Erikson's formulation of adolescence in the 1950s, which drew attention to the importance of the community in providing both the cultural institutions and, ultimately, the recognition essential to identity formation, can easily accommodate the insertion of another phase in contemporary society.

> Societies offer, as individuals require, more or less sanctioned intermediary periods between childhood and adulthood, called institutionalized *psychosocial moratoria*, during which a lasting pattern of "inner identity" is scheduled for relative completion. (Erikson 1956, p. 66)

How does the decade of the 20s figure into the intrapsychic developmental progression elucidated in this book? What do these new findings reflect about the internal experience and developmental transformations of the 20s? The lack of any clear biological markers, at either the decade's beginning or its end, highlights the psychosocial or psychocultural transformation involved (Cote 2006; Staples and Smarr 1991). Unlike adolescence, which is initiated by the momentous physiological events of puberty, emerging adulthood has no new developmental impetus that arises from bodily and mental novelties. Nonetheless, *emerging adulthood* describes a period of psychological development, especially in relation to the complex challenge of adaptation to the cultural changes of the last half-century. Although proponents recognize the Western society–specific appearance of this phase, they suggest that the impact of societal changes has caused a shift in the consensual linkage of behavior and age, which, by implication, drives internal developmental pace (Neugarten et al. 1965); societal expectations of "age-appropriate" milestones create psychological pressure to achieve them on society's schedule.

As noted above in the section "Introduction to Emerging Adulthood," some of the challenges and conflicts formerly ascribed to adolescence do seem to figure significantly in this next phase. However, there is little doubt that these challenges and conflicts are experienced differently by people in their 20s. Rather than extend the parameters of adolescence, the notion of emerging adulthood or the odyssey years recognizes that these conflicts have a biphasic dimension. Emerging adulthood as a developmental phase illuminates a moment in contemporary Western society wherein formerly emancipated youth return home and struggle to "become someone"; the tasks formerly ascribed to adolescence must be extended, revisited, and re-sized for the adult world. In other words, the identity work of college and the degree of autonomy from the family of origin, both supported by geographic distance and the "independent" living of the college campus, erode as the 21- or 22-year-old moves back home and gropes toward a meaningful career and personal commitments. The processes are gradually finalized as the commitments central to adulthood are made (Emde 1985). Moreover, the solutions to developmental challenges introduced during this phase, whether they are adaptive or maladaptive, can have a profound impact on the individual's future adaptation; for example, substance use peaks in the mid-20s and can harden into chronic addiction (Tucker et al. 2005).

Criteria of Emerging Adulthood

1. Identity/role exploration
2. Instability
3. Internal focus
4. Feeling neither adolescent nor adult
5. Sense of new possibilities but growing anxiety as age 30 approaches

IS COLLEGE GRADUATION THE KEY?

Regardless of the merits of the currently mandated "college-for-all" policy, it has unwittingly contributed to a pool of disappointed 20- to 30-year-olds (Rosenbaum 2011; Rosenbaum and Person 2003); recent reports indicate that 39% of freshmen at 4-year colleges and 68% of students entering 2-year colleges do not have their degrees 6 years later (Attewell et al. 2011). These young men and women seem to hit a dead end in their chosen path, emerging without a degree and without vocational training in an economy that offers a diminishing array of well-paying manufacturing jobs and that increasingly requires advanced education for employment. As described in Coupland's (1991) book *Generation X,* these young people often end up in a "McJob"—a "low-paying, low-prestige, low-benefit, no-future job in the service sector" (p. 5)—which they endure without enthusiasm or future aspirations in order to support themselves. As these individuals move through their 20s, these jobs threaten to become their lifetime employment and heighten a feeling of disaffection. Although this outcome is certainly structural, in the sense that it reflects societal constraints and pressures, it has a profound effect on the confidence of the emerging adult in contemplating the future. Some of these individuals, of course, settle into jobs or join and/ or begin their own start-up businesses, discover their true calling, and develop a strong sense of occupational identity ahead of their college-attending peers.

The late adolescent who completes college presumably has the opportunity to resolve crucial developmental conflicts; the college experience provides the moratorium described by Erikson (1956) in which the struggle for identity is conducted in a remarkably adult-free and relatively consequence-free atmosphere. Despite the respite it provides, however, the passage through college follows its own progressive sequence of attitudes toward the future and gradually turns the attention of the imminent graduate to the questions of emerging adulthood. As graduation approaches, the students with a prescribed trajectory proceed, if they have done well, to graduate school, military service, or other "next-step" programs that may lead directly to careers or may simply further extend the education-to-work transition. Other students, for reasons of inadequate preparation, personal immaturity, or squandered opportunities for identity exploration, arrive at graduation without a game plan (Erikson 1956). After spending a few years in the workforce, many of these students, especially women, return to school with a specific agenda to train themselves for better jobs (Rampell 2011). It seems that, at least for women in the first decade of the twenty-first century, emerging adulthood has become a "back-to-school" era.

• **See the video "Young Adult Male, Age 25." Because this young man's choice to go to art school for college was determined by the "free ride" he was able to get there, he had no developed career path. The death of his mother was a loss of his primary support and guidance. His progress illustrates the importance of mentoring, however brief and serendipitous, in helping an emerging adult set goals for the future.**

Evidence, however, suggests that high school and college graduates looking for work "mill about" equivalently (Tanner 2006), and job exploration is often more thorough without the constraints of college or postgraduate education that can feel like a commitment. Nonetheless, as demonstrated in the following vignette, there is a modicum of self-esteem associated with the milestone accomplishment of college, especially if it transcends the student's family background.

Jen was the first in her family to attend college and hoped to find a professional way out of her small home town and working class family. She had been popular, active in extracurricular activities, and a good student during high school, winning admission to the urban campus of her excellent state university. Once there, she felt set back by her relative lack of sophistication and found that she missed her high school friends and boyfriend, all of whom were attending the local community college. She followed their activities on Facebook and felt out of place at her school. Returning to college unhappily after winter break of her freshman year, she was immediately summoned home because her mother had been diagnosed with breast cancer. She took a semester's leave to help her father in his small business and to accompany her mother to her chemotherapy treatments. This was certainly not what she had imagined herself doing. To her chagrin, Jen found that she was as embarrassed and uncomfortable with her high school friends as she had been with her new college crowd. She parted ways with her boyfriend. Her mother did well after a rocky and difficult course. In the meantime, Jen shouldered increasing responsibilities in her father's business and began to think that she might as well stay put. At this point her high school friends were graduating from community college and some were planning to continue at the state university for a bachelor's degree. Following their progress on Facebook, Jen began to feel completely out of sync and disappointed in her life. She was supposed to be headed for "bigger things" and had never imagined herself working in her dad's business. Her broad horizon had collapsed.

Jen's interest in medicine had been stimulated by the contact with doctors during her mother's treatments, although she felt that they were not always very attentive to their patients' suffering. The idea of returning to college and embarking on a premed course was at once inspiring and daunting, but her old confidence returned and carried her forward. She sampled some basic science courses along with a few required freshman courses to complete a bachelor's degree locally. Once again an outsider, she was shocked at the level of competition among the premed students she encountered. Even while worrying that she was "just running" from the challenge, she decided that 22 years old was too old to start from scratch. She was impatient to get on with a career where she knew she would succeed. She began looking into a 2-year nursing school program that, should she excel, would qualify her to take the licensure exam and become a registered nurse. Jen admitted that she felt this was settling for a lesser career; she spent the first year feeling disappointed in her classmates and the level of the coursework. However, during her first summer internship, she developed a relationship with a practicing nurse whose dedication, humanity, and intellectual breadth impressed Jen deeply. With her guidance, Jen became increasingly engaged in her training, honing her interests and discovering that nursing could be stimulating and engaging. At the point of completing her associate nursing degree, she decided to apply to a program to seek a master of science in nursing, a degree that her mentor said would give her both status and better remuneration within the field. At 26, she was admitted to an accelerated program. She planned to specialize in oncological nursing. By graduation, she saw nursing as a noble calling, one that conferred respect and self-worth through hard work and dedication.

PROLONGED ADOLESCENCE?

As noted earlier, some of the psychological tasks previously assigned to the close of adolescence are now cited as fundamental to emerging adulthood. How, then, can a normative postadolescent phase be distinguished from a prolongation of the adolescent process itself? The theorist of adolescence Peter Blos (1954, 1979), who developed the concept of the "second individuation," delineated a specific clinical entity in young men in whom the attenuation of the adolescent crisis is a form of psychopathology. *Prolonged adolescence* is characterized by an inability to renounce the position of the admired child of doting parents when forced to grapple with demands to prove oneself in the adult world. Despite insistence on autonomy and respect, the prolonged adolescent does not demonstrate the capacity or determination to steer an independent course forward in any area; he wants the unconditional praise he received in childhood while still insisting on the privileges of adulthood. Instead of an active transitional period, adolescence becomes a static state persisting well into the 20s. These are young men who appear to be unconflicted about their paralysis and have traditionally sought treatment only when they observe their peers leaving them behind or when parental support is finally withdrawn.

Blos's (1979) description of the clinical features of prolonged adolescence is similar to "identity diffusion," the term used by Erikson (1956) and subsequently Kernberg (2006) to identify individuals who fail to resolve the identity crisis of adolescence and typically present in clinical settings with severe personality disorders (see Chapter 9). It also shares features with Cote's (2006) proposed "youthhood," defined as an indefinitely prolonged identity moratorium with origins in the economic circumstances of contemporary Western society, the late modern "anomic" and "fragmented developmental context" that fails to facilitate identity consolidation and internal predilections (Cote 2006, p. 91). All of these are clinical syndromes and should be distinguished from the generational phenomenon called emerging adulthood as a normative phase. Prolonged adolescents, with their perpetual youthhood and personality disorders characterized by identity diffusion, may blend into the culture of emerging adulthood, but they are different from the normative group by virtue of their evident psychopathology. Instead of undertaking an active process, prolonged adolescents show a determination *not* to resolve adolescent issues; they do not commit to "self-defining representations of self, role relationships, and core values" (Wilkinson-Ryan and Westen 2000, p. 529), they do not confront the requirement that they make choices, and they manifest stasis in their progression toward attaining intimate relationships and meaningful work. The following vignette describes a young man whose stalled trajectory is typical in prolonged adolescence.

> Eugene, now age 24, had been a highly regarded actor in his small, supportive high school where his mother taught. He was the star of every school production and made his way through the academics, despite learning disabilities and attentional problems, with the help of a dedicated faculty. He was able to gain admission to an excellent moderate-sized liberal arts college,

chosen in part because of the academic support available on campus. However, during college Eugene had two separate episodes, extending over a 3-year period, of gradual shutdown in his academic performance, even while continuing to participate actively in theater productions on campus and in the community. In the first such episode, his nonattendance led to a forced medical leave, but the second resulted in expulsion. Following this blow, he continued to live in off-campus housing with other students and to perform in college shows through the conscious or unknowing collusion of the drama faculty. Outside of his family, Eugene told no one of his status. He "acted" as if he were attending classes, and when his peers graduated, he pretended he graduated with them but chose not to walk the ceremony. This "illusion" became the central organizing feature of his day-to-day life; the longer it continued, the more preoccupied he was about exposure of his facade. The lie infiltrated his romantic life and employment and became the rationale for a suspension of all effort. Most importantly, he made no moves to connect to the world of theater—no auditions and no acting classes—due to his worry about being "found out." When confronted about his apparent passivity both in regard to earning a living and especially in regard to an acting career, he was visibly offended and stated, "This is the most important thing to me. You just don't understand. I am an actor."

Eugene's clinical picture resembles some aspects of the normative emerging adult's typical trajectory. Many students drop out or take many years or even decades to complete their undergraduate education, such that only one-third of individuals ages 25–29 years possess college degrees, despite the increase in college attendance in the United States (Arnett 2004, p. 125). The obstacles to the pursuit of meaningful work are economic, social, and intrapsychic, because the paths to employment are more circuitous than in the past, and many emerging adults have not used their high school or college experience to forge a direct route to a career. However, the kind of narcissistic entitlement, inconsistent self-representation, and primitive denial implied in the vignette are not typical for young adults. All emerging adults grapple with issues of identity and the requirement to renounce grandiose ideals. However, their preoccupations with questions of authenticity, competence, and responsibility reflect a sincere struggle to resolve unsettled conflicts in regard to core psychological issues, which ultimately include their integration into society.

• **See the video "Young Adult Male, Age 26." This young man followed the prescribed path through high school to attend college but discovered that he had no interest in that form of education. After returning home and feeling undirected for a year or two, he found a work environment in which he felt stimulated to grow and excel. For him, relationships take a back seat until a career identity is firmly established.**

THE SUBJECTIVE EXPERIENCE OF THE EMERGING ADULT

A crucial difference between adolescence and young adulthood is reported to be a shift in the inner experience of self. While late adolescents are certainly observing and even fearing the future ahead, most do not feel unsure about their status in relation to it; although they no longer consider themselves children, they commonly refer to themselves as "kids." The future seems vast and unlimited. However, 21- to 30-year-olds gradually feel too old to consider themselves kids, or boys and girls; the use of that terminology feels awkward at least some of the time.

The sense of internal inconsistency and division has been documented in a number of studies (Shulman et al. 2005) and reflects unevenness in the process of settling into defined adult roles at the same time that there is an urgent feeling that important choices must be made. Such unevenness corresponds to the psychodynamic observation that ego consolidation progresses inconsistently through the 20s, with different aspects of mental structure lagging behind others (Escoll 1987) and with the contemporary developmental idea that life course transitions involve the interplay of multiple systems, each with its own developmental pace (Hendry and Kloep 2007). For example, maturation of the capacity to tolerate competition and succeed in the context of academic settings may well precede the delineation of long-term commitment to a professional goal, or the impulse control and judgment to manage risky behavior such as alcohol or cocaine misuse may lag behind stabilization of ego capacities and attitudes sufficient to pursue a career, thus jeopardizing burgeoning professional status. Internal distress over such unevenness can be heightened by the acceleration in the experience of time (Colarusso 1991) as these young adults approach age 30.

The emerging adult of today is often uneasy and uncertain about the future, while nonetheless fully cognizant of this widespread and well-publicized generational phenomenon that normalizes uncertainty (at least in Western society). Although some surveys show sustained optimism still highly endorsed at age 24 (Arnett 2004), there is divergence in the research assessing the state of mind of the emerging adult. Whereas some studies indicate improvement in depressive symptoms, conflict with parents, and overall confidence in concert with the increased autonomy and decision making of individuals in their mid-20s (Arnett 2004; Galambos et al. 2006), others suggest that as age 30 looms, the level of "anxiety, depression, and even despair" increases (Bynner et al. 1997, p. 128). Clinical experience supports the idea that age 30 is contemplated as a marker; the future is now. However, the emerging adult is not defensively complacent, but rather openly concerned about how to navigate the crucial steps leading to the transformation into productive adulthood: how to find a stable relationship, how to find mean-ingful work, and how to rely on internal decision making and internal values and goals to achieve a sense of personal agency—in short, how to assume full responsibility for a full life.

As adolescents move out of the family and into the world and as they de-velop the cognitive capacities for abstraction and meta-analysis, they often experience disillusionment with their "implicit family ideology" (Barnett 1971, p. 113). The world order, the sense of right and wrong, the hierarchy of values, and the terms of intimate relationships are conveyed in myriad ways to family members and are only subject to conscious reckoning as the young person's cognitive capacities and access to differences accrue. *Recentering,* which involves the emerging adult's assumption of self-determina-tion around these meaningful and value-laden beliefs and choices, introduces a qualitatively different source of conflict in relationship to par-ents, even while the young person still depends on the parents for support (Tanner 2006). Ultimately, this recentering process establishes firm bound-aries in regard to parental influence; the emerging adult's stabilization of identity and a self-experience approximates the adult form, achieving "inde-pendence of parental control, expression of own goals and preferences, and assumption of responsibilities" (Cohen et al. 2003, p. 660). The following vi-gnette demonstrates this process of recentering.

> Marie was raised in a small town in the Midwest, the third child of hardwork-ing parents with a small family-owned service business. From a very early age, she was discovered to be an amazing musician. Her parents were big fans of country music, and her brother, 6 years older than Marie, had a keyboard. She was able to listen to a tune and re-create it almost as soon as she could reach the keys. Her parents knew very little about classical music, but Marie's school music teacher assured them that she was very talented. They bought an up-right piano and devoted a disproportionate share of their limited resources to providing her with music training. In their excitement, they readily grafted the culture of serious classical musicianship onto the family activities, trying to at-tend concerts and listen to famous recordings. In high school, she traveled over 2 hours daily to attend a performing arts school. She played at every fam-ily event and occasion and eventually developed a little business playing music at parties and dances. She was the pride of the family and her town. As a high school junior, Marie competed in a local university-sponsored piano festival, where she won the precollege solo piano competition, participated in master classes, and performed at the university-wide award ceremony. Despite her success, Marie was always anxious about performing and was treated by her pediatrician for her stage fright with propranolol as needed; she took this in stride and there was little comment about it.
>
> Marie chose to attend a conservatory on the East Coast; however, sepa-rated from the enthusiastic atmosphere of her family and town, she felt de-

flated and daunted by the competition and the exacting expectations of her teachers. Now, she was afraid to play for faculty or classmates and felt she needed daily propranolol to survive. She was increasingly unhappy and unfocused. To her parents' dismay, she decided in midyear to apply for transfer out of the conservatory to a small liberal arts school in a nearby city. When she arrived there, she began to look back at her musical career with anger and disillusionment, even feeling at times that she had been treated like a "performing monkey." She did not ask her parents for financial help and grew distant from them for several years. She was determined "never again" to come under their sway; she lived in a tiny space (actually a closet) in the tenement apartment of a classmate and supported herself through school by working as a barista in a popular coffee shop. There, she met her boyfriend, Jared, a law student, and they developed a warm and loving relationship.

Marie decided in college that she would like to write about the performing arts, and she landed a desk job at an online events magazine, a start-up company of recent graduates from her program. Although it was undeniably boring, the job promised future opportunities to actually attend concerts and do reviews. However, as one year dragged into the next, Marie was unhappy, physically "a wreck" from frequent migraines and carpal tunnel syndrome, and felt trapped in her job. She had to keep working to survive, but she felt completely lost in terms of career and was envious but proud as Jared moved forward in his profession and landed a job as a law clerk. At least, she thought, she was increasingly committed to Jared, and *he* was successful. Jared came from a very different home environment, with successful professional parents and high-achieving siblings. Marie was deeply impressed by the shared intellectual interests in Jared's family and grew closer to them. Jared's father was a dedicated amateur oenophile, and over the course of her relationship with Jared, Marie was inspired by his dad to read about wine and viticulture. She also accompanied him to tastings and showed a real talent for understanding and appreciating the complexity of wine. Following the advice of Jared's father, she discussed her new interest with her parents, who agreed to contribute to the cost of the Sommelier Society of America's certification course and exam. Although this is a notoriously difficult program, she excelled; while studying, she developed her connections in the world that Jared's father had introduced to her. With "a little help from her friends," she landed a sommelier job at an up-and-coming restaurant, joining the small but growing group of women in head sommelier positions. Her parents were very impressed and grateful to Jared and his family, promised not to mention the piano anymore, and were invited East to visit, meet Jared's family, and come to a fabulous dinner at Marie's place of work. Marie was 29 years old, finally in a career she loved, and reconciled to her parents, who gave their blessing to her marriage to Jared.

IDENTITY

As described in Chapter 9, the concept of identity is an aspect of subjective experience that involves the interface with society. The adolescent identity crisis is understood as a psychosocial one, and requires the recognition and affirmation of the environment. Although formation of identity has been designated the task of late adolescence, Blos (1962) suggested that what he called "post-adolescence" is the time when adult identity is consolidated. Following the period of exploration, identity achieves "harmonization" as final choices in regard to love and work are settled (p. 149). Supporting this idea from a life-span perspective, the adult narrative sense of self is primarily centered on "benchmark memories" from the period between ages 20 and 29 years when enduring choices with long-term repercussions are made (Elnick et al. 1999).

In the early years of emerging adulthood, however, a new kind of disillusionment threatens: disillusionment with the only recently formed sense of identity. As in the preceding vignette about Marie, identities forged and reinforced in high school, and even those overhauled significantly through college, do not necessarily translate into adult roles; aside from the lucky few, the star football players, actors, artists, musicians, and intellectuals of the college campus are now dealing with the daunting task of reconfiguring themselves to fit into the adult world. This is documented in studies that describe the potential for continuity and discontinuity in the young person's trajectory, with some individuals able to make use of transitions to reinvent themselves and others unable to or obstructed from making use of new opportunities for psychological or circumstantial reasons (Schulenberg et al. 2004). There are those fortunate individuals whose remarkable talents, connections, structured career paths, or luck have pole-vaulted them into a career; some of these trajectories are deeply gratifying and feel like a "fit" with native abilities and aspirations. However, for those young adults whose earlier adolescent successes do not lead directly to adult ones, the sense of discouragement and loss is a more or less constant companion. The college basketball scholarship student and star not quite talented enough to be drafted into the professional leagues is often left feeling that he is a disappointment not only to himself but also to his family and community. The star of her college drama department who never successfully ignites a career on the stage is often dogged by a sense of failure in subsequent career choices. Thus, the identity crisis of the earlier phase, which may have been satisfactorily resolved within a smaller community, is now revisited when the individual moves into the larger adult world.

Unfortunately, contemporary social structures offer less support and guidance than 50 years ago, and the older generation is uniquely ill equipped to advise today's young adults, since the older individuals are unfamiliar with the technology, the social networking, and the changes in career paths in contemporary society (Beyers and Seiffge-Krenke 2010; Konstam 2007). In addition, the subjective experience of emerging adults as they pass into their 20s is that they are increasingly liberated from, if not altogether independent of, control by parents and other institutional mentors. Although this is typically a boon to an improved relationship with parents (Galambos et al. 2006), it can result in a further loss of guidance.

Identifications with parents become more compelling in emerging adulthood, because young adults are approaching the age of their parents as remembered from early childhood. The confluence of memory, current experience, and the history of struggle with identifications with parents can heighten both the determination to be different and the recognition of strong identificatory ties. Because of the cultural shift in the average age of marriage and childbearing, most emerging adults are as old as their parents were when they were born. This can add an element of rueful recognition to long-standing disappointments with parental decisions and behavior, as these emerging adults realize how ill equipped they themselves feel to make important choices, especially in regard to child rearing. In optimal circumstances, such awareness can lead to reduction of tension and revision of the internal parental representations and to deeper self-reflection about relationship and work decisions.

Surveys assessing the young adult's state of mind diverge as to the degree to which these circumstances contribute to destabilization or even unhappiness. Part of the disagreement may be due to the way the cohort is defined; as suggested above (see "The Subjective Experience of the Emerging Adult"), the level of concern about the future may actually peak in the late 20s, thus certainly after Arnett's cutoff of 24 years. Arnett and other thinkers impressed with the improved mental state of the young adult emphasize that the internal maturation occurring through the 20s enhances confidence and mood; greater autonomy liberates emerging adults from the ongoing deleterious effects of negative family life and identifications. Improved self-regulation and refinement of goals fuel optimism and promise eventual success (Arnett 2004, 2007). However, manifestos such as *Quarter Life Crisis*, written for and by emerging adults, suggest that many are in a protracted struggle to achieve identity and suffer from "overwhelming senses of helplessness and cluelessness" (Robbins and Wilner 2001, p. 4). For these eyewitnesses, disappointment or disillusionment is a palpable feature of the emerging adult experience. Because the environment must provide crucial scaffolding for identity, the nature of the individual's immediate surround and the larger society figure significantly in this evolving feature of mental life; current social supports matter for self-esteem maintenance (Galambos et al. 2006). However, some contributions to successful identity resolution are ideally sustained and sustaining through this period, because they rest on an internal, psychological foundation: a sense of competence, the integration of personal ideals and goals, and the feeling of confidence that one will fulfill a future—perhaps not the one of childhood dreams, but a valuable one nonetheless.

"The Second Individuation" Revisited

As discussed in Chapter 8, the concept of the second individuation, with modifications, remains useful in considering the adolescent process. The shift in the subjective sense of self, which can be such a painful aspect of young adulthood, is counterbalanced by a mature rapprochement with the parents. Although the relationship with family was affected by the adolescent's need to establish his or her own internal "ideology," to become immersed in the peer culture, and to develop self-selected values, young adulthood presents new opportunities to revisit the relationship with parents and to reengage as an adult. In families where the adolescent movement toward autonomy proceeded without significant disruption of the attachment, the parents remain an essential source of guidance, and the quality of their marital relationship can serve as a model (Bell et al. 1996).

The individual progress of the individuation process plays an important role as backdrop to multiple developmental systems in emerging adulthood, including educational achievement, occupational prestige, and intimate relationships (Tanner 2006). The balance between optimal distance and closeness seems to be the overarching principle, reinforcing the idea that a secure attachment is the foundation for a successful individuation process. Individuation requires both parental facilitation and the adolescent's ego maturation. From the side of the parents, their tolerance of conflict and negativity, ongoing availability for counsel and advice, and simultaneous encouragement of autonomy (especially by fathers [Scharf and Mayseless 2008]) are factors that promote individuation and self-esteem (Allen et al. 1994). Parents' constraining interactions (e.g., controlling, withholding, or overindulging) inhibit their children's ego development toward maturity (Stierlin 1974). In fact, in regard to ego development, evidence of maturity is typically accompanied by striving toward self-sufficiency, which in turn facilitates adaptation and achievement following college (Tanner 2006, p. 29). The establishment of a life plan or weltanschauung (Jacobson 1961; Tanner 2006) has been considered a central component of the individuation process that in turn supports the harmonization of identity; this idea was part of Piaget's (1972) original description of the cognitive capacities for abstraction and symbolic thought achieved in adolescence. The life plan may differ significantly from the values of the family of origin without requiring its repudiation; for today's emerging adults, the future in a world transformed by technology often makes the parental model obsolete.

The important distinction between the late adolescent search for an alternative idealized adult (Chused 1987) and the emerging adult's readiness to realistically assess, and if possible admire, his or her own parents rests on the degree to which the process toward autonomy and differentiation has progressed internally. In this context, the unrelated mentor can greatly facilitate the late adolescent's struggle to find his or her own agency and make his or her own choices. Some careers may have been adequately negotiated without relying on parental input because models present themselves in the course of their unfolding. However, among young adults who have not chosen a highly structured career path such as medicine or the law, there remain the momentous decisions that will determine the future and reconfigure the subjective experience of identity. For these choices, the emerging adult often relies on the emotional support provided by parents; even if the older generation is admittedly unfamiliar with the realities of contemporary culture, there is a far greater likelihood that today's emerging adults were raised by two working parents with experience of various types in the working world. Contacts, encouragement, and the provision of a sounding board are the reconsidered rightful domain of the parents. In a study addressing optimal parenting in emerging adulthood, "parenting clusters" were identified: uninvolved, controlling-indulgent, authoritative, and inconsistent. Emerging adult outcomes benefited least from controlling-indulgent parents and most from authoritative ones (i.e., parents who present a point of view that is clear but not domineering) (Nelson et al. 2011). Moreover, if parents can sustain a collaborative relationship or "parenting alliance" (Cohen and Weissman 1984), even in situations of divorce, their mutually respectful conversation and balance is a source of inspiration and confidence about internalizing their feedback in regard to both choosing a profession and choosing a mate.

Individuation and the Return Home

Individuation remains a useful formulation for a nuanced appreciation of the emerging adult, especially if understood in relation to attachment patterns as described in Chapter 9. In fact, rather than being in conflict, these two dimensions can be understood as deeply intertwined and especially at play as the young adult "child" struggles to establish an autonomous, independent identity. This process is greatly complicated by the likelihood that young adult children have either remained home through their early 20s or must return to the parental home, at least temporarily, after college or during financially stressful periods. The return home can be a regressive experience for both parents and children, because the transition from parent-child to adult-adult dynamics is often rocky. The specific relationships of the emerging adult to the same- and opposite-sex parents and to the parents as a couple have reverberations in many of the conflicts of this phase: how to manage identifications, how to integrate the images of the parental couple as a representation of a love relationship, and how to transform the parent-child relationship into an adult relationship even while still depending on the parents.

The fate of the marital couple with grown children is certainly part of the picture, because the emerging adult who leaves home at 18 may find a new set of circumstances upon returning. Parental divorce, remarriage, and reconfigurations of the family home can be surprisingly disturbing to adult children. The notion of "secure base" seems especially relevant as the emerging adult relies on parental stability to scaffold his or her own moves toward autonomy. The college graduate who is required to achieve autonomy and independence in a hurry because his room has been converted into a guest room, storage space, or gym can feel resentful, even if he had no intention of returning home. Or the young woman whose widowed father has remarried and whose room is now occupied by a step-sibling can experience her forays into independent living as a banishment. There is comfort for these emerging adults in having a familiar place to return to, even if they have no conscious desire to resume their dependent status.

Current relationships between parents and emerging adult children, even if mature, do not necessarily correct the deleterious effects of a developmental history of disturbed attachment to parents or negatively tinged internal working models established earlier in life. There is evidence to suggest that core vulnerabilities of emerging adults—"low self-esteem, lack of purpose in life, poor life satisfaction, romantic relationship problems, and psychological distress"—are correlated with "troubled ruminations about parents" due to childhood feelings of rejection from one or both parents (Schwartz and Finley 2010, p. 88). Even when there is a foundation of positive identifications, secure attachment, and idealization of parents, the passage through adolescence usually heightens ambivalence and the search for alternative, less fraught objects of admiration and aspiration. As adolescents move into the transitional period of emerging adulthood, they are usually able to better appreciate their parents as adults, especially if the parents have evolved toward a comparable recognition. The parents can be observed as personalities with vulnerabilities and idiosyncrasies as well as strengths and wisdom. This facilitates a more genuine and mutual acceptance, and initiates a phase of the parent-child relationship that, ideally, is both realistic and admiring. Similar shifts can occur in sibling relationships; the emerging adult is potentially capable of more nuanced and objective assessments of brothers and sisters when released from the remnants of childish rivalry, dependence, and/or forced distance from parents. The sibling competitions can similarly evolve into mutual recognition and respect, although elements of the old struggles can of course persist throughout life.

Tasks of Emerging Adulthood

- Finalization of identity
- Commitment to intimate relationship
- Clarification of personal goals and values
- Establishment of career path
- Realignment vis-à-vis parents and family of origin toward equality and mutual respect

MOTHERS AND FATHERS, FRIENDS AND LOVERS, MEN AND WOMEN

In families where the adolescent movement toward autonomy proceeded without significant disruption of attachment, parents remain an essential source of guidance, and the quality of their relationship with each other can serve as a model (Bell et al. 1996). Secure attachment to parents has a modest but reliable connection to the capacity to develop intimate relationships in emerging adulthood. Nonetheless, a diminution in closeness over the course of adolescence seems to be a prerequisite for adequate individuation and the capacity to form an intimate peer relationship (Seiffge-Krenke et al. 2010).

Young men and women grapple with their specific relationship with each parent based on their complex developmental histories, the role the parent played throughout their childhood, and the way that gender and gender stereotypes were handled in the family and the surrounding culture. Contemporary dynamic thinking has raised many important questions about binary categorization of male and female, mother and father, son and daughter, and has illuminated the "fluidity" and idiosyncratic construction of gender in development (Harris 2008). As children become adult men and women, they are compelled to grapple anew with their own gender representations and their multiply determined ideas about their gender roles. In this arena, cultural conventions and transformations exert powerful influence; widely available and effective contraception has revolutionized women's opportunity to fulfill the gender role of their preference and led to a decline in the birth rate in Western societies. Similarly, changes in social policy (such as how taxation and welfare policy affect homemakers) influence how men and women anticipate their gendered adult choices (Hakim 2011). These cultural trends in turn introduce tension between generations. Contemporary adult development during this phase may be less significantly at odds with the parent generation than in the parents' own young adulthood; for example, the dual-income family with a mother and father sharing the roles of providers and caretakers is a fairly common childhood paradigm for the current twenty-somethings in industrialized countries. This model has repercussions on both men's and women's anticipated conflicts between work and family; as a consequence, men and women are more congruent with each other among today's emerging adults than historically. In prior generations, women entering the workforce diverged from their mothers' trajectories (Cinamon 2006) and often elicited parental disapproval. Today, generational conflicts seem to coalesce around the desire for and timing of parenthood, the changing face of feminism (see, e.g., Kramer 2011), homosexuality, and the meaning of marriage. These are arenas of considerable disagreement between generations that are highlighted as young people consider life partners and careers.

For young women, the relationship to the mother is inevitably reworked during each developmental phase. In young adulthood, the balance between attachment and dependency on the one hand and the ongoing striving for autonomy and differentiation into her own person on the other hand takes on a new layer of meaning as the young woman considers her future course. The current events in the young woman's life influence the nature of the mother-daughter relationship significantly during this phase (Notman 2006); her unique odyssey can become the arena for competition, guidance, or alienation depending on its manifest similarities to or differences from her mother's life course, both historically and in the recent past. For example, the emerging adult woman who anticipates postponement of motherhood into her 30s can come under some pressure from her own mother's wishes and example (Gordon et al. 2005). Similarly, the young woman who eschews the feminist principles of her mother and seeks to restore "family centering" may be felt to imply that her mother's choices were reactionary (Hakim 2011). The young woman whose parents divorced in her early adulthood may experience her own progress toward a committed relationship as an additional blow to her single and lonely mother. Indeed, the recognition of the daughter's achievement of her own contemporary version of mature womanhood, active sexuality, and success in romance can heighten her mother's reactions of envy, vicarious pleasure, or disapproval, depending on her own psychology and personal history. Sexuality is, in a sense, the great "differentiator" throughout the history of the mother-daughter relationship; the mother's sexual partnership draws her out of the exclusive mother-daughter bond in infancy, and subsequently the daughter draws away from their intimate connection to have her own private life of sexual fantasy, masturbation, and ultimately sexual activity and intimacy. Nonetheless, the earliest mother-daughter "love affair" forms a basis for funda-

mental feminine identifications and for all future tender and affectionate relationships for males and females alike (Klockars and Sirola 2001).

Moreover, the daughter's search for a meaningful romantic relationship
in her 20s takes on a more consequential intent and may lead to a greater understanding of her mother's choices. The latter's success or failure in establishing an enduring marriage and the nature of the partnerships observed in
parents and their friends are contemplated with a greater appreciation of the
complexity of relationships. The mother's course can be seen as an inspiration or source of anxiety. Young women whose mothers have had multiple
marriages can harbor a jaundiced view of the possibilities of a sustained and
loving relationship, but often actively disavow the traits they associate with
their mothers' failures and hope for a different outcome. If the relationship
between mother and daughter shifts toward "friendship," it may prove surprisingly uncomfortable for the daughter, who is typically made anxious by
"girlfriend" confidences. Despite the maturity of the daughter, there is still
an experienced need to maintain a parent-child boundary and a wish to be
spared responsibility for the mother's conflicts and unhappiness.

The emerging adult woman's relationship to her father is similarly delicately balanced between childhood and adulthood; although the awkwardness
between the adolescent girl and her father has abated, there is still an expectation of a firm boundary. Despite the vast variability in father-daughter relationships and the role of the daughter's ultimate sexual orientation, the father's
appreciation of her as a maturing woman is important in both her sense of
herself as attractive and desirable and her capacity to tolerate "erotic excitement" (Tessman 1982, p. 224). The fact that the emerging adult of today is
typically the child of two working parents has diminished the father's exclusive
contribution to "endeavor excitement" (Tessman 1982, p. 225)—that is, the
excitement of being out in the world, competing, and achieving—but the father certainly is central to the values the young woman internalizes in regard
to her importance as a productive person. Her experience of her father while
in her 20s, as she gropes toward adult decisions, has the potential to evolve toward an easier warmth and mutually respectful dialogue especially if her father himself progresses toward a less authoritarian stance.

The childhood history of the father-daughter relationship can also reverberate through her development as an intimate partner. Distance from the
father seems to account for the ambivalent, anxious component of love relationships, at least in part, and has been correlated with short-term relationships characterized by emotional extremes, intense preoccupation, and
jealousy (Seiffge-Krenke et al. 2010).

Young men shift in their relationships to parents in similar ways; their history of identifications and attitudes toward work and love coalesce under the

same pressure to take definitive steps toward adult commitments. Of course, the trajectory of each relationship up to this phase has a powerful shaping effect, as do contemporary cultural shifts that define masculinity and adult manhood. The young man, presumably more capable of assessing his father realistically, nonetheless harbors old idealizations, as well as disappointments and resentments. In optimal circumstances, these can be reprocessed to create a more balanced representation that facilitates the son's individuation and supports his self-esteem. Despite readiness for an adult relationship, and similar to the mother-daughter relationship, the young adult man still has a psychological need for the father to remain a father and not a "pal" on equal footing. Moreover, the father's role in preserving optimism about adulthood remains significant. As the young man closes in on life choices and examines whether he measures up, the contribution of the father who, despite the travails of his own adulthood, can convey the importance of cultural values and confidence in his son and in society, cannot be underestimated. In subcultures with a high percentage of absent fathers, the toll on young men's lives is extraordinarily high (see Banks and Oliviera 2011). Although this is not a simple correlation and does not identify specific psychological sequelae, there is no doubt that fathers' presence or absence is a factor in the fate of late adolescents and young adult men; optimal solutions to their absence, both intrapsychic and societal, often include provision of father substitutes, such as mentors, as we have mentioned throughout the discussion of adolescence through emerging adulthood. As described in Chapter 9, the mid- to late adolescent as well as the young adult often seeks an alternative, self-selected role model to support the recrafting of goals and ideals differentiated from parents. In more privileged sectors, these are often provided as part of the social fabric (e.g., college advisors and coaches); when such positive role models are not available, the young man is likely to seek his own, either through the idealization of distal heroes, such as sports celebrities, or of proximal ones, which, depending on socioeconomic factors, can range from charismatic neighborhood criminals to revered community activists to local war heroes. However, the integrity of the father's own life—his morality, work ethic, and sexual history—forms the developmental foundation of the son's internal ego ideal (Milrod 1990), even when the son actively rebels or chooses a different approach. In young adulthood, when adolescent conflicts have abated and a more mature assessment is possible, the potential for self-reflection in regard to past idealizations is much greater and can contribute to the modifying of identifications. In this regard, we believe that although the foundation for the superego and ego ideal is established in childhood, it is not immune from the ongoing impact of experience and maturation.

The mother-son relationship in emerging adulthood plays an important role as well. For boys raised by single mothers—a configuration that comprises

50% of black households—the mother-son relationship is crucial for development of values and positive images of masculinity (Lawson Bush 2004). Even an absent parent is represented, consciously or unconsciously, in mental life; these representations are an amalgam of internal fantasy plus pieces of information provided and attitudes conveyed about the absent parent by the available parent and other involved relatives. These representations are the basis of identifications and mental development, especially in regard to sense of self and superego evolution. In addition, the mother-son relationship seems to bear directly on the emerging adult male's anticipation of parenting. The desire for children in men is affected by the current relationship to both parents, but much more so by the attachment history in regard to mothers. "Buds of parenting" and the sense of future competence as a parent are correlated with a history of security and closeness with mothers. Indeed, Sroufe and colleagues' longitudinal study (2005), frequently referenced in this book, underscores the reverberations of early attachment on all intimate relationships.

For the young man who has not been fortunate enough to connect to a personally satisfying field of endeavor, the 20s are a time of growing anxiety as the bankruptcy of meaningless jobs or misguided identifications becomes more evident. The increasingly urgent need to "figure it out" is unfortunately often met with little in the way of pragmatic guidance; aside from the societal and generational factors, the intrapsychic determinants, which evolve in relation to a more fragmented and confusing picture of career possibilities, are often the core problem. The following vignette illustrates these themes.

> Mal's childhood experience was deeply affected by his father's minimal role in his life after his parents' relationship ended when he was 3 years old. His father, Patrick, was a local sports hero who was offered an excellent, very public job (not as an athlete) in the sports world that relocated him to another city. Patrick's efforts to stay in close contact with Mal and his mother ended after about a year, when he became involved with another woman. Mal was raised by his mother, Beverly, and his maternal grandparents in an urban environment; they "got by" but were never completely secure financially and were unwilling, for reasons of pride, to ask Mal's increasingly successful father for regular help. Patrick's monetary contributions were random and unpredictable, not something that could be counted on. Mal was bitterly aware of his father's lucrative career and fame. He was resentful and defensive for his mother and was frustrated by his own desire for more of Patrick's attention, because he viewed his father with cynicism as a "typical deadbeat dad" who abandoned the family. Mal would like to be able "to do without him." Visits were limited to 1–2 weeks in the summer, when Mal felt mostly offended and peripheralized by his father's entourage. Despite the presence of a series of interested women over the years, Patrick did not remarry and no half-siblings appeared. Mal was distressed that he found him-

self intermittently preoccupied with the possibility of other children; it pained him to admit that he feared a usurper, because he didn't want to care. He was similarly bothered that his father did not encourage Mal to use his well-known surname, which felt like a pointed snub; Mal's name was his mother's. Their relationship was, according to Mal, superficial and "meaningless."

As Mal matured, his own growing athletic ability in a different sport began to interest Patrick. When Mal was recruited to play for a Division 1 university, his father began to reach out and made regular appearances at the school. Mal was irritated and embarrassed but also felt his stock rise on campus. He handled his feelings of hypocrisy with a shrug and mentioned Patrick's visits only occasionally to his mother and grandparents.

Mal's own sports career started with great promise but then declined precipitously in his sophomore year. He got caught up in the privileges and perks of being an athlete at his school, which included easy sex and a lot of drinking; from the perspective of his coach, Perry, Mal lost sight of the work involved in being successful in his sport. Perry voiced his concern that Patrick's campus appearances had a negative effect on Mal's investment in being an athlete. Beverly and her family were increasingly put off by what seemed like Mal's worsening character and arrogance; he reminded them of Patrick.

When the situation became dire, Perry sat down with Mal at the beginning of senior year and told him that his chances to contribute to his team and/or to be drafted into a professional league rode on a change in his attitude. He needed to give the sport his attention. Perry pointed out that Mal was trying to live his father's life except that Patrick kept up his performance and was a hardworking professional in his current sports role. Perry's "tough love" had an impact: Mal felt disgusted with himself and actually did cut back on his raucous behavior. However, he didn't seem to have the heart to pull himself together athletically. He graduated as a middle-level player, without professional prospects.

Mal spent the next year at his mom's home doing very little, feeling intermittently down on himself, hanging out with his "do-nothing" high school friends and avoiding contact with his father. Beverly finally got angry and threatened to kick him out if he didn't start contributing to the household. Mal turned to his father, asking if he could stay with him and maybe find an occupation connected to his father's sports-related activities. This quickly led to a crisis in their relationship, as Mal was deeply disappointed in what felt like his father's grudging help and lack of real interest, now that Mal had "nothing special" to offer. It was humiliating to ask his mother if he could return home, but she did not "rub it in," because she was sensitive to his new level of disillusionment with his father. Very soon after this fiasco, Mal called his old coach Perry and asked for guidance. Unlike his father, Perry spent hours talking with him—about his relationship to the sport, to his father, and to his future. Perry, who appreciated the complications of having a father like Patrick—"super successful and super disappointing," encouraged Mal to spend a semester as assistant coach on campus; pay would be minimal, but he could live with Perry and his family and so his expenses would be small. One semester extended to two as Mal increasingly valued his role as coach and mentor to young players. Although his relationships with women remained undeveloped well into his 20s, when he finally met someone who sustained his interest, his feeling of responsibility and self-determination grew. He was ultimately hired to a permanent position at his alma mater and took a deep pleasure in his own mentoring skills.

As Mal's narrative suggests, the need for emerging adults "to get their own lives in order" often takes precedence over seeking a life partner (Arnett 2004, p. 101). Contemporary twenty-somethings are delaying marriage while figuring themselves out. Their search for a suitable partner is often based on feelings of similarity and shared interests; the gender divide in leisure activities is increasingly rare, and couples tend to spend more time together outside of the workplace than ever before. Contemporary research supports the familiar idea that friendships decline somewhat in importance as intimate relationships develop into commitments (Barry et al. 2009). Given that the personal capacities required in friendships are similar to those necessary for a romantic relationship, especially the capacity to rely meaningfully on others (called *interdependence*—a capacity associated with adulthood), it seems that friendships help prepare individuals for romantic relationships but then become less relevant for tasks of adulthood that follow soon after. Certainly, friendships undergo reconfiguring to accommodate the preferences of the romantic partner and the "time of life" concerns of friends whose marital commitment and childbearing do not correspond. However, as age 30 looms, emerging adults, men and women alike, experience more urgency about marriage and move decisively toward commitment: by age 34, 7 out of 10 have "tied the knot" (Settersten and Ray 2010, p. 31).

As illustrated by Mal's struggles, reworking both representations of family and the current relationships with individual parents can have powerful repercussions not only on identity but on the emerging adult's own confidence about entering into a meaningful long-term relationship. Contemporary culture tolerates intermediate steps such as cohabitation, which presumably allows emerging adults necessary role exploration in this crucial arena before commitment. Today, cohabiting is a typical premarital step; fully two-thirds of young adults cohabit with a romantic partner before marriage (Arnett 2004). Although such a preamble to marriage would seem to serve as a useful trial period, evidence suggests that premarital cohabitation is not associated with better marital quality, and that quality is decidedly worse if nonmarital births occur (Tach and Halpern-Meekin 2009). Marital commitment would appear to introduce requirements for specific role adaptations, which reverberate with fantasies originating in childhood concerning the meaning of adult relationships, weddings, and, inevitably, oedipal conflicts. Indeed, the wedding ritual can be experienced as relationship altering—disruptive to some couples and cementing to others as they assume roles associated with their parents. Of course, parenthood itself inevitably shifts prior friendships and relationships.

Sibling Relationships

Sibling relationships are subject to fluctuations throughout development and perhaps most profoundly during emerging adulthood (Conger and Little 2010; Scharf et al. 2005).

Physical and Cognitive Development

Finally, we revisit the question of whether emerging adulthood is "developmental" in the strict sense of an underlying biologically driven program, observable in physical changes, cognitive transformation, and/or the emergence of new capacities. One could certainly argue that mental structure is fully established by the end of adolescence and no significant biological changes occur subsequently, save those associated with decline. However, for many people it is only in their 20s when they undergo the subtle but nonetheless notable physical changes that are typically experienced as the culmination of pubertal development and its evolution into the adult form. Particularly for "late bloomers," but even among average developers, the consolidation of pubertal changes reaches its full expression through the early 20s. Secondary sex characteristics such as chest hair; fully filled-in facial hair; muscular development, strength, and endurance; breast configuration; and fat distribution take on the mature adult form (McAnarney et al. 1992; Neinstein et al. 2000). The emerging adult "fills out" and loses the fresh and nubile appearance of late adolescence (Colarusso 1991).

Because of the wide variability of growth rates, pubertal changes, and early evidence of aging (e.g., graying, hair loss, weight gain), physical development in the 20s can range from insignificant to transformational. But as the 20s come to a close, most individuals experience their physical selves, which had formerly been inexorably pushing them forward, as gradually settling into their adult shape and function. This change is often associated with the shocked recognition of a parent in the physical self, which can be greeted with pleasure or dismay but most often with a premonitory sense of finality: "This is the body I will have, and my parent shows the way that body ages." Emerging adults' history of conflict over identifications can be heightened by their physical transformation and by the environmental response.

Cognitively, the standard Piagetian developmental progression to formal operations, said to reach completion in adolescence, has been recognized as an underestimation of subsequent cognitive growth, especially as young adults begin to focus on what interests them: "the aptitudes of individuals differentiate progressively with age" (Piaget 1972/2008, p. 44). The completion and refinement of formal operations become increasingly dependent on environmental nutriment, suggesting that the emerging adult must become immersed in his or her area of special interest in order to come into his or her own cognitively. Here again, the environment takes a major role in the ongoing refinement of activity-dependent connectivity through the late myelination processes described in Chapter 8.

Many scholars would argue that all these changes are variations on the multifaceted achievement of adulthood, which is unevenly accomplished across domains within and across individuals. They would propose that there is continued refinement and consolidation of the adult form throughout life, and that no new developmental phase need be invented to distinguish this era.

Key Concepts

Hailed as the new developmental phase of the twenty-first century, emerging adulthood has become a focus for sociologists, youth theorists, and social commentators. Nonetheless, significant disagreement exists among these thinkers about whether the period, variously situated between ages 18 and 24 or between ages 21 and 30, is a legitimate developmental era; alternative views suggest that the social changes of postindustrial Western culture have introduced conditions conducive to postponement of the so-called markers of adulthood—such as independent living, marriage, career permanence, and the bearing and rearing of children—and to the loss of traditional pathways to achieve these that were available in the past. In addition, some developmentalists and sociologists suggest that the term *emerging adult* refers to individuals who represent a small segment of Westen postindustrial society at a unique moment—namely the children of affluent parents who are willing to support their offspring in their search for adulthood—and believe that this generational phenomenon is unlikely to recur because the next generation, today's emerging adults, will not have the resources to indulge their own young adult children. These critics argue further that the notion of emerging adulthood is grounded in a dated conceptualization of development as a series of chronological phases, with little recognition of the complex interaction of culture, families, economics, individual psychology, growth and development, and so on, and with little appreciation of the huge variability in domains within individuals (Hendry and Kloep 2007).

According to Arnett, an important theorist and originator of the term *emerging adulthood,* there are five criteria for this stage: 1) identity or role explorations, 2) instability, 3) self-focus, 4) feeling in-between, and 5) a widening of possibilities (Arnett 2004, p. 55). His position is complicated by the fact that he places emerging adulthood in the age range from 18 to 24 years, which many would argue is more accurately seen as late adolescence, the traditional time frame for identity and role exploration. However, there is no doubt that many of today's twenty-somethings are still exploring: their career options, their sexual orientation, their political and religious beliefs, their feelings and attitudes toward having children of their own, their commitment to partners, and many other facets of adult life. They are nonetheless simultaneously engaging in risky behaviors that seem to indicate that one foot is still in adolescence. As these young people contemplate their autonomous, self-determined life choices and begin to settle into partnerships of their own, their attitudes about responsible self-management mature and their relationships with parents shift conclusively toward equality.

- The subjective experience of people ages 21–30 is in many ways the most sensitive measure of their struggle to achieve adulthood. They feel simultaneously not quite ready to be an adult and yet no longer a "kid." The emerging adult typically describes both a degree of uncertainty about the future and a fearful recognition that the future has arrived.

- Role exploration, described as the central task of emerging adulthood (Arnett 2000), differs from the comparable adolescent experience due to the sense of urgency that important decisions must be made.

- Risky behaviors, especially excessive alcohol use, actually peak during this phase but wane as age 30 approaches.

- Selective identifications with parents and individuated worldviews evolve over the course of emerging adulthood, leading to the gradual focusing and refinement of interests, the development of expertise, personal philosophy, and enduring commitments.

- No dramatic physical, neurological, psychological, or cognitive transformation occurs in emerging adulthood, but this period does usually encompass the attainment of full maturation in all these arenas and increased specialization in mental capacities. However, maturation does not necessarily progress smoothly; uneven physical and ego development throughout the 20s makes for uneven accomplishment of the markers of adulthood.

REFERENCES

Abrams S: The psychoanalytic process: the developmental and the integrative. Psychoanal Q 59:650–677, 1990

Adatto CP: Ego reintegration observed in analysis of late adolescents. Int J Psychoanal 39:172–177, 1958

Allen JP, Hauser ST, Eickholt C, et al: Autonomy and relatedness in family interactions as predictors of expressions of negative adolescent affect. J Res Adolesc 4:535–552, 1994

Arnett JJ: Young people's conceptions of the transition to adulthood. Youth Soc 29:3–23, 1997

Arnett JJ: Emerging adulthood: a theory of development from the late teens through the twenties. Am Psychol 55:469–480, 2000

Arnett JJ: Emerging Adulthood: The Winding Road From the Late Teens Through the Twenties. Oxford, UK, Oxford University Press, 2004

Arnett JJ: The developmental context of substance use in emerging adulthood. J Drug Issues 35:235–253, 2005

Arnett JJ: Suffering, selfish, slackers? Myths and reality about emerging adults. J Youth Adolesc 36:23–29, 2007

Arnett J, Taber S: Adolescence terminable and interminable: when does adolescence end? J Youth Adolesc 23:517–537, 1994

Attewell P, Heil S, Reisel L: Competing explanations of undergraduate noncompletion. Am Educ Res J 48:536–559, 2011

Banks D, Oliviera A: Young men's initiative: report to the mayor from the chairs. August 2011. Available at: http://www.nyc.gov/html/om/pdf/2011/young_mens_initiative_report.pdf. Accessed October 15, 2012.

Barnett J: Dependency conflicts in the young adult. Psychoanal Rev 58:111–125, 1971

Barry CM, Madsen SD, Nelson LJ, et al.: Friendship and romantic relationship qualities in emerging adulthood: differential associations with identity development and achieved adulthood. J Adult Dev 16:209–222, 2009

Bell KL, Allen JP, Hauser ST, et al: Family factors and young adult transitions: educational attainment and occupational prestige, in Transitions Through Adolescence: Interpersonal Domains and Context. Edited by Graber JA, Brooks-Gunn P, Brooks AC. Mahwah, NJ, Erlbaum, 1996, pp 345–366

Beyers W, Seiffge-Krenke I: Does identity precede intimacy? Testing Erikson's theory on romantic development in emerging adults of the 21st century. J Adolesc Res 25:287–415, 2010

Blos P: Prolonged adolescence: the formulation of a syndrome and its therapeutic implications. Am J Orthopsychiatry 24:733–742, 1954

Blos P: On Adolescence: A Psychoanalytic Interpretation. Glencoe, IL, Free Press of Glencoe, 1962

Blos P: Prolonged male adolescence, in The Adolescent Passage: Developmental Issues. New York, International Universities Press, 1979, pp 37–53

Brooks D: The odyssey years. New York Times, October 9, 2007. Available at: www.nytimes.com/2007/10/09/opinion/09brooks.html?_r=0. Accessed October 15, 2012.

Bynner J: Rethinking the youth phase of the life-course: the case for emerging adulthood? J Youth Stud 8:367–384, 2005

Bynner J, Ferri E, Shepherd P: Twenty-Something in the 1990s: Getting On, Getting By, Getting Nowhere. Aldershot, UK, Ashgate, 1997

Chused JF: Idealization of the analyst by the young adult. J Am Psychoanal Assoc 35:839–859, 1987

Cinamon RG: Anticipated work-family conflict: effects of gender, self-efficacy, and family background. Career Dev Q 54:202–215, 2006

Cohen P, Kasen S, Chen H, et al: Variations in patterns of developmental transitions in the emerging adulthood period. Dev Psychol 39:657–669, 2003

Cohen RS, Weissman SH: The parenting alliance, in Parenthood. Edited by Cohen RS, Cohler BJ, Weissman SH. New York, Guilford, 1984

Colarusso CA: The development of time sense in young adulthood. Psychoanal Study Child 45:124–144, 1991

Conger KJ, Little WM: Sibling relationships during the transition to adulthood. Child Dev Perspect 4:87–94, 2010

Cote JE: Emerging adulthood as an institutionalized moratorium: risks and benefits to identity formation, in Emerging Adults in America: Coming of Age in the 21st Century. Edited by Arnett JJ, Tanner JL. Washington DC, American Psychological Association, 2006, pp 85–116

Coupland D: Generation X: Tales for an Accelerated Culture. New York, St. Martin's Press, 1991

Elnick AB, Margrett JA, Fitzgerald JM, et al: Benchmark memories in adulthood: central domains and predictors of their frequency. J Adult Dev 6:45–59, 1999

Emde RN: From adolescence to midlife: remodeling the structure of adult development. J Am Psychoanal Assoc 33(suppl):59–112, 1985

Erikson EH: The problem of ego identity. J Am Psychoanal Assoc 4:56–121, 1956

Escoll PJ: Psychoanalysis of young adults: an overview. Psychoanalytic Inquiry 7:5–30, 1987

Furstenberg FF: On a new schedule: transitions to adulthood and family change. Future Child 20:67–87, 2010

Galambos NL, Barker ET, Krahn HJ: Depression, self-esteem, and anger in emerging adulthood: seven-year trajectories. Dev Psychol 42:350–365, 2006

Gordon T, Holland J, Lahelma E, et al: Imagining gendered adulthood: anxiety, ambivalence, avoidance and anticipation. European Journal of Women's Studies 12:83–103, 2005

Hakim C: Women's lifestyle preferences in the 21st century: implications for family policy, in The Future of Motherhood in Western Societies: Late Fertility and Its Consequences. Edited by Beets G, Schippers J, teVelde ER. The Hague, The Netherlands, Springer, 2011, pp 177–195

Hall GS: Adolescence: Its Psychology and Its Relations to Physiology, Anthropology, Sociology, Sex, Crime, Religion and Education. New York, D Appleton, 1904

Harris A: Gender as Soft Assembly. London, Routledge, 2008

Hendry LB, Kloep M: Conceptualizing emerging adulthood: inspecting the emperor's new clothes? Child Dev Perspect 1:74–79, 2007

Horowitz A, Bromnick R: "Contestable adulthood": variability and disparity in markers for negotiating the transition to adulthood. Youth Soc 39:209–231, 2007

Jacobson E: Adolescent moods and the remodeling of psychic structure in adolescence. Psychoanal Study Child 16:164–183, 1961

Kernberg OF: Identity: recent findings and clinical implications. Psychoanal Q 75:969–1003, 2006

Klockars L, Sirola R: The mother-daughter love affair across the generations. Psychoanal Study Child 56:219–237, 2001

Konstam V: Emerging and Young Adulthood: Multiple Perspectives, Diverse Narratives. New York, Springer-Verlag, 2007

Kramer J: Against nature: profiles. New Yorker, July 25, 2011, p 44

Lawson Bush V: How black mothers participate in the development of manhood and masculinity: what do we know about black mothers and their sons? J Negro Educ 74:381–391, 2004

McAnarney ER, Kreipe RE, Orr DP, et al: Textbook of Adolescent Medicine. Philadelphia, PA, WB Saunders, 1992

Milrod D: The ego ideal. Psychoanal Study Child 45:43–60, 1990

Neinstein L, Gordon CM, Katzman DK, et al: Handbook of Adolescent Health Care. Philadelphia, PA, Lippincott Williams & Wilkins, 2000

Nelson LJ, Padilla-Walker LM, Christensen KJ, et al: Parenting in emerging adulthood: an examination of parenting clusters and correlates. J Youth Adolesc 40:730–743, 2011

Neugarten BL, Moore JW, Lowe JC: Age norms, age constraints, and adult socialization. Am J Sociol 70:710–717, 1965

Notman MT: Mothers and daughters as adults. Psychoanalytic Inquiry 26:137–153, 2006

Piaget J: Intellectual evolution of adolescence to adulthood (reprint of Hum Dev 15:1–12, 1972). Hum Dev 51:40–47, 2008

Rampell C: Instead of work, younger women head to school. New York Times, December 28, 2011, p A1

Robbins A, Wilner A: Quarterlife Crisis: The Unique Challenges of Life in Your Twenties. New York, Tarcher/Putnam, 2001

Rosenbaum J: The complexities of college for all: beyond the fairy-tale dreams. Sociol Educ 84:113–117, 2011

Rosenbaum JE, Person AE: Beyond college for all: policies and practices to improve transitions into college and jobs. Professional School Counseling 6:352–260, 2003

Scharf M, Mayseless O: Late adolescent girls' relationships with parents and romantic partner: the distinct role of mothers and fathers. J Adolesc 31:837–855, 2008

Scharf M, Shulman S, Avigad-Spitz L: Sibling relationships in emerging adulthood and in adolescence. J Adolesc Res 20:64–90, 2005

Schulenberg JE, Bryant AL, O'Malley PM: Taking hold of some kind of life: how developmental tasks relate to trajectories of well-being during the transition to adulthood. Dev Psychopathol 16:1119–1140, 2004

Schwartz SJ, Finley GE: Troubled ruminations about parents: conceptualizations and validation with emerging adults. J Couns Dev 88:80–91, 2010

Seiffge-Krenke I, Overbeek G, Vermulst A: Parent-child relationship trajectories during adolescence: longitudinal associations with romantic outcomes in emerging adulthood. J Adolesc 33:159–171, 2010

Settersten RA Jr, Ray B: What's going on with young people today? The long and twisting path to adulthood. Future of Children 20:19–41, 2010

Shulman S, Feldman B, Blatt S, et al: Emerging adulthood: age-related tasks and underlying self processes. J Adolesc Res 20:577–603, 2005

Sroufe LA, Egeland B, Carlson E, et al: The Development of the Person: The Minnesota Study of Risk and Adaptation From Birth to Adulthood. New York, Guilford, 2005

Staples HD, Smarr ER: Bridge to adulthood: the years from eighteen to twenty-three, in The Course of Life, Vol 4: Adolescence. Edited by Greenspan S, Pollack G. Madison, CT, International Universities Press, 1991

Stierlin H: Psychoanalytic approaches to schizophrenia in the light of a family model. Int Rev Psychoanal 1:169–178, 1974

Tach L, Halpern-Meekin S: How does premarital cohabitation affect trajectories of marital quality? J Marriage Fam 71:298–317, 2009

Tanner JL: Recentering during emerging adulthood: a critical turning point in life span human development, in Emerging Adults in America: Coming of Age in the 21st Century. Edited by Arnett JJ, Tanner L. Washington, DC, American Psychological Association, 2006, pp 85–116

Tessman LH: A note on the father's contribution to the daughter's ways of loving and working, in Father and Child: Developmental and Clinical Perspectives. Edited by Cath S, Gurwitt A, Ross JM. Boston, MA, Little, Brown, 1982, pp 219–240

Tucker JS, Ellickson PL, Orlando M, et al: Substance use trajectories from early adolescence to emerging adulthood: a comparison of smoking, binge drinking, and marijuana use. J Drug Issues 35:302–332, 2005

Wilkinson-Ryan T, Westen D: Identity disturbance in borderline personality disorder: an empirical investigation. Am J Psychiatry 157:528–541, 2000

CHAPTER 11

The Role of Developmental Thinking in Psychodynamic Psychotherapy

In this chapter, we briefly revisit our central thesis that an informed understanding of development is foundational for psychodynamic work. In fact, we believe that knowledge of development can serve the clinician in every interaction. Patients who consult with mental health professionals have myriad agendas and disorders; there certainly are diagnostic groups that neither seek nor benefit from the psychodynamic exploration of "meanings, unconscious ideas, and hidden motives" (Wolff 1996, p. 369). However, even in work with patients who request and are best served by purely behavioral interventions, therapists' grounding in the solid understanding of development enhances their expertise and navigation through the inevitable transference/countertransference dynamics and resistance to change that arise in every form of therapy. Appreciation of the impact of prior history, the universal tendency to repeat and re-create versions of past relationships, the presence of pockets of naïve cognition based on childhood mentation, and the role of specific defenses in managing past trauma are all crucial to deeper understanding of the person in the consulting room, whatever therapeutic modality is deemed suitable.

THE PAST, THE PRESENT, AND DEVELOPMENTAL AWARENESS

For psychodynamic therapy, the therapist's developmental theory, familiarity with phase-related mental organizations, and sensitivity to central developmental themes become the organizing backdrop for a comprehensive picture of the patient. As psychodynamic clinicians interested in the experience of the patient both inside and out of the consulting room, we work to integrate developmental events and presenting symptoms with the picture we see unfolding in the therapeutic relationship. Past and present circumstances and experience, unconscious fantasy, ongoing impact of attachment security, physical attributes and the pace of their developmental emergence, and many more factors are woven not only into the patient's self-representation and overall mental life, but also into the fabric of patient-therapist interaction. From this vantage point, *the present predicts the past* (Hartmann and Kris 1945; Tuch 1999); the patient's present set of expectations and modes of relating, as best revealed in the relationship with the therapist, illuminate important elements of the past, as filtered through experience. Is it necessary, however, to make connections between the here-and-now and the patient's past to achieve the goals of a psychodynamic treatment? And is it necessary to know anything about development to do that?

Upon examination, these two related questions are complex indeed. Not only do therapists from different schools disagree in regard to both the goals of treatment and the relevance of developmental knowledge, but patients also differ in their preferred forms of relief and their interest in their own histories. Furthermore, patient and therapist in a given therapeutic encounter may differ in significant but unformulated ways about what they think will help and how the present problems are grounded in the past. Patients seek relief from suffering, but their ideas, usually unconscious, about how this is to be achieved are not necessarily the same as the therapists'. Patients who are eager to understand themselves in relation to their past often seek redress for childhood privation or gratification for unmet childhood needs from the therapist. They may be excessively attached to their version of their history and reluctant to reconsider cherished ideas about their past experience and how it shaped them. Such fixed narratives are often a significant and tenacious component of their current adaptation and contribute to resistance to treatment. For example, the patient who tells the story of her life as a saga of lonely independence due to unreliable others, from parents to current spouse, can prove highly resistant to recognizing her contribution to her disappointments and her own refusal to make use of opportunities for help, including the therapy. Most patients, such as the man described in the following vignette, come to us with well-established ways of thinking about how they came to be the people they are; one important task of psychotherapeutic treatment is to raise questions about that version, to take a second look, and to facilitate more reflective, psychologically minded personal narratives.

Ross, a man age 28, sought therapy for recurrent difficulties in his romantic relationships. He currently had, by his description, a very attractive girlfriend who, he felt, was intellectually inferior and embarrassed him. He wondered if this had something to do with him in some way, as he reluctantly recognized that it was a pattern in his adult life: he inevitably discovered, sooner or later, that his girlfriends were lacking in sophistication, education, and culture. In the very first session, this young man spontaneously presented his history with the introduction, "My parents divorced when I was three. It was the best thing that could have happened. It taught me to be self-sufficient and made my relationship with my mother very close." He went on to say that time spent with his father was always a lot of fun; his father was an affluent, prominent intellectual who took him on wonderful vacations where he learned how to ski and scuba dive and where he got to socialize with "important people." In contrast, he and his mother lived in relative poverty; his mother had a clerical job, and he was required to work after school and on weekends to supplement their meager income. His father had remarried a very sophisticated socialite and showed palpable disdain for his ex-wife, her professional limitations, and her straitened circumstances. The patient described his self-satisfaction in adolescence working as a hot dog vendor at the baseball park near his home; he frequently served his classmates and, on a few occasions, sold hot dogs to his father and his father's new family. When, as a high school student, he showed considerable promise academically, his father took more interest in him and even agreed to pay his college tuition.

This story of his father's grudging participation in his upbringing, condescension toward his mother, and, by extension, disdain for the son (until he "proved" his mettle), was offered neutrally; the patient presented it without irony as a tale of plucky self-sufficiency. These experiences taught him a lot, he insisted, and he "wouldn't have had it any other way." In fact, he treated his female therapist's wish to examine this story dismissively; she just didn't understand the "advantages of being disadvantaged." Nonetheless, as she repeatedly showed him the impact of the past on his current adaptation, he became aware that these childhood experiences were painful and humiliating and that they reverberated throughout his life. Exploration of the transference further illuminated his disdain for his therapist, providing the opportunity to reflect in the here and now on his childhood coping strategies and the character deformation that ensued. Ultimately, he was able to recognize his identification with his father (a form of *identification with the aggressor*) resulting in his own largely unconscious contempt for his mother—an attitude that had been previously contained by and deflected onto his girlfriends, and now onto the therapist. He also began to understand his historical need for his Panglossian perspective and became aware of his anger both at his father for his arrogance and indifference and at his mother for the submissiveness that had led her to accept grossly inequitable terms in the divorce proceedings.

Although this young man rued the loss of the sunny picture of his life story, he understood its defensive purposes in the course of his 3 years of treatment. His new story, which emerged gradually in therapy, was more coherent, even if less sanguine. Understanding the desperate childhood anxiety behind his identification with his abandoning father allowed him to tolerate an examination of his present-day hostility toward women, which consciously he found appalling and at odds with his philosophical, political, and moral convictions. His growing capacity to feel compassion, not only for the little boy he was but also for his overwhelmed mother, made this deep vein of increasingly conscious hostility more and more ego-dystonic. After much working through of these issues with his therapist, he gradually came to recognize his love for and wish to commit to his girlfriend.

Certainly, some patients do not dwell on their histories and rarely refer to past experiences unless prompted. Although the concept that *childhood experience has a role in personality* is part of the general culture, many patients interested in their maladaptive patterns do not offer useful historical data and do not make use of speculations or hypotheses regarding the effects of their childhoods. This may be especially true of our youngest and oldest patients; children do not readily volunteer memories of their (brief) earlier lives, and many older adults experience themselves at a significant remove from childhood. Moreover, some contemporary thinkers view the elucidation of past experience as unnecessary, because the here and now provides ample data for self-exploration and psychotherapeutic change. However, we contend that the *therapist's* thorough grounding in developmental thinking is essential to listening to any patient; it informs his or her own deepening understanding of the unfolding relationship, the patient's choices and ways of experiencing the world, tenacious aspects of maladaptation, repetitive dynamics both within and outside of the therapy, and so on.

We also believe that most adults, however young or old, have an interest in a coherent life story. Historical narratives are building blocks of identity and lend a distinctive cast to present-day experience and convictions about the future. Patients often articulate that they want to better understand themselves and make sense of behavior that is self-defeating or causes pain to others. Giving meaning and coherence to baffling current patterns by placing them in a historical context is crucial to the success of treatment for many reasons: it facilitates more compassionate and less defensive self-reflection, promotes the integration of the sense of self and identity, reduces reflexive destructive behaviors developed to manage self-esteem and avoid threat, and greatly enhances the self-awareness that is a true marker of effective therapy. Indeed, in addition to the aim of achieving a more *mentalized* picture of the childhood self and important love-objects, the recognition by patients that they are essential contributors to their past and present is a crucial piece of psychotherapeutic success; their endowment, their self-regulation, their cognitive profile, their experience, and their defensive needs to protect their narcissistic balance all interface with the environment throughout development, producing both the past incarnations and the current picture.

The following example shows how a patient who felt chronically out of place in every setting of her life began to have a new perspective on this persistent self-experience when she understood more about how it developed, how it supplied masochistic pleasure, and how it was woven through her history and current choices.

> Gretchen, a married professional woman, felt chronically awkward and unfeminine; despite her self-description as "a tall, attractive graduate of an Ivy League school," she worried about her capability and power as a woman. This was only compounded by the fact that she had a long, albeit successful, struggle with infertility. Now the mother of twins, she was dissatisfied in her marriage and her job as a mid-level executive in a private equity company. Although her own marriage was "okay," she found herself powerfully attracted to her married boss, who was immensely successful and charismatic, but well known to be a philanderer.
>
> From her earliest recollection she was frustrated by her beautiful South American mother's self-absorption and self-satisfaction. She recalled having had recurrent tantrums during which she screamed for her mother, who was focused on preparing elaborate dinner and dancing parties. The patient's father was a very successful banker who had a history of intermittent self-defeating behaviors that cost him considerably in hard-won status and reputation. The fallout was often publicly humiliating to the family; as a very visible executive in a prominent banking institution, her father was fired unceremoniously due to inappropriate social behavior when the patient was 6 and had a well-publicized affair when she was 17. Despite these incidents, he continued to resurrect himself. He was highly critical and demanding of his only child, but as she did well in the various phases of her development, he showed a growing interest in and even excitement about her accomplishments and her late-blooming beauty.
>
> Always "a foot taller" than her peers and "skinny as a beanpole," she did not show any sign of secondary sexual development until menarche at age 17. When she was 11, her family moved to a neighboring town that was the storied home of affluent, aristocratic families. She entered her new middle school as a gawky, athletic, somewhat ethnic-looking girl who was out of sync with her cliquish, exceedingly precocious classmates. Despite the fact that she gradually made lasting friends in this environment, she felt that she was always one step behind them. She was entirely excluded from the dating loop and remained a virgin until her sophomore year of college.
>
> The patient came into treatment just as her affair with her boss began. She rapidly developed a profoundly ambivalent attachment to her boss, characterized by jealousy of his wife and other lovers (many of whom she encountered in professional settings), disparagement of him as a liar and philanderer, and a sexual passion she had never before experienced. Despite his

reliable professional behavior, he was unpredictable, repeatedly disappointing, and frustrating in their relationship. She felt preoccupied with his refined, glamorous wife, whom she viewed as far more feminine than she herself was. She read minute shifts in his tone or attentiveness as indications of a new lover or renewed dedication to his wife. Her own marriage felt increasingly dull and her husband infantile. She was anxiously aware that she was risking both her family and her career in this affair, but her fixation on her boss only intensified.

Patients recreate and repeat in the present their experiences and identifications with significant figures from their childhood; the present illuminates events of the past and, most importantly, the patient's continuous reworking of such events in mental life and subsequent experience. In this woman's case, her delayed puberty and physical attributes interfered with her self-representation as a desirable woman, despite her rational understanding that she was in fact quite striking. Her father's affairs (about which she was aware from her earliest memories) felt degrading to her mother, for whom she too had some degree of disdain. However, his affairs were also part of her own feelings of triumph and despair, as she became conscious of her father's excited interest in her in the midst of his many affairs. Her marital situation recapitulated her parents' with a gender reversal—she disparaged her husband and cheated on him—at the same time that her affair with her boss represented an oedipal triumph and defeat rolled into one. Notably, her two representations of her father were split, so that her husband was the "loser" and her boss was the elusive, charismatic but unattainable man. Her brinksmanship in regard to both her family and her job was a guilty identification with her father's self-destructiveness. Certainly, this affair also served to diminish the importance of her male therapist, whom she treated in a "professional" manner. Although it was difficult to bring the transference into her awareness, examination of this "neutral" stance unmasked the same hypersensitivity and excitement in the transference; gradually, she revealed her pattern of "stalking" the therapist's wife on the Internet. Work in this arena facilitated a deeper understanding of connections to her childhood familial triangle and shifted the balance of intensity toward the treatment relationship where it could be worked on.

Sroufe's (2005) longitudinal study underscores that attachment categorization observed in early childhood is recognizable in subsequent relationships over the course of development. However, attachment patterns accrue complexity over the course of life, infiltrated by sexuality, guilt and need for punishment, competition, and so on—in short, the whole array of nuanced emotion. One-on-one therapy unpacks this connection in a far more elaborated and specific way, discovering the reverberations of the patient's historical relationships in current ways of engaging, in conditions for sexual arousal, in attitudes toward friends and lovers, in repeating patterns of object choice, and in the unfolding treatment relationship.

CONTEMPORARY RELEVANCE OF DEVELOPMENTAL CONCEPTS

As noted in Chapter 1, "A Psychodynamic Developmental Orientation," there are a few ideas ubiquitous in psychodynamic literature that rely on developmental concepts or reflect a kind of shorthand for developmental shifts. Some of these have been carried forward from earlier formulations and, on examination, seem anachronistic and dated. Others continue to be useful but require a reconceptualization in contemporary terms. These include the following:

1. *The idea that development introduces conflict and disequilibrium and can produce symptoms.* For example, toddler tantrums and adolescent risky behaviors, within limits, are expectable and usually correct themselves. When this does not happen—that is, when a developmental disruption does not reequilibrate—then psychopathology ensues. Sources for this failure to maintain progressive movement include all the contributions that have been delineated in this book: endowment (including problematic thresholds and the delay or absence of "emerging capacities" due to physiological or experiential causes), environment demand, impact of trauma, and others.

2. *The categorization of oedipal (higher-level) versus preoedipal (primitive) psychopathology, personality disorder, or level of ego functioning.* Historically, this terminology has been used to distinguish neurotic from borderline or psychotic disturbances. Clearly rooted in the outdated idea that the continuum of psychopathology corresponds to the continuum of development (Westen 1990), this terminology promotes a linear conceptualization of developmental contributions to adult psychopathology. Contemporary thinking does not support such a view, but the terminology remains prevalent and should be understood to designate primitive (in regard to type of psychopathology, not childhood) versus better modulated, smoothly integrated capacities or states. For example, "primary process thinking"—that is, the mode of psychic functioning manifested in dream life that is illogical, pictorial, and internally contradictory—is not the same thing as the thinking of an infant, toddler, or oedipal-age child. It is "primitive" because it is preemptory and associational and because it defies the ordinary rationality commensurate with the individual's maturity.

3. *The use of the term "regression."* Certainly, children can "regress" under stress in the form of (usually temporary) relinquishment of developmental milestones, as occurs, for instance, when a 4-year-old's recent toilet training unravels under the stress of a sibling's birth or an adolescent attributes all restraint to authoritarian parents and loses sight of her own moral quandaries. However, such behavior is not simply a return to a prior level of functioning because it is now a symptomatic expression of conflict and occurs in a person recently capable of a more mature level who is using an old behavior to express feelings in the present crisis. The term *regression* is often used with the also outdated notion of *fixation* to a prior psychosexual stage; together, regression and fixation imply linear backward slides to a previous childhood moment of deprivation or overstimulation, like a time machine that dials back to re-create the past as it once as. In our view, mental life should be understood as "a complex and largely unconscious 'horizontal' present" (Dowling 2004, p. 192) in which prior modes of coping remain dormant but present, although inevitably transformed in the course of development and in the present moment. The mind of the present can invoke remnants of these modalities that were used in the past if they serve a present purpose, but only as reinterpreted by current mental life. "Regression" never faithfully replicates thinking or feeling from the past (Inderbitzen and Levy 2000).

4. *The theorizing of mother-infant paradigms for the patient-therapist relationship.* Contemporary theorizing among attachment researchers, infant observers, and some relationalists and intersubjectivists relies heavily on observations of mother-infant interaction; some of these thinkers tend to understand patient-therapist interactions as re-creations of paradigms observed in mother-infant dyads. If we are correct that there is no "past relationship" buried intact and available to reinvoke, then any similarities must be understood to indicate present-day access to certain nonverbal modes of behavior (which have also been reworked and reintegrated at various developmental points) for the purpose of grappling with present-day experience.

Trauma and Resilience: Understanding Childhood Experience in the Adult Patient

As suggested in Chapter 1, we believe that understanding developmental progression and the sequential mental organizations that assume dominance in different phases provides an invaluable lens into the present, just as the present illuminates the impact and meaning of the past. Importantly, we believe that early experience is foundational, but it is not everything; development contains multiple opportunities for deviations and corrections. This means that a good beginning, while enormously salubrious, is not the only determining factor. Certainly, traumatic experience, a surprisingly common feature of childhood even in the most carefully monitored circumstances, can have lifelong repercussions and deform developmental progression.

In this regard, there is a growing body of research on human resilience intended to illuminate the factors that allow certain children to overcome adversity and trauma and to achieve relatively positive psychological adaptation (Masten and Narayan 2012; Mastan and Obradovic 2006; Rutter 2006). Consistent with our view of development as a multifactorial interactive process, resilience is not a quality that resides in the individual alone but rather reflects the nature of the interaction between a complex individual, the environment, and the current environmental stressor. Moreover, these interacting systems are not static entities; as we have attempted to show in this book, even a very young child is a product of all previous development, including attachment history as well as past exposure to stress that can "steel" or "sensitize" the individual to subsequent trauma (Rutter 2006, p. 2). Furthermore, resilience is not always apparent in the moment of adversity, because protection may ensue from subsequent experience. Protection itself derives from multiple sources, including "supportive and effective caregiving (preferably by established attachment figures in a child's life), problem solving systems, self-regulation and social-regulation systems, motivational/reward systems underlying self-efficacy, and hope and belief systems that convey a sense of meaning" (Masten and Narayan 2012, p. 249). Again, these are all complex and evolving systems with multiple iterations in the course of development.

An ear educated to recognize the cadences of childhood and the reverberations of childhood events, from the traumatic to the quotidian, in the adult personality is one that is more attuned to the patient in the consulting room. This does not mean that adult patients reproduce the interactions of the mother-baby dyad in the relationship with the therapist, nor does it support the notion of a linear regression in the patient's inner life as manifested in the transference. With rare exceptions, there is nothing in mental life that has not been subjected to revision, if simply by virtue of being remembered or re-created in the present—a present that is at a distance from the actual occurrence, whether measured in seconds or years. These resonances, when recognized, yield new insights for the therapist by highlighting the importance in the present moment of a past one that powerfully influenced subsequent personality development. Such accumulated connections deepen the shared growing appreciation of the patient's mind and contribute to the patient's experience of being understood and helped.

REFERENCES

Dowling S: A reconsideration of the concept of regression. Psychoanal Study Child 59:191–210, 2004

Hartmann H, Kris E: The genetic approach in psychoanalysis. Psychoanal Study Child 1:11–30, 1945

Inderbitzen LB, Levy ST: Regression and psychoanalytic technique: the concretization of a concept. Psychoanal Q 69:195–223, 2000

Masten AS, Narayan AJ: Child development in the context of disaster, war, and terrorism: pathways of risk and resilience. Annu Rev Psychol 63:227–257, 2012

Masten AS, Obradovic J: Competence and resilience in development. Ann NY Acad Sci 1094:13–27, 2006

Rutter M: Implications of resilience concepts for scientific understanding. Ann NY Acad Sci 1094:1–12, 2006

Sroufe LA, Egeland B, Carlson E, et al: The Development of the Person: The Minnesota Study of Risk and Adaptation From Birth to Adulthood. New York, Guilford, 2005

Tuch RH: The construction, reconstruction, and deconstructions of memory in the light of social cognition. J Am Psychoanal Assoc 47:153–186, 1999

Westen D: Toward a revised theory of borderline object relations: contributions of empirical research. Int J Psychoanal 71:661–693, 1990

Wolff P: The irrelevance of infant observations for psychoanalysis. J Am Psychoanal Assoc 44:369–392, 1996

Index

Page numbers printed in **boldface** type refer to tables.

emerging adults and relationship
with, 303–304, 305–306
moral development of toddlers
and feared loss of approval by,
52–53
preadolescence and relationships
with daughters, 188–189
role of discourse with child in
emotional development during
oedipal phase, 77–78
Mother-infant relationship
attachment of infant and, 33–35
developmental concepts in
psychodynamic psychotherapy
and, 324
introduction to infancy and, 21–22
patient-therapist relationship and, 5
role of temperament in, 28–30
Motor skills, and toddlers, 36–38, 66
Motor vehicles. *See* Driving
Mourning, and adolescent love
experience, 264

Narcissism, and role of shame and guilt
in superego formation 127, 128
Narratives
oedipal phase and capacities for,
76–77, 86
oedipal themes in, 133–134
pretend play and, 86
psychodynamic psychotherapy and,
320
National Comorbidity Survey
Replication, 273
Negative oedipal complex, 109
Neglect, mother-infant relationship
and childhood experience of, 25
Neural deficits, and learning disorders,
165
Newborns, and development during
first weeks of life, 26–27
"No," and toddlers, 53, 64–65
Normative crisis, and preadolescence,
179

Obesity, rates of in children, 171
Object constancy, and oedipal phase,
74, 79–80
Object permanence, and toddlers,
62–64
Object removal, and adolescence, 229–
230, 262
Obsessional tendencies, in latency
phase, 145
Obsessive-compulsive disorder, 145
Oedipal complex. *See also* Oedipal
phase
adoption and, 122–124
contemporary view of siblings and,
117–119
contemporary views on and
variations of, 110–116, 131–
132
effect of divorce on, 120
Freud's theory of, 106–110
identity development and,
124–126
single-parent families and,
121–122
universal fantasy and, 132–134
use of term, 111–112
Oedipal configuration, 112
Oedipal constellation, 106, 112
Oedipal phase. *See also* Oedipal
complex
development of pretend play and
role of imagination in, 84–91
introduction to concept of, 73–74,
105–106
mentalization capacities and, 79–84
preoperational thinking and, 91–94
role of language in development
during, 74–78
superego formation during, 74,
95–97
Operational thinking, and
preadolescence, 179
Orality, as mode of learning for
infants, 31